Textbook of Lifestyle Medicine

Textbook of Lifestyle Medicine

LABROS S. SIDOSSIS, PHD
Rutgers, The State University of New Jersey
New Brunswick, NJ, USA

STEFANOS N. KALES, MD, MPH
Cambridge Health Alliance/Harvard Medical School
Cambridge, MA, USA

WILEY Blackwell

The right of Labros S. Sidossis and Stefanos N. Kales to be identified as the authors of this work has been asserted in accordance with law.

Registered Office(s)
John Wiley & Sons, Inc., 111 River Street, Hoboken, NJ 07030, USA
John Wiley & Sons Ltd, The Atrium, Southern Gate, Chichester, West Sussex, PO19 8SQ, UK

Editorial Office
9600 Garsington Road, Oxford, OX4 2DQ, UK

For details of our global editorial offices, customer services, and more information about Wiley products visit us at www.wiley.com.
Wiley also publishes its books in a variety of electronic formats and by print-on-demand. Some content that appears in standard print versions of this book may not be available in other formats.

Limit of Liability/Disclaimer of Warranty
The contents of this work are intended to further general scientific research, understanding, and discussion only and are not intended and should not be relied upon as recommending or promoting scientific method, diagnosis, or treatment by physicians for any particular patient. In view of ongoing research, equipment modifications, changes in governmental regulations, and the constant flow of information relating to the use of medicines, equipment, and devices, the reader is urged to review and evaluate the information provided in the package insert or instructions for each medicine, equipment, or device for, among other things, any changes in the instructions or indication of usage and for added warnings and precautions. While the publisher and authors have used their best efforts in preparing this work, they make no representations or warranties with respect to the accuracy or completeness of the contents of this work and specifically disclaim all warranties, including without limitation any implied warranties of merchantability or fitness for a particular purpose. No warranty may be created or extended by sales representatives, written sales materials or promotional statements for this work. The fact that an organization, website, or product is referred to in this work as a citation and/or potential source of further information does not mean that the publisher and authors endorse the information or services the organization, website, or product may provide or recommendations it may make. This work is sold with the understanding that the publisher is not engaged in rendering professional services. The advice and strategies contained herein may not be suitable for your situation. You should consult with a specialist where appropriate. Further, readers should be aware that websites listed in this work may have changed or disappeared between when this work was written and when it is read. Neither the publisher nor authors shall be liable for any loss of profit or any other commercial damages, including but not limited to special, incidental, consequential, or other damages.

Library of Congress Cataloging-in-Publication Data Applied for

[PB: 9781119704423]

Cover Design: Wiley
Cover Image: Cover Illustration © Eleni Chrysikou

Set in 9.5/12.5pt SourceSans Pro by Straive, Pondicherry, India

SKY5EAE53EF-90FD-4B61-9246-B0C61878A840_122121

Dedication

To our loving and supportive parents and families. They taught us, continue to inspire us, and make us work hard, because they know that physical exertion is good for our health! This book would not have been possible without you.

Contents

About the Authors

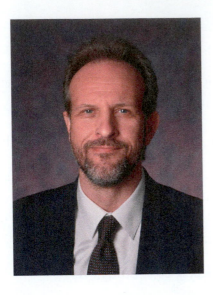

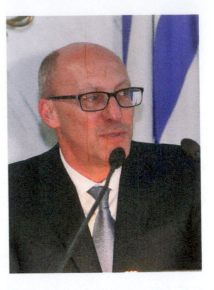

Dr Labros S. Sidossis, PhD, FTOS, FAHA, FNAK is a Distinguished Professor and Chairperson of the Department of Kinesiology and Health and Professor of Medicine at the Robert Wood Johnson Medical School at Rutgers University. He is also a founding member and the first President of the Mediterranean Lifestyle Medicine Institute (https://medlifestyle.org).

His research over the past 30 years has focused on the role of lifestyle factors in the pathophysiology, prevention, and treatment of various noncommunicable diseases, including obesity, insulin resistance, and dyslipidemias. His studies have been funded by the US National Institutes of Health, the American Diabetes Association, the Shriners Hospitals for Children, the European Union, and the industry. His 200+ publications in peer-reviewed journals have been cited >15,000 times.

Dr. Sidossis has been an inspiring teacher for undergraduate and graduate students in the fields of nutrition, physical activity, and health. He has developed and taught numerous undergraduate and graduate courses in these disciplines in the European and US universities, and has published four textbooks.

Dr. Stefanos N. Kales, MD, MPH, FACP, FACOEM is Professor of Medicine, Harvard Medical School; Professor & Director of the Occupational Medicine Residency, Harvard Chan School of Public Health; and Chief of Occupational Medicine /Employee Health, Cambridge Health Alliance, a Harvard-affiliated system. He has participated in medical and public health activities on five continents resulting in over 200 publications and wide recognition internationally. He is a faculty member in Harvard's Cardiovascular Epidemiology Program and its Division of Sleep Medicine.

Dr. Kales has received numerous honors, including the Kehoe and Harriet Hardy Awards for outstanding scientific contributions. He has organized several groundbreaking Mediterranean Diet/Lifestyle Conferences (Harvard Chan 2014, Halkidiki-Greece 2017 and Harvard's Radcliffe Institute 2019). Dr. Kales leads by example, following a Mediterranean diet, practicing regular physical fitness and good sleep hygiene. Based on the scientific evidence, he is convinced that lifestyle measures are the most accessible and cost-effective of chronic disease prevention and control.

Preface

We are thrilled to share this book with you. It is the product of more than 50 years of combined research, practice, and teaching on modifiable lifestyle factors affecting human health. We have been struggling in the lab, classroom, clinic, and workplace for years to understand the epidemiology and pathophysiology of some of today's most common diseases (e.g., obesity, type 2 diabetes mellitus, hypertension, and dyslipidemia) and to find nonpharmacological ways to prevent and mitigate these disorders. Our work has contributed a small fraction to the tremendous progress that has been accomplished during the past few decades by many excellent labs, research institutions, and centers around the world, led by brilliant colleagues, investigators, teachers, and clinicians.

We have tried to evaluate, understand, organize, and translate all this knowledge into clinical practice and share it with you. You will be the judge if we have succeeded in this endeavor. Our main goal was not only to provide accurate and trusted knowledge to undergratuate and graduate students but also to make available the tools for current and future clinicians to translate this knowledge into best practices.

Lifestyle factors and the way individuals conduct their lives have recently received great attention, since these factors are modifiable and, therefore, may be subject to considerable intervention and improvement. Many healthy lifestyle choices – such as sensible diets, adequate physical activity, avoiding tobacco use, moderate alcohol intake, good social life, and stress-reduction – have been associated with lower risks of obesity, insulin resistance, hypertension, dyslipidemia, and other chronic diseases, which are considered the major public health concerns of our time. Therefore, scientific research on the lifestyle factors that may have negative (unhealthy lifestyle) or positive (healthy lifestyle) effects on health has intensified during the past 20 years.

The findings are very encouraging; even small changes toward healthier lifestyle choices can translate into substantial health benefits. The clinical implications are so significant that the first professional organizations to promote lifestyle changes as a primary means to treat diseases were formed. In 2004, the American College of Lifestyle Medicine (ACLM) was formed to provide education and certification to health professionals who want to use lifestyle changes as the foundation of transformed and sustainable health-care systems. Soon after, many similar organizations were formed around the world (e.g., Lifestyle Medicine Global Alliance, European Lifestyle Medicine Council, European Lifestyle Medicine Organization, British Society of Lifestyle Medicine, Australasian Society of Lifestyle Medicine). According to the ACLM, "Lifestyle Medicine is the use of a whole food, plant-predominant dietary lifestyle, regular physical activity, restorative sleep, stress management, avoidance of risky substances, and positive social connection as a primary therapeutic modality for treatment and reversal of chronic disease."

We do not consider ourselves the ultimate authorities in all the scientific areas covered in this book. But this is exactly the main message of our book: metabolic health is a multifaceted entity requiring a multidisciplinary approach. No one can be an expert in all components of lifestyle: diet, physical activity, stress, sleep, substance use and abuse. However, it is crucial for all health-care professionals who treat patients suffering from chronic diseases to understand the importance of lifestyle choices and help patients to best utilize those choices to their own benefit.

The book is divided into four units to present these complex subjects in a clear and concise manner.

Unit I: Lifestyle Choices and Human Health begins by providing the basic knowledge necessary to introduce students and scientists with diverse backgrounds to this relatively new area of research and practice and the related terminology: healthy lifestyle, wellness, and lifestyle medicine. Next it presents in detail the characteristics and principles of healthy and unhealthy lifestyle choices.

Unit II: Healthy Diets presents the history of how our nutrition habits, the most studied of all lifestyle factors, evolved to what they are today, and discusses the methods scientists have used to evaluate the connections among food, health, and disease. Subsequently, we present several of the world's most important dietary models/patterns, followed by billions of people. Finally, we finish this unit with one of the best-known and evidence-based eating patterns, the Mediterranean dietary pattern. One-day sample meal plans for all dietary models/patterns are presented in Appendix B.

Unit III: From Mediterranean Diet to Mediterranean Lifestyle describes the major milestones in the development of our current understanding of building and maintaining health and well-being. We can no longer consider diet as the sole determinant of health. We now recognize that other lifestyle factors (physical activity, sleep, stress management, social life, substance use and abuse) are equally important; furthermore, it is the synergistic effect of all these factors that leads to a healthy lifestyle, a life not only with less disease but a state of physical, mental, and social well-being.

Unit IV: Mediterranean Lifestyle in Clinical Practice presents four case studies, each devoted to one of the prominent features of the metabolic syndrome: obesity, type 2 diabetes mellitus, hypertension, and dyslipidemia. For each case, we present a detailed, step-by-step description of the methods a clinician should use to evaluate a patient's lifestyle. Next, we describe general treatment protocols utilizing lifestyle modifications pertinent to the specific disorders. We hope that this section will become a useful tool in the hands of clinicians when managing patients utilizing lifestyle medicine as the first, and possibly most important, line of defense against noncommunicable diseases, before resorting to prescription drugs with possible side effects.

The book has six distinctive features:

1. It is inclusive of all the major lifestyle factors affecting human health.

2. It has a textbook format and can be used for undergraduate and graduate teaching.

3. It uses the unique and evidence-based perspective of the traditional Mediterranean lifestyle as the gold standard of a healthy lifestyle. A plethora of scientific evidence supports the notion that the traditional Mediterranean diet/lifestyle is one of the healthiest diet/lifestyle patterns. The 2015 Dietary Guidelines for Americans identify the Healthy Mediterranean-Style Eating Pattern/Lifestyle as probably the healthiest and easiest to follow.

4. The "Take-Home Messages" at the end of each chapter denote the most important points of the chapter.

5. The "Key Points" throughout the book help the reader focus on important points.

6. Finally, to assist the reader/student in comprehending the presented material, at the end of each chapter we present a list of "Self-Assessment Questions" with answers provided in Appendix A.

We hope that this book will become a valuable resource to students in medical and health-related disciplines, and to health professionals such as nutritionists, exercise physiologists, psychologists, addiction specialists, sleep therapists, athletic trainers, physicians, nurses, and other health professionals who are using or considering using lifestyle changes to prevent and treat noncommunicable diseases. The Clinical Cases section provides specific practical tools to assist with everyday practice in the clinic; the materials presented apply to most noncommunicable diseases of today (e.g., cardiovascular disease, autoimmune diseases, stroke, most cancers, chronic kidney disease, osteoarthritis, osteoporosis), not only the specific examples we are presenting.

We are indebted to Christina Katsagoni, PhD; Michael Georgoulis, PhD; Elena Bellou, PhD; Anastasia Diolintzi, PhD; Anastasia Papadimitriou, PhD; Glykeria Psarra, PhD; Amalia Sidossis, MD; and Ioanna Katsaroli, MS. These talented young scientists contributed tremendously to this book by offering ideas regarding book format and content, conducting thorough literature reviews, drafting and editing sections or chapters, and offering constructive criticism throughout the writing of this book. Special thank you to Christina and Michael for their invaluable help during the final stages of book editing. We would not be able to do it without them. Ms. Dafni Kyriakou was quick and effective as always in book formatting. We would also like to thank the Wiley team for their dedication and professionalism: James Watson, Anne Hunt, Tom Marriott, Cheryl Ferguson, P. Sathishwaran, and their colleagues. Finally, we would like to thank Sarah Brown for proofreading our book.

Last but not least, we want to thank our families for their continuous love and support.

LABROS S. SIDOSSIS, PHD
Princeton, New Jersey, USA

STEFANOS N. KALES, MD, MPH
Cambridge, Massachusetts, USA

Abbreviation List

(F)PG	(fasting) plasma glucose
(He)FH	(heterogenous) familial hypercholesterolemia
(hs)CRP	(high-sensitivity) C-reactive protein
(N)REM	(non-)rapid-eye-movement
(S/D)BP	(systolic/diastolic) blood pressure
(V)LCD	(very) low-calorie diet
(V)LDL(C)	(very) low-density lipoprotein (cholesterol)
AACE	American Association of Clinical Endocrinologists
ACC	American College of Cardiology
ACE	American College of Endocrinology
ACLM	American College of Lifestyle Medicine
ACS	acute coronary syndrome
ACSM	American College of Sports Medicine
AD	Alzheimer's disease
ADI	acceptable daily intake
ADP	air displacement plethysmography
AHA	American Heart Association
AHI	apnea-hypopnea index
ALT	alanine transaminase
APA	American Psychological Association
APAQ	Athens Physical Activity Questionnaire
Apo	apolipoprotein
ApoB	apolipoprotein B
ARIC	Atherosclerosis Risk Communities
ASCVD	atherosclerotic cardiovascular disease
ATP	Adult Treatment Panel
BIA	bioelectrical impedance analysis
BIS	bioelectrical spectroscopy
BMI	body mass index
BMR	basal metabolic rate
BP	blood pressure
BW	body weight
CBT	cognitive–behavioral therapy
CDC	Centers for Disease Control and Prevention
CE	cholesterol esters
CETP	cholesterol ester transfer protein
CFG	Chinese Food Guide
CG	control group
CHD	coronary heart disease
CHNS	China Health and Nutrition Survey
CKD	chronic kidney disease
CLOCK	circadian locomotor output cycles kaput
CM	chylomicron
CNS	central nervous system
COPD	chronic obstructive pulmonary disease
CRD	chronic respiratory disease
CRP	C-reactive protein
CT	computed tomography
CVD	cardiovascular disease
DALY	Disability-Adjusted Life Years
DASH	Dietary Approaches to Stop Hypertension
DASH-CF	DASH with chicken and fish
DASH-P	DASH with lean pork
DEXA	dual-energy X-ray absorptiometry
DHA	docosahexaenoic acid
EAPC	European Association of Preventive Cardiology
EAS	European Atherosclerosis Society
EAT	Eating Among Teens
EEG	electroencephalograph
eGFR	estimated glomerular filtration rate
EPA	eicosapentaenoic acid

EPA	energy required for physical activity
EPIC-NL	European Prospective Investigation into Cancer and Nutrition
EPIDIAR	Epidemiology of Diabetes and Ramadan
ESC	European Society of Cardiology
EVOO	extra-virgin olive oil
FDA	Food and Drug Administration
FFA	free fatty acids
FFQ	food frequency questionnaire
FTO	fat-mass obesity
GDM	gestational diabetes mellitus
GDS	Geriatric Depression Scale
GI	glycemic index
GL	glycemic load
GWAS	genome-wide association study
HbA1c	glycated/glycosylated hemoglobin
HDL(C)	high-density lipoprotein (cholesterol)
HEI	Healthy Eating Index
HF	heart failure
HF-DASH	high-fat DASH
HL	hepatic lipase
HOMA-IR	Homeostatic Model Assessment of Insulin Resistance
HPA	hypothalamic-pituitary-adrenal
HPV	human papilloma virus
HR	heart rate
HRQoL	health-related quality of life
HRR	heart rate reserve
IDF	International Diabetes Federation
IDL(C)	intermediate-density lipoprotein (cholesterol)
IHD	ischemic heart disease
IHME	Institute for Health Metrics and Evaluation
IL-1β	interleukin-1β
IL-6	interleukin-6
IL-18	interleukin-18
IMT	intima-media thickness
IOOC	International Olive Oil Corporation
IPAQ	International Physical Activity Questionnaire
IR	insulin resistance
ISAAC	International Study on Allergies and Asthma in Childhood
LCD	low-calorie diet
LDL	low-density lipoprotein
Lp(a)	lipoprotein a
LPL	lipoprotein lipase
MCI	mild cognitive impairment
MDG	Mediterranean diet group
MedD	Mediterranean diet
MedL	Mediterranean lifestyle
MEST	mesoderm-specific transcript
MET	metabolic equivalent of task
MetS	metabolic syndrome
MI	motivational interviewing
MI	myocardial infarction
MLG	Mediterranean lifestyle group
MRI	magnetic resonance imaging
MRS	magnetic resonance spectroscopy
MUFA	monounsaturated fatty acid
NAFLD	nonalcoholic fatty liver disease
NASH	nonalcoholic steatohepatitis
NCD	noncommunicable disease
NCEP	National Cholesterol Education Program

NEAT	nonexercise activity thermogenesis
NEFAs	non-esterified fatty acids
NHLBI	National Heart, Lung and Blood Institute
NHS	Nurses' Health Study
NICE	National Institute for Health and Care Excellence
NIH	National Institutes of Health
NSF	National Sleep Foundation
NWI	National Wellness Institute
OGTT	oral glucose tolerance test
OSA	obstructive sleep apnea
PA	physical activity
PAE	physical activity expenditure
PCA	principal component analysis
PCOS	polycystic ovary syndrome
PCP	primary care physician
PD	Parkinson's disease
PF	physical fitness
PKU	phenylketonuria
PL	phospholipid
PREDIMED	Prevencion con Dieta Mediterranea
PSQI	Pittsburgh Sleep Quality Index
PSS	Perceived Stress Scale
PUFA	polyunsaturated fatty acid
QoL	quality of life
RA	rheumatoid arthritis
RCT	randomized controlled trial
REE	resting energy expenditure
REM	rapid eye movement
ROS	reactive oxygen species
RPE	rating of perceived exertion
SAS	Zung Self-Rating Anxiety Scale

SCN	suprachiasmatic nucleus
SCORE	Systematic Coronary Risk Evaluation
SCS	Seven Countries Study
SENECA	Survey in Europe on Nutrition and the Elderly Concerted Action
SFA	saturated fatty acid
SNP	single-nucleotide polymorphism
STP	systolic blood pressure
SUN	Seguimiento Universidad de Navarra
T1/2DM	type 1/2 diabetes mellitus
TAG	triacylglycerol
TC	total cholesterol
TEE	total energy expenditure
TEF	thermic effect of food
TFA	trans fatty acid
TG	triglycerides/triacylglycerols
TIA	transient ischemic attack
TLC	Therapeutic Lifestyle Changes
TNF-α	tumor necrosis factor-α
TRL	triglyceride-rich lipoprotein
ULSAM	Uppsala Longitudinal Study of Adult Men
UNESCO	United Nations Educational, Scientific and Cultural Organization
USDA	United States Department of Agriculture
VO_2max	maximal aerobic capacity
VOO	virgin olive oil
WC	waist circumference
WELL	Wellbeing, Eating and Exercise for a Long Life
WHO	World Health Organization

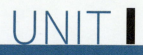

Lifestyle Choices
and Human Health

CHAPTER 1

Basic Concepts

Health, Wellness, and Lifestyle

Day by day, what you choose, what you think and what you do is who you become.
Heraclitus (Ancient Greek, pre-Socratic, Ionian philosopher)

Health is considered the most valuable asset of our lives and central to human happiness. According to Hippocrates (Ancient Greek physician, also known as the Father of Medicine), "A wise man should consider that health is the greatest of human blessings, and learn how, by his own thought, to derive benefit from his illnesses." Defining health is not as straightforward as it may seem; various definitions have been given through the years, gradually incorporating many aspects of human life.

Early definitions conceptualized health primarily as the absence of disease. The World Health Organization (WHO) was the first to introduce a more holistic definition of health in 1948: "Health is a state of complete physical, mental and social well-being and not merely the absence of disease or infirmity." This more inclusive concept of health, which encompasses the multifaceted nature of human beings, has recently gained ground. The suggestion that health has a positive component, instead of just the absence of a negative one, i.e., illness, gradually led to the use of other terms, such as wellness and well-being.

> **Key Point**
>
> "Health is a state of complete physical, mental and social well-being and not merely the absence of disease or infirmity." WHO

Wellness can be described as optimal health in all three dimensions – body, mind, and spirit – within the limits of one's hereditary and personal traits. The term *wellness* was added in the WHO Health Promotion Glossary in 2006 to describe "the optimal state of health of individuals and groups, with two focal concerns: the realization of the individual's fullest potential physically, socially, spiritually, and economically, and the fulfilment of one's role expectations in the family, community,

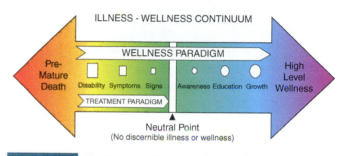

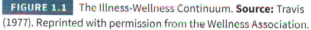

FIGURE 1.1 The Illness-Wellness Continuum. **Source:** Travis (1977). Reprinted with permission from the Wellness Association.

place of worship, workplace, and other settings." Figure 1.1 illustrates the Illness-Wellness Continuum proposed by John W. Travis According to this view, wellness is not just the absence of disease, but it incorporates the individual's mental and emotional health. The right side of the Continuum reflects degrees of wellness. Individuals can move further to the right, toward health and wellness, through awareness, education, and growth. The left side of the Continuum reflects degrees of illness or worsening states of health, reflected by signs, symptoms, and disability. This approach underlined that traditional Western medicine typically treats injuries, disabilities, and symptoms, to bring the individual to a "neutral point" but not to achieve a high level of wellness.

The National Wellness Institute (NWI) introduced the "Six Dimensions of Wellness" model that includes physical, occupational, social, intellectual, spiritual, and emotional parameters (Figure 1.2). According to this model, the feature of consciousness is critical in achieving and maintaining wellness. It gives the impetus to opt for choices, which will enhance a person's maximal capabilities. In

> **Key Point**
>
> "Wellness is an active process through which people become aware of, and make choices toward, a more successful existence." NWI

Textbook of Lifestyle Medicine, First Edition. Labros S. Sidossis and Stefanos N. Kales.
© 2022 John Wiley & Sons Ltd. Published 2022 by John Wiley & Sons Ltd.

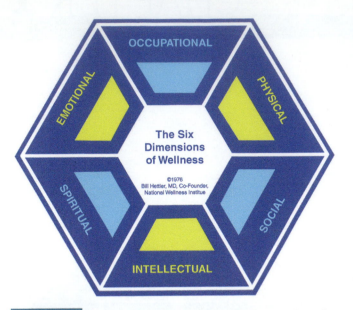

FIGURE 1.2 Six Dimensions of Wellness Model. ©1976 Bill Hettler, MD. **Source:** Reprinted with permission from the National Wellness Institute, Inc. (2020).

addition, wellness is characterized by positiveness – a complex condition that incorporates balance and harmony in lifestyle, environmental, mental, and spiritual features. According to the NWI, "Wellness is an active process through which people become aware of, and make choices toward a more successful existence."

The holistic character of wellness integrates the effects of frequent physical activity, sound dietary habits, self-reliance, and determination but also self-confidence, assertiveness, mental creativity, and inventiveness, along with the eagerness to share one's virtues with others. For optimal health, a person is expected to be physically able to fulfill everyday activities without disproportionate tiredness or stress. To this end, *physical wellness* can be achieved by the adaption of health-promoting practices, such as regular physical activity, healthy dietary and sleeping habits, and the rejection of the detrimental ones (e.g., undue stress, excessive alcohol intake, and use of tobacco or other substances).

Occupational (or vocational) wellness pertains to the satisfaction gained in the workplace, in balance with personal life. Employment is associated with personal satisfaction and life enrichment comparable with someone's goals, values, and lifestyle, offering unique skills and talents that are meaningful and rewarding. Furthermore, being socially involved (i.e., *social wellness*) means being harmoniously related to other people and efficiently sustaining positive intimate bonds with family, friends, and colleagues. *Emotional wellness* refers to the trait of self-consciousness and the state of being in harmony with oneself, as well as coping with life's adversities and expressing one's feelings in a constructive way. *Spiritual wellness* delineates the state of living peacefully by achieving concordance between ethical principles and course of action in combination with creativity. In a similar way, *intellectual wellness* refers to the adeptness of being receptive to different views and

perspectives, and constructively encompassing them in future decision-making, not only on a personal level but also while interacting with the social environment in an attempt to improve it. In addition, the *environmental dimension* refers to the acknowledgment of the effect that people exert on their environmental surroundings (i.e., air, water, and land) and the adoption of such practices that sustain and preserve the environment. Finally, the term *financial wellness* refers to the sense of satisfaction when people manage to live within their means. This involves making the appropriate financial decisions, setting realistic goals, and preparing to meet their short- and long-term needs.

The assessment of the various aspects of well-being is subjective. It depends on the perceived views a person holds, rather than his or her actual abilities. For example, a person might have a very important job, but the perception and satisfaction might be negative, whereas another person with a less important job might be more satisfied with his or her work. Therefore, healthy thinking and positive outlook are essential features to ensure overall wellness.

> **Key Point**
>
> Healthy thinking and positive outlook are essential features to ensure overall wellness.

Given the important role of health throughout life, scientific research has, from very early on, been focused on factors that could affect health. The genetic background has been acknowledged to be crucial to an individual's health. For example, heritability estimates for type 2 diabetes mellitus (T2DM) range from 20% to 80%. High estimates for the heritability of obesity have also been proposed (typically >70%). However, the exposure to an obesogenic environment is necessary for the development of T2DM and obesity, suggesting that the genetic background is important, but several other environmental/lifestyle factors may also exert a cumulative effect on human health.

> **Key Point**
>
> The genetic background is important, but several other environmental/lifestyle factors may also exert a cumulative effect on human health.

Lifestyle choices and the way the individuals conduct their lives have recently received great attention, since these factors are modifiable and, therefore, may be subject to intervention and improvement. Lifestyle factors that may affect health include habits, attitudes, tastes, moral standards, economic level, activities, interests, opinions, and values. It is a constellation of motivations, needs, and wants, influenced by factors such as culture, family, reference groups, and social class. Many unhealthy lifestyle choices, such as poor diet, physical inactivity, tobacco use, excessive alcohol intake, and excessive stress have been associated with the development of many chronic diseases. Therefore, scientific research on the lifestyle factors that may have negative (unhealthy lifestyle) or positive (healthy lifestyle) effects on health has intensified over the last decades.

Key Point

Even small changes toward healthy lifestyle choices can translate to significant benefits in the prevention and treatment of chronic diseases.

The findings are very encouraging; even small changes toward healthy lifestyle choices can translate to significant benefits in the prevention and treatment of chronic diseases. The clinical significance is so obvious that a few years ago the first professional organizations to promote lifestyle changes as a means to prevent and treat diseases were formed. In 2004 the American College of Lifestyle Medicine (ACLM) was formed to provide education and certification to health professionals who wanted to use lifestyle changes as the foundation of a transformed and sustainable health-care system. According to the ACLM, "Lifestyle Medicine is the use of a whole-food, plant-predominant dietary lifestyle, regular physical activity, restorative sleep, stress management, avoidance of risky substances, and positive social connection as a primary therapeutic modality for treatment and reversal of chronic disease."

Soon after the ACLM was formed, many similar organizations were formed (e.g., Lifestyle Medicine Global Alliance, European Lifestyle Medicine Council, European Lifestyle Medicine Organization, British Society of Lifestyle Medicine, Australasian Society of Lifestyle Medicine), demonstrating the global realization of the benefits of lifestyle medicine.

Key Point

"Lifestyle Medicine is the use of a whole-food, plant-predominant dietary lifestyle, regular physical activity, restorative sleep, stress management, avoidance of risky substances, and positive social connection as a primary therapeutic modality for treatment and reversal of chronic disease." ACLM

Take-Home Messages

- Wellness is the holistic integration of an individual's physical, mental, and spiritual health.
- The "Six Dimensions of Wellness" are physical, occupational, social, intellectual, spiritual, and emotional wellness.
- Healthy thinking and positive outlook are essential features to ensure overall wellness.
- Several parameters such as the genetic background and environmental and lifestyle factors affect human health.
- Lifestyle choices, as modifiable factors, may have negative (unhealthy lifestyle) and positive (healthy lifestyle) impact on health.

Self-Assessment Questions

1. How has the definition of health evolved through the years?
2. Give the definition of wellness according to the NWI.
3. What are the Six Dimensions of Wellness according to the NWI?
4. Physical wellness can be achieved through:
   a. regular physical activity
   b. healthy dietary habits
   c. adequate sleep
   d. the rejection of detrimental habits (e.g., undue stress, excessive alcohol intake, and use of tobacco or other substances)
   e. all of the above
5. Emotional wellness refers to:
   a. the satisfaction gained in the workplace, in balance with personal life
   b. the trait of self-consciousness and the state of being in harmony with oneself as well as coping with life's adversities and expressing one's feelings in a constructive way
   c. being harmoniously related to other people and efficiently sustaining positive intimate bonds
   d. the adeptness of being receptive to different views and perspectives, and constructively encompassing them in future decision-making
   e. the sense of satisfaction when someone manages to live within his or her means
6. Which components of the unhealthy lifestyle have been associated with the development of chronic diseases?
7. Give the definition of lifestyle medicine.

Bibliography

Birrell, F.N., Pinder, R.J., and Lawson, R.J. (2021). Lifestyle medicine is no Trojan horse: it is an inclusive, evidence-based, and patient-focused movement. *Br. J. Gen. Pract.* 71 (708): 300. doi: 10.3399/bjgp21X716201.

Frates, E.P. and Bonnet, J. (2016). Collaboration and negotiation: the key to therapeutic lifestyle change. *Am. J. Lifestyle Med.* 10 (5): 302–312. doi: 10.1177/1559827616638013.

Frates, E.P., Morris, E.C., Sannidhi, D. et al. (2017). The Art and science of group visits in lifestyle medicine. *Am. J. Lifestyle Med.* 11 (5): 408–413. doi: 10.1177/1559827617698091.

Kent, K., Johnson, J.D., Simeon, K. et al. (2016). Case series in lifestyle medicine: a team approach to behavior changes. *Am. J. Lifestyle Med.* 10 (6): 388–397. doi: 10.1177/1559827616638288.

Lalley, N.A., Manger, S.H., Jacka, F. et al. (2021). The Mind-Body Well-being Initiative: a better lifestyle for people with severe mental illness. *Australas Psychiatry*, 1039856220978864. doi: 10.1177/1039856220978864.

Lawson, R. (2020). British Society of Lifestyle Medicine: founding principles and current achievements. *Am. J. Lifestyle Med.* 14 (3): 286–288. doi: 10.1177/1559827619867627.

Masic, I. (2015). Determinants of health and health concepts according to WHO targets. *Int. J. Biomed. Health* 3: 16–21.

National Wellness Institute (NWI). (2020). The Six Dimensions of Wellness. www.nationalwellness.org.

Phillips, E.M., Frates, E.P., and Park, D.J. (2020). Lifestyle medicine. *Phys. Med. Rehabil. Clin. N. Am.* 31 (4): 515–526. doi: 10.1016/j.pmr.2020.07.006.

Saper, R.B. (2017). Integrative medicine and health. *Med. Clin. N. Am.* 101 (5): xvii-xviii. doi: 10.1016/j.mcna.2017.07.002.

Smith, B.J., Tang, K.C., and Nutbeam, D. (2006). WHO health promotion glossary: new terms. *Health Promot. Int.* 21 (4): 340–345.

Stoewen, D.L. (2017). Dimensions of wellness: change your habits, change your life. *Can. Vet. J.* 58 (8): 861–862.

Travis, J.W. (1977). *Wellness Workbook: A Guide to Attaining High Level Wellness.* Wellness Resource Center.

Travis, J.W. and Ryan, R.S. (2004). *The Wellness Workbook: How to Achieve Enduring Health and Vitality*, 3e. Random House Digital.

CHAPTER 2

The Lifestyle Disease Epidemic

Global Burden and Risk Factors

Lifestyle diseases are diseases linked to the way people live their lives and represent a leading threat to human health and human development. They are chronic conditions that do not result from an acute infectious process. They are noncommunicable diseases (NCDs), they have a prolonged course, they are not cured spontaneously, and a complete cure is rarely achieved. Finally, lifestyle diseases may result from a combination of genetic, physiological, environmental, and behavioral factors. NCDs include cardiovascular diseases (CVDs; e.g., coronary heart disease [CHD] and stroke), cancer, chronic respiratory disease (CRD), type 2 diabetes mellitus, chronic neurologic disorders (e.g., Alzheimer's, dementia), arthritis/musculoskeletal diseases, and unintentional injuries (e.g., from traffic accidents). According to the World Health Organization (WHO), NCDs cause more deaths than all other causes combined, and NCD deaths are projected to increase from 38 million in 2012 to 52 million by 2030. Figure 2.1 shows the proportion of deaths by cause among people who were 70 years and older.

Globally, approximately 45% of all NCD deaths occur before the age of 70 years. Figure 2.2 shows the country-dependent probability of dying from the four main NCDs between the ages of 30 and 70 years.

In general, NCDs have a multifactorial etiology. Risk factors include certain aspects of lifestyle as well as environmental and genetic determinants. It is well known that genetic predisposition alone cannot explain all the disease risk; lifestyle and environmental factors are also key contributors.

> **Key Point**
>
> NCDs cause more deaths than all other causes combined.

> **Key Point**
>
> NCDs have a multifactorial etiology. Risk factors include certain aspects of lifestyle as well as environmental and genetic determinants.

Genetic Background and NCD Development

Genetic predisposition has been acknowledged to have a significant contribution to the incidence of NCDs. A number of mutations in the coding regions of the human genome have been considered as causative factors for various NCDs. Nonsynonymous nucleotide substitutions result in missense, nonsense, or frameshift changes in protein coding sequence; this may lead to loss-of-function or gain-of-function in certain proteins that have linked with specific disease phenotypes. However, the vast majority of single-nucleotide polymorphisms (SNPs) are distributed throughout the human genome, in the noncoding regions. Therefore, it is difficult to establish a causal relationship between the allelic variants originating from SNPs and the disease phenotype.

The relationship between heritable genetic traits and metabolic morbidity has been accrued through genome-wide association studies (GWASs), which examine similarities in the entire DNA sequence of different people, as regards specific SNPs, and the presence of certain diseases across this population. Data from GWASs have shown that SNPs are preferentially concentrated in functional genomic regions, namely enhancer elements, DNase hypersensitivity regions, and epigenetically important chromatin markers, playing a crucial role in the development of a variety of diseases, including cancer, stroke, and cerebrovascular diseases. Moreover, the epigenetic modifications in the form of DNA methylation lay among the most critical processes that could change gene expression, while at the same time leaving intact the nucleotide sequence (please refer to Chapter 3 for more information about the epigenetic mechanism).

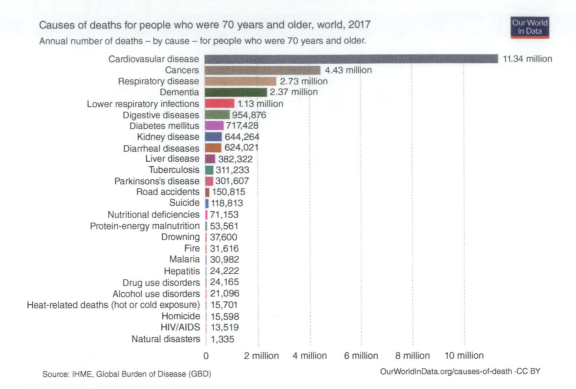

FIGURE 2.1 Results of the Global Burden of Disease Collaborative Network, Global Burden of Disease Study 2017. Institute for Health Metrics and Evaluation (IHME) (2018).

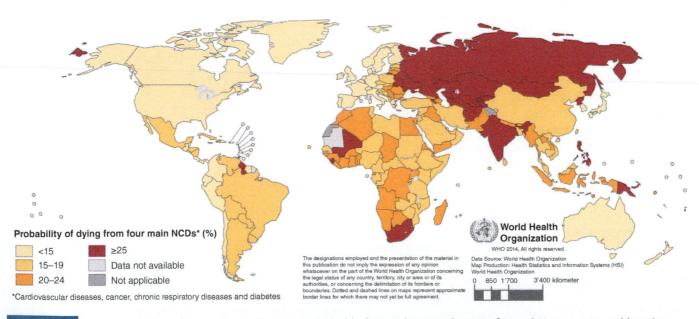

FIGURE 2.2 Probability of dying from the four main noncommunicable diseases between the ages of 30 and 70 years, comparable estimates, 2012. **Source:** Reprinted with permission from WHO Library Cataloguing-in-Publication Data Global Status Report on Noncommunicable Diseases, 2014 ed.

Diet, physical activity, sleep patterns, and stress have been shown to significantly affect the development of many NCDs. These factors can influence pathogenetic pathways and even gene expression, and therefore may positively or negatively affect the development of a disease. In the following paragraphs, we are presenting the epidemiology of the most important NCDs and the effect of the modern lifestyle. The protective role of several other lifestyle aspects in NCDs will be presented in Unit III.

Obesity: Epidemiology and Impact of Modern Lifestyle

The prevalence of obesity has nearly doubled since 1980. More than 39 million children under the age of 5 were overweight or obese in 2020; 13% of adults in the world were obese in 2020, whereas 39% were overweight. The prevalence of obesity varies significantly between countries (Figure 2.3.).

This "globesity" phenomenon may have contributed to the rise in the global incidence of major NCDs. Obesity often leads to adverse effects on blood pressure (BP), cholesterol, triacylglycerols (TAGs), and insulin resistance (IR). The risk of CHD, ischemic stroke, and type 2 diabetes mellitus (T2DM) increases steadily with increasing body mass index (BMI).

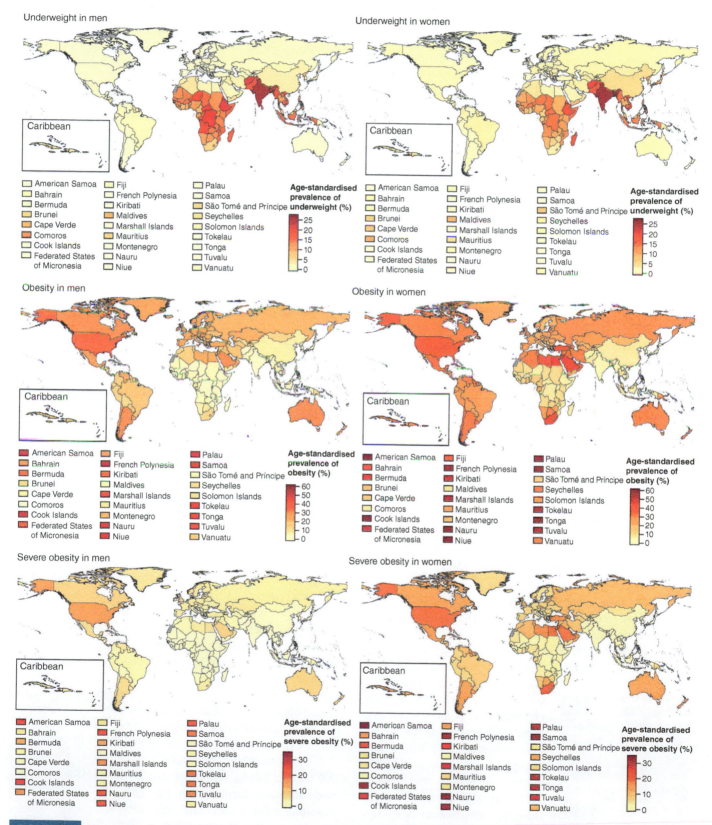

FIGURE 2.3 Age-standardized prevalence of underweight, obesity, and severe obesity by sex and country in 2014. Underweight (BMI < 18.5 kg/m²); obesity (BMI ≥ 30 kg/m²); and severe obesity (BMI ≥ 35 kg/m²). **Source:** NCD Risk Factor Collaboration (2016).

Overweight and obesity have also been associated with several types of cancer – namely, breast, colon, prostate, endometrium, kidney, and gall bladder cancer. Furthermore, overall mortality rates seem to be higher among severely obese individuals compared to the general population.

The genetic background plays a crucial role in the development of obesity and obesity-associated comorbidities. However, genes cannot be changed. Among several modifiable risk factors, physical inactivity, unhealthy diet, sleep deprivation, and chronic stress overload are the main contributors of overweight and obesity. These lifestyle behaviors not only acutely affect weight status but may also cause epigenetic modifications; i.e., these habits hold the potential to affect the expression of certain genes in the long term, which, in turn, can influence the predisposition to some chronic diseases.

Obesity is the consequence of a long-term energy imbalance, whereby energy intake is higher than energy expenditure. A dramatic change in the way people consume food, ingest drinks, and move has been recorded during the past decades. A significant increase in the consumption of energy-dense foods and simple sugars has been recorded worldwide. At the same time physical activity has decreased, due to the sedentary character of the working environment, changes in transportation, and urbanization. Moreover, short sleep duration (i.e., less than 7 hours/day) has been associated

with an increase in BMI and the risk for developing obesity. Hormonal changes seen with sleep deprivation could potentially increase food intake and contribute to weight gain. The increase of the glucocorticoid stress hormone cortisol may also play a role in the development of obesity by increasing the appetite with a preference for energy-dense foods ("comfort food").

Overall, these unhealthy lifestyle behaviors and habits seem to be the result of environmental and social changes associated with the lack of supportive policies in sectors such as health, agriculture, education, transportation, urban planning, environment, distribution, and food trade. Although their involvement in the pathogenesis of obesity has not been fully elucidated, it is now clear that social and environmental factors may influence food intake and energy expenditure more than the internal regulatory mechanisms that regulate people's weight. Moreover, the human body has been programmed to preserve energy, and this has deleterious

TABLE 2.1   Technological clashes with our biology.

Biology	Technology
Sweet preferences	Cheap caloric beverage revolution
Thirst and hunger/satiety mechanisms not linked	Caloric beverage revolution
Fatty food preference	Edible oil revolution – high-yield oilseeds, cheap removal of oils
Desire to eliminate exertion	Technology in all phases of movement/exertion

Source: Popkin et al. (2012).

effects when people are found in an obesogenic environment (Table 2.1). The proclivity of an individual to these environmental influences is affected by genetic and other biological factors.

Cardiovascular Disease: Epidemiology and Impact of Modern Lifestyle

CVDs include ischemic heart disease (IHD), stroke, heart failure and peripheral arterial disease, and a number of cardiac and vascular conditions, such as cerebrovascular disease, rheumatic heart disease, and congenital heart disease. It has been estimated that heart attacks and strokes account for over 85% of CVD death events. The events themselves are generally acute in nature and result from an obstruction of blood flow to the heart or brain due to the chronic accumulation of lipid deposition on the inner walls of the blood vessels. In addition, strokes can also occur as a consequence of a brain blood vessel bleeding or because of the presence of blood clots.

CVDs have emerged as the primary cause of death around the globe. According to the 2019 Heart Disease and Stroke Statistics report from the American Heart Association, someone dies of CVD every 38 seconds. Nearly 80% of premature deaths, i.e., death events among people under 70 years old, have been recorded in low-to-middle-income countries, with 37% being attributed to CVDs. Underdeveloped or developing countries suffer high rates of CVD mortality, whereas high-income industrialized countries and some regions in Latin America show the lowest CVD mortality.

Similar to other major NCDs, CVD burden can be attributed to modifiable risk factors such as unhealthy diet, sedentariness, tobacco smoking, obesity, hypertension, dyslipidemia, T2DM, and excessive alcohol consumption. The variation in the presence of those lifestyle risk factors between countries may explain the difference in CVD burden observed among the countries.

Diabetes Mellitus: Epidemiology and Impact of Modern Lifestyle

According to the WHO, diabetes mellitus is defined as "a metabolic disorder of multiple etiology, characterized by chronic hyperglycemia (high blood sugar) with disturbances of carbohydrate, fat, and protein metabolism resulting from defects in insulin secretion, insulin action, or both." Diabetes mellitus is classified into type 1 (T1DM; insulin-dependent) and type 2 diabetes mellitus (T2DM; non-insulin-dependent or adult-onset). While the main feature of T1DM is the defective production of insulin (by the pancreas) and the requirement of daily administration of insulin, T2DM is characterized by inefficient use of insulin from the body.

T1DM cannot be prevented, and we still do not fully understand what causes the disease. Furthermore, it is still under investigation whether environmental factors could trigger the destruction of the body's insulin-producing cells. On the other hand, T2DM development and progression are affected by genetic and environmental factors; exposure to an obesogenic environment, characterized by sedentary behavior, increased stress, and excessive energy consumption, is known to exert an effect on preexisting genetic factors.

The prevalence of T2DM has dramatically increased since the 1980s, affecting more than 430 million people, compared to 108 million about three decades ago. The increase in diabetes cases is more evident in low- to middle-income countries. According to the World Health Organization, more than 1.5 million people worldwide died due to diabetes in 2019. The Centers for Disease Control and Prevention (CDC) estimated that almost 80.000 deaths occur each year due to diabetes in the United States. The WHO projects that by 2030, diabetes mellitus will be the seventh most important cause of mortality.

Diabetes mellitus can progressively lead to a host of other metabolic abnormalities affecting the heart, blood vessels, eyes, kidneys, and nerves. It has been shown that individuals suffering from diabetes mellitus have two to three times higher risk for developing CVDs compared to their nondiabetic counterparts. Furthermore, reduced blood flow and nerve damage (i.e., neuropathy) in the lower extremities can substantially exaggerate the occurrence of foot ulcers and infection, even leading to amputation of the lower limbs. Chronic impairments in the small blood vessels of the retina (i.e., retinopathy) can gradually lead

> **Key Point**
>
> Diabetes mellitus can progressively lead to other metabolic abnormalities affecting the heart, blood vessels, eyes, kidneys, and nerves.

to blindness; approximately 3% of all blindness cases worldwide could be attributed to diabetes. Finally, diabetes mellitus constitutes one of the major causes of renal failure.

Cancer: Epidemiology and Impact of Modern Lifestyle

Cancer covers a wide spectrum of diseases whose typical characteristic is abnormal cellular growth, exceeding the normal rate of cellular proliferation. Other terms used for cancer include *malignant tumors* and *neoplasms*. According to the WHO, cancer constitutes the second-leading cause of death on a global scale – one out of six death events occurring globally is attributed to cancer. Epidemiological data show that males are mostly affected by lung, prostate, colorectal, stomach, and liver cancers, whereas females are more susceptible to breast, colorectal, lung, cervix, and stomach malignancies.

In addition to the health burden of the disease, cancer incurs a significant economic burden, over 1.5 trillion US dollars in 2020. Given that 30–50% of cancer incidence may be preventable, it is obvious that we should urgently employ preventive strategies to constrain cancer incidence. Raising public awareness regarding the risk factors associated with cancer development and providing people with sufficient information and resources to enhance compliance with healthy lifestyle behaviors stand at the forefront of cancer prevention. The major risk factors for cancer onset include consumption of tobacco products, excessive alcohol intake, unhealthy body weight, physical inactivity, and certain infections and occupational/environmental chemical exposures.

> **Key Point**
>
> The major risk factors for cancer onset include use of tobacco products, excessive alcohol intake, unhealthy body weight, physical inactivity, and certain infections and occupational/environmental chemical exposures.

Tobacco use accounts for approximately six million deaths on an annual basis. At least 50 of the chemicals contained in tobacco have a well-established causal effect on cancer development. Tobacco smoking causes malignancies in lung, esophagus, larynx, mouth, throat, kidney, bladder, pancreas, stomach, and cervix. Second-hand smoking can also cause lung cancer. Additionally, smokeless tobacco products, such as oral or chewing tobacco, have been shown to cause oral, esophageal, and pancreatic neoplasms. Interestingly, the majority of smokers globally (i.e., 80% of 1 billion) live in regions of low or middle income.

Other lifestyle-related factors associated with cancer onset include unhealthy dietary habits, being physically inactive, and obesity. Obesity has been linked to esophageal, colorectal, breast, endometrial, and kidney malignancies. Excess alcohol intake increases the risk of malignancies developed in the oral cavity, pharynx, larynx, esophagus, liver, colorectum, and breast.

There is a dose–response relationship between alcohol intake and cancer development, and the risk of several cancer types is further exacerbated when increased alcohol consumption is combined with smoking. Alcohol use accounted for about 6% of all cancers and 4% of all cancer deaths in the United States in 2020.

Infection-related factors, exposure to carcinogens derived from occupational environment or environmental pollution, and ultraviolet and ionized radiation can also increase the risk for developing cancer. Infectious agents such as helicobacter pylori, human papilloma virus (HPV), hepatitis B and C, and Epstein–Barr virus accounted for 20% of cancer cases in 2020, and their prevalence was substantially greater in developing countries. Air, water, and soil contamination with carcinogens plays a role in the total burden of the disease. Contamination of foods with carcinogenic chemicals, such as aflatoxins and dioxins, is another

means by which humans are exposed to carcinogens. Exposure to occupational carcinogens mainly affects specific population groups whose working environment incurs exposure to carcinogenic chemicals, such as asbestos. Exposure to ionized and ultraviolet radiation can also aggravate the risk of developing certain types of neoplasms. There is a dose–response relationship between the extent to radiation exposure and risk of carcinogenesis, and a greater risk of cancer onset when the exposure occurs at a young age.

More than 80% of US healthcare costs are spent in the treatment of preventable chronic diseases and conditions, such as T2DM, obesity, osteoporosis, heart disease, hypertension, stroke, and many types of cancer. Preventing even a small fraction of chronic disease cases could significantly improve people's health and alleviate the pressure on healthcare systems around the world.

> **Key Point**
>
> Preventing even a small fraction of chronic disease cases could significantly improve people's health and alleviate the pressure on health-care systems around the world.

Take-Home Messages

- NCDs, also known as chronic diseases, usually have a long duration, and they are the result of a combination of genetic, physiological, environmental, and behavioral factors.
- There are four types of NCDs: CVDs (e.g., heart attacks and stroke), cancers, CRDs (e.g., chronic obstructive pulmonary disease and asthma), and diabetes.
- The genetic predisposition of a disease explains only part of the disease risk, while lifestyle factors such as unhealthy diet, physical inactivity, excessive stress, and environmental factors (e.g., access to health-care systems) are also key contributors.

- The "globesity" phenomenon has an important contribution to the global incidence of most major NCDs.
- The human body has been programmed to preserve energy, and this has deleterious effects when people are found in an obesogenic environment.
- Exposure to an obesogenic environment affects the onset of T2DM, irrespective of existing genetic factors.
- It has been estimated that up to 50% of cancer incidence is preventable.

Self-Assessment Questions

1. List the types of NCDs.
2. Which are the main adverse effects of obesity?
3. Why is the prevalence of obesity rising in modern societies?
4. Genome-wide association studies:
   a. assess how genes can be modified to combat chronic diseases
   b. examine similarities in the entire DNA sequence of different people, as regards specific SNPs, and the presence of a certain abnormality across this population
   c. investigate interactions between diet and genes
   d. investigate how people with a certain genetic background respond to different dietary manipulations (e.g., increased saturated fat intake)
   e. none of the above

5. Which of the following are modifiable risk factors for obesity?
   a. diet
   b. genes
   c. age
   d. sex
   e. physical activity
   f. stress
   g. all of the above
6. T1DM is characterized by:
   a. defects in liver glucose production
   b. inefficient use of insulin from the body
   c. defective production of insulin
   d. inability of glucose transportation in the adipose tissue
   e. a and b
   f. none of the above

7. What is T2DM, and how is lifestyle linked to its development?
8. Which of the following are possible consequences of diabetes?
    a. cardiovascular disease
    b. retinopathy
    c. kidney failure
    d. nerve damage
    e. amputation of lower limbs
    f. all of the above
9. Which of the following are CVDs?
    a. stroke
    b. cancer
    c. heart failure
    d. diabetes
    e. ischemic heart disease
    f. asthma
10. Which are the main contributors to CVDs?
11. Which are the major risk factors for cancer onset?
12. Excess alcohol intake increases the risk of malignancies developed in:
    a. the lungs
    b. the oral cavity
    c. the brain
    d. the larynx
    e. the liver

Bibliography

American Diabetes Association. (2020). Classification and diagnosis of diabetes: standards of medical care in diabetes–2020. *Diabetes Care* 43 (Suppl 1): S14–S31.

Anastasiou, C.A., Yannakoulia, M., Pirogianni, V. et al. (2010). Fitness and weight cycling in relation to body fat and insulin sensitivity in normal-weight young women. *J. Am. Diet Assoc.* 110 (2): 280–284.

Benjamin, E.J., Muntner, P., Alonso, A. et al. (2019). Heart disease and stroke statistics–2019 update: a report from the American Heart Association. *Circulation* 139 (10): e56–e528.

Chatterjee, S., Khunti, K., and Davies, M.J. (2017). Type 2 diabetes. *Lancet* 389 (10085): 2239–2251.

Cooper, C.B., Neufeld, E.V., Dolezal, B.A., and Martin, J.L. (2018). Sleep deprivation and obesity in adults: a brief narrative review. *Br. Med. J. Open Sport Exerc. Med.* 4 (1): e000392.

Global Burden of Disease Cancer Collaboration Authors. (2019). Global, regional, and national cancer incidence, mortality, years of life lost, years lived with disability, and disability-adjusted life-years for 29 cancer groups, 1990 to 2017: a systematic analysis for the global burden of disease study. *JAMA Oncol.* 5 (12): 1749–1768.

Hruby, A. and Hu, F.B. (2015). The epidemiology of obesity: a big picture. *Pharmacoeconomics* 33 (7): 673–689.

Hruby, A., Manson, J.E., Qi, L. et al. (2016). Determinants and consequences of obesity. *Am. J. Public Health* 106 (9): 1656–1662. doi: 10.2105/AJPH.2016.303326.

Institute for Health Metrics and Evaluation (IHME). (2018). *Findings from the Global Burden of Disease Study 2017*. Seattle, WA: IHME. http://ghdx.healthdata.org/gbd-results-tool.

International Diabetes Federation. (2020). Type 2 diabetes prevention. https://idf.org/our-activities/care-prevention/prevention.html.

Krekoukia, M., Nassis, G.P., Psarra, G. et al. (2007). Elevated total and central adiposity and low physical activity are associated with insulin resistance in children. *Metabolism* 56 (2): 206–213.

Ley, S.H., Ardisson Korat, A.V., Sun, Q. et al. (2016). Contribution of the nurses' health studies to uncovering risk factors for type 2 diabetes: diet, lifestyle, biomarkers, and genetics. *Am. J. Public Health* 106 (9): 1624–1630.

Li, Y., Gu, M., Jing, F. et al. (2016). Association between physical activity and all cancer mortality: dose-response meta-analysis of cohort studies. *Int. J. Cancer* 138 (4): 818–832.

Mahabir, S., Willett, W.C., Friedenreich, C. et al. (2018). Research strategies for nutritional and physical activity epidemiology and cancer prevention. *Cancer Epidemiol Biomarkers Prev.* 27 (3): 233–244. doi: 10.1158/1055-9965.EPI-17-0509.

Mensah, G.A., Roth, G.A., and Fuster, V. (2019). The global burden of cardiovascular diseases and risk factors: 2020 and beyond. *J. Am. Coll. Cardiol.* 74 (20): 2529–2532.

Nassis, G.P. and Sidossis, L.S. (2009). Thighs and heart disease. Exercise, muscle mass, and insulin sensitivity. *Br. Med. J.* 339: b4249.

National Cancer Institute. (2017). Tobacco. www.cancer.gov/about-cancer/causes-prevention/risk/tobacco.

NCD Risk Factor Collaboration. (2016). Trends in adult body-mass index in 200 countries from 1975 to 2014: a pooled analysis of 1698 population-based measurement studies with 19.2 million participants. *Lancet* 387 (10026): 1377–1396.

Popkin, B.M., Adair, L.S., and Ng, S.W. (2012). Global nutrition transition and the pandemic of obesity in developing countries. *Nutr. Rev.* 70 (1): 3–21.

Rehm, J., Soerjomataram, I., Ferreira-Borges, C., and Shield, K.D. (2019). Does alcohol use affect cancer risk? *Curr. Nutr. Rep.* 8 (3): 222–229.

Schols, A. and Sidossis, L.S. (2011). Abnormal body composition and early biomarkers of metabolic complications. *Curr. Opin. Clin. Nutr. Metab. Care* 14 (6): 517–519.

Schwenk, R.W., Vogel, H., and Schurmann, A. (2013). Genetic and epigenetic control of metabolic health. *Mol. Metab.* 2 (4): 337–347.

Shekhar, H.U., Chakraborty, S., Mannoor, K., and Sarker, A.H. (2019). Recent advances in understanding the role of genomic and epigenomic factors in noncommunicable diseases. *Biomed. Res. Int.* 2019: 1649873.

van der Valk, E.S., Savas, M., and van Rossum, E.F.C. (2018). Stress and obesity: are there more susceptible individuals? *Curr. Obes. Rep.* 7 (2): 193–203.

World Health Organization. (2017). Cardiovascular diseases (CVDs). https://www.who.int/news-room/fact-sheets/detail/cardiovascular-diseases-(cvds).

Yu, E., Rimm, E., Qi, L. et al. (2016). Diet, lifestyle, biomarkers, genetic factors, and risk of cardiovascular disease in the nurses' health studies. *Am. J. Public Health* 106 (9): 1616–1623.

CHAPTER 3

Components of an Unhealthy Lifestyle

Unhealthy Diets

Research has long linked specific nutrients (e.g., refined carbohydrates and added sugars, saturated and trans fatty acids [TFAs] and sodium), foods and food groups (e.g., sweets, sugary soft drinks, red meat, and processed meats), and specific dietary patterns (e.g., Western diet) with a number of diseases and conditions: CVD, cancer, diabetes, hypertension, liver and gallbladder diseases, and obesity. Moreover, diets low in whole grains, fruits and vegetables, nuts and seeds, and ω-3/ω-6 fatty acids seem to be the leading dietary risk factors of mortality the last two decades.

Regarding specific nutrients, high TFA intake increases the risk of all-cause mortality, total CHD, and CHD mortality. Historically, studies on saturated fatty acids (SFAs) suggest positive associations with total and low-density lipoprotein (LDL) cholesterol, coagulation markers, insulin resistance, and inflammation. Some studies have suggested that a long-term diet high in SFAs could increase the risk for CVD and some cancers. However recent data do not fully support a direct connection between SFA and CVD.

An increased amount of dietary salt is an important risk factor for the development of hypertention and increased overall CVD risk. On the other hand, there is an inverse relation between fiber intake and all-cause mortality. According to the WHO, approximately 3% of deaths worldwide are attributable to low fruit and vegetable consumption. Insufficient intake of fruits and vegetables increases the risk for gastrointestinal cancer, ischemic heart disease, and stroke. Most of the benefit of consuming fruits and vegetables comes from reduction in CVD risk, but fruits and vegetables also prevent cancer. Moreover, high consumption of red and processed meat has been associated with all-cause mortality and with several types of cancer, diabetes, and CVD mortality. However, the consumption of whole-grain cereals has been linked to improvements of metabolic syndrome (MetS) and its components: obesity, dyslipidemia, hypertension, and hyperglycemia or T2DM. According to the World Cancer Research Fund, up to 40% of cancers can be prevented by improving diet and increasing physical activity.

Therefore, shifting our diet from animal-based foods to predominantly plant-based foods may result in better health outcomes. In the following sections, we will focus on the most important components of an unhealthy diet.

Excess Caloric Intake

Experimental studies have demonstrated that excess caloric intake can adversely affect insulin sensitivity and plasma glucose, insulin, and triglyceride levels, all positively linked to obesity. Even 1 week of hypercaloric feeding may result in elevated fasting plasma insulin, glucose, and triglyceride levels and to exacerbated insulin response, without any weight gain. These findings suggest that the observed metabolic disturbances during excess caloric intake are not necessarily linked to obesity.

> **Key Point**
>
> Observed metabolic disturbances during excess caloric intake are not necessarily linked to obesity.

Epidemiological data suggest that intake of energy-dense foods (i.e., more than 225–275 kcal/100 g of food), consumers' exposure to large serving sizes, and overeating may contribute to obesity and, therefore, increase the risk for the development of chronic diseases. Overeating has also been associated with increased aging rate and decreased lifespan. According to the "rate-of-living/oxidative damage" theories, lifespan extension is linked to low energy metabolism, low reactive oxygen species (ROS) production rates, low molecular damage, and slow aging. Long-term caloric restriction studies in humans show persistent metabolic slowing accompanied by reduced oxidative stress, evidence supporting the "rate-of-living/oxidative damage" theories of mammalian aging.

Textbook of Lifestyle Medicine, First Edition. Labros S. Sidossis and Stefanos N. Kales.
© 2022 John Wiley & Sons Ltd. Published 2022 by John Wiley & Sons Ltd.

Saturated Fatty Acids

Key Point

It is now generally accepted that the effects of SFA on CVD depend mainly on what replaces them in the diet.

It is now generally accepted that the effects of SFAs on CVD depend mainly on what replaces them in the diet. For example, the substitution of omega-3 polyunsaturated fatty acids (PUFAs) and monounsaturated fatty acids for SFAs might reduce CHD risk. On the other hand, replacing SFA with carbohydrates has mixed results over the CVD risk, while there is some evidence suggesting that whole grains but not refined carbohydrates reduce CVD risk.

In populations following Western dietary habits, it has been shown that when 5% of the energy derived from SFAs is replaced by PUFAs, LDL cholesterol concentrations decrease. In turn, this change can generate a decrease in CHD occurrence and deaths. Males from the Health Professionals Follow-up Study and females from the Nurses' Health Study (NHS) were followed prospectively for 24–30 years; people with the highest consumption of PUFAs had 20% lower CHD risk compared to those who consumed a diet low in PUFAs. Notably, for every 5% decrease of energy coming from SFAs, the CHD risk decreased by 25% when an equal amount of energy was replaced by PUFAs. Similarly, combined scientific data from randomized controlled trials (RCTs) have demonstrated that individuals with increased PUFA intake, instead of SFAs, were 20% less likely to develop CHD, compared with those following a higher SFA diet. The protective effect against CHD incidence was 10% for every 5% of energy replacement by PUFAs, and the magnitude of this beneficial effect was contingent on the duration of the intervention.

Mixed results have been reported when total carbohydrates replace SFA, showing either no overall benefit, reduction, or even increased CVD risk. However, when separating whole grains from refined carbohydrates, isocaloric substitution of whole grains for SFA is associated with a decreased risk of CHD; CHD risk does not change in the case of isocaloric substitution of refined starches/added sugars for SFA.

Current guidelines recommend decreasing saturated fat intake to improve blood lipids and reduce cardiovascular risk. Dairy products have been thought to increase the risk of CVD, due to their high SFA, cholesterol, and calorie content. Indeed, most of the existing dietary guidelines for the prevention and management of cardiometabolic risk recommend low-fat or nonfat dairy consumption. However, robust evidence from prospective studies shows no increase or even a small benefit in CVD risk from high dairy consumption (e.g., yogurt and cheese). The potential mechanisms of the

Key Point

Robust evidence from prospective studies shows no increase or even a small benefit in CVD risk from high dairy consumption.

attenuating effects of dairy foods remain to be fully elaborated but seem to involve food matrix effects on fat bioavailability, changes in the gut microbiome, and glucose, insulin, and other hormonal responses.

Trans Fatty Acids

TFAs are present in foods such as meat and dairy products from ruminant animals (i.e., cattle, sheep, goats, and camels). However, more TFAs are generated during the manufacturing process of partially hydrogenated vegetable and marine oils, such as margarines, confectionary fats, and fat spreads. Foods that commonly contain margarine (such as deep-fried foods, baked goods, and snacks) are therefore high in TFAs. Compared to animal fats, hydrogenated vegetable oils are more stable and less likely to become rancid during repeated deep-frying processes and have greater stability at room temperature. Thus, they are widely used for commercial purposes.

However, TFA intake has been positively and robustly associated with increased risk of CHD and related mortality. The Zutphen Elderly Study showed a positive correlation between intake of TFAs and 10-year risk for CHD. It was shown that for every 2% increase in TFA-derived energy at baseline, there was 28% greater risk to develop CHD within the next decade. In the NHS, the 20-year CHD risk for the women with high trans-fat intake was associated with 1.3-fold, i.e. 130% greater risk, compared to their counterparts with the lowest TFA intake, particularly the younger women.

The underlying mechanism by which TFAs increase CVD risk is probably related to changes in lipoprotein profile. Even moderate levels of TFA intake may lead to increased LDL concentrations, while high-density lipoprotein (HDL) concentrations usually decrease. A meta-analysis of RCTs exploring the impact of either naturally occurring or industrially produced TFAs on plasma LDL to HDL ratio revealed that, independently of their source, all TFAs can lead to an increase in the LDL to HDL ratio. However, others have challenged these findings; they suggested that the high variability in types of oils and interventions used in the various studies precludes drawing safe conclusions on the effect of specific types of TFAs on lipoproteins levels and CHD risk (i.e., naturally occurring or industrially produced TFAs). Indeed, a systematic review and meta-analysis of prospective studies found that industrially produced but not naturally occurring TFAs are associated with increased risk of CHD.

Interestingly, growing evidence supports the notion that specific animal-derived TFAs not only do not have detrimental health effects but may also be beneficial for human health. The naturally occurring trans-palmitoleic acid, mainly found in

Key Point

Industrially produced but not naturally occurring TFAs are associated with increased risk of CHD.

whole-fat dairy products, was associated with reduced CHD mortality, while no association was found with the industrially produced TFAs in a 10-year study by Kleber and co-workers. Finally, in a 2016 systematic review and meta-analysis authorized by the WHO, it was found that the replacement of total or industrial TFAs with either monounsaturated fatty acids (MUFAs) or PUFAs results in improvements in the lipid and lipoprotein profiles, which further lead to the reduction of CVD risk.

Another mechanism through which high TFA consumption can add to the CVD risk is by increasing inflammation and endothelial dysfunction. Data from the Nurses' Health Study I (NHS-I) have shown that women who were free of CVD, cancer, and diabetes at baseline and who consumed a diet high in TFAs were more likely to have increased levels of inflammation and endothelial dysfunction. The positive relationship between TFA intake and systemic inflammation was also evident in an NHS-II cohort; a modest mitigation of this association after controlling for serum lipid levels led to the hypothesis that TFAs impact on serum lipids may act as mediator of this positive association. In 2018, the WHO published an action package to reduce TFA use in the global food supply called the "REPLACE action package." Based on a six-step strategy, each country should implement actions to eliminate the industrially produced TFAs.

> **Key Point**
>
> Each country should implement actions to eliminate the industrially produced TFAs.

Carbohydrates and Dietary Fiber

The evidence linking simple carbohydrate-rich foods with CHD is quite strong. High intake of refined carbohydrates, especially sugar-sweetened beverages, has been consistently associated with increased risk of CHD. However, the characterization of carbohydrates according to their glycemic load (GL) may be a better way to categorize carbohydrates for predicting CHD risk, compared to the more simplistic categorization into "simple" and "complex" carbohydrates. Consumption of high GL meals has been associated with increased CHD incidence in female subjects followed prospectively for 10 years. Interestingly, those consuming a high GL diet had twice the likelihood to develop CHD, compared with those refraining from a high GL diet. In the NHS (76,000 female subjects), refined carbohydrates were associated with increased coronary heart disease, presumably due to increased dietary GL.

> **Key Point**
>
> Consumption of high GL meals has been associated with CHD incidence in female subjects followed prospectively for 10 years.

Dietary fiber intake seems to be beneficial for human health. A meta-analysis of 185 prospective studies yielded a 15–30% reduction in all-cause and cardiovascular mortality, T2DM, and colorectal cancer in individuals with the highest dietary fiber intake, compared with those in the lowest consumption category. In the same meta-analysis, 58 clinical trials were separately analyzed, showing significantly lower body weight, systolic blood pressure, and total cholesterol in people in the high dietary fiber category compared to the lower fiber category. The best outcomes were observed when daily intake of dietary fiber was 25–29 g. In another meta-analysis of 17 prospective studies from 1997 to 2014, it was found that for every 10 g/day increase in fiber intake, there is a 10% decrease in all-cause mortality.

> **Key Point**
>
> For every 10 g/day increase in fiber intake, there is a 10% decrease in all-cause mortality.

According to the 2015–2020 dietary guidelines for Americans, the adequate daily intake of fiber is 14 g/1000 cal, or approximately 25 g/day for women and 38 g/day for men.

Foods and Food Groups

High red meat consumption, and especially processed meat like bacon, sausages, salami or other cold cuts, may increase the risk for chronic diseases (e.g., T2DM and cardiovascular diseases) and certain cancers, including colorectal cancer. Red meat consumption has also been associated with elevated blood pressure and all-cause mortality.

There are several possible mechanisms by which red meat may increase mortality risk. Saturated fat, cholesterol, and heme iron in red meat may stimulate certain atherosclerotic processes and therefore affect the onset of the aforementioned chronic diseases. Moreover, it has been found that people who consume large quantities of meat may consume fewer fruits and vegetables, which have been shown to decrease cardiovascular risk.

During the high-temperature cooking processes of red meat, several potential carcinogens, such as polycyclic aromatic hydrocarbons and heterocyclic amines, are formed, increasing the risk of cancer. Also, the high sodium content in processed meat has been shown to increase the risk for stomach cancer, hypertension, and vascular stiffness. The World Cancer Research Fund recommends no more than three portions of red meat per week, which is equivalent to no more that 350–500 g (cooked weight or 525–750 g raw weight), and minimal consumption of processed meat.

However, a systematic review of 12 randomized trials with 54,000 subjects suggested that diets restricted in red meat may have little effect on cardiometabolic

> **Key Point**
>
> Diets restricted in red meat may have little effect on cardiometabolic outcomes, cancer incidence, and mortality.

outcomes and cancer incidence and mortality. Apparently, the effect of red meat consumption on human health is mediated by many other factors, mainly the specific genetic and lifestyle characterists of each individual.

Dietary Patterns

The Western dietary pattern is generally characterized by high intakes of red and processed meat, refined grains/carbohydrates, fast food, eggs, high-sugar drinks and sweets/desserts, and low intake of fruits and vegetables. According to the INTERHEART study, a standardized case-control study with participants from 52 countries (i.e., 5761 cases and 10,646 controls), an unhealthy diet increases CVD risk by 30%. Western-type diets are considered a major risk factor for developing hypertension due to their high content of salt and have been linked to arterial stiffness. Findings from the ATTICA study in Greece suggest that the sodium content of processed foods can be several-fold higher compared to similar homemade meals; this difference may explain, at least in part, the increased CVD risk in people eating processed foods.

The Western dietary pattern has also been associated with an increased risk for MetS, general and central obesity, and higher BMI and waist circumference in several countries. The Atherosclerosis Risk Communities (ARIC) study followed the dietary patterns of 3782 participants (aged 45–64 years) for 9 years; those with the highest Western dietary pattern scores had 18% greater risk of developing MetS compared to those with the lowest scores. Other prospective data have shown similar associations between Western-type diets and the prevalence of obesity in adults.

A large body of literature suggests that such an unhealthy dietary pattern may also increase the risk of developing T2DM via exacerbating insulin secretion and insulin resistance. Furthermore, Western-type diets increase the production of ROS, promote low-grade inflammation, and abnormally activate the sympathetic nervous system and the renin-angiotensin system. Finally, high-fat diets seem to alter the structure of the microbiome even in the absence of obesity; these changes have been associated with metabolic diseases, including cancer, T2DM, and others.

Physical Inactivity

Inactivity is defined as doing less physical activity (PA) than the recommended levels. In 2021, the recommendation for children and youth aged 5–17 was to do at least 60 minutes of moderate- to vigorous-intensity PA daily, preferably aerobic and performed as play. For adults, the 2021 recommendations call for at least 150 minutes of moderate-intensity aerobic PA per week, or at least 75 minutes of vigorous-intensity aerobic PA throughout the week, or an equivalent combination of moderate- and vigorous-intensity activity.

More than one in four adults globally (~1.5 billion people) were physically inactive in 2018. Women were less active than men (32% men were active vs. 23% women). Citizens from high-income countries were more inactive (37%) compared with citizens from middle-income and low-income countries (16%). Older adults were less active than younger adults (Figures 3.1 and 3.2a and b).

Regarding the pediatric population, 81% of adolescents aged 11–17 years did not meet physical activity recommendations in 2010. Adolescents from the Southeast Asia region showed the lowest prevalence of insufficient PA (74%), whereas the highest were observed in the Asian Pacific region, the Eastern Mediterranean region, and the Sub-Saharan African region (92%, 89%, and 85%, respectively). Globally, adolescent girls were generally less active than adolescent boys, with 85% vs. 78% not meeting WHO recommendations. Furthermore, the prevalence of inactivity was highest in the upper-middle-income countries and lowest in the lower-middle-income countries, for all age groups.

The high prevalence of physical inactivity globally is attributed to insufficient participation in PA during leisure time and an increase in sedentary behavior during occupational, domestic, and transportation activities. Research into the correlates (i.e., factors associated with activity) or determinants (i.e., those with a causal relationship) has proliferated in the past two decades, mostly focused on individual-level factors in high-income countries, and has shown that age, sex, health status, self-esteem, and motivation are associated with PA. However, recently developed ecological models suggest that various components of the social and physical environment, e.g., urban planning, transportation systems, parks, and trails, significantly affect our daily physical activity.

Modern urbanization has resulted in environmental changes that are thought to discourage participation in PA in all domains, such as an increase in violence, high-density traffic, and air pollution, as well as a lack of parks, sidewalks, and sports/recreation facilities. The aforementioned factors might explain, at least in part, the lower prevalence of physical inactivity in low- and lower-middle-income countries, due to maintenance of work and transport-related PA, and the higher prevalence observed in higher-income countries, where the increased automation of life creates opportunities for sedentariness.

Inactive adults have 20–30% increased risk of all-cause mortality, compared to those who engage in at least 150 minutes of moderate-intensity PA per week (Figure 3.3). A study by Lee et al. in 2012 revealed that physical inactivity can be deemed responsible for 6% of the burden of disease from coronary heart disease, 7% of T2DM, 10% of breast cancer, and 10% of colon cancer. Moreover, it was estimated that physical inactivity causes 9% of premature mortality, or more than 5.3 million of the 57 million deaths that occurred worldwide in 2008; if inactivity were

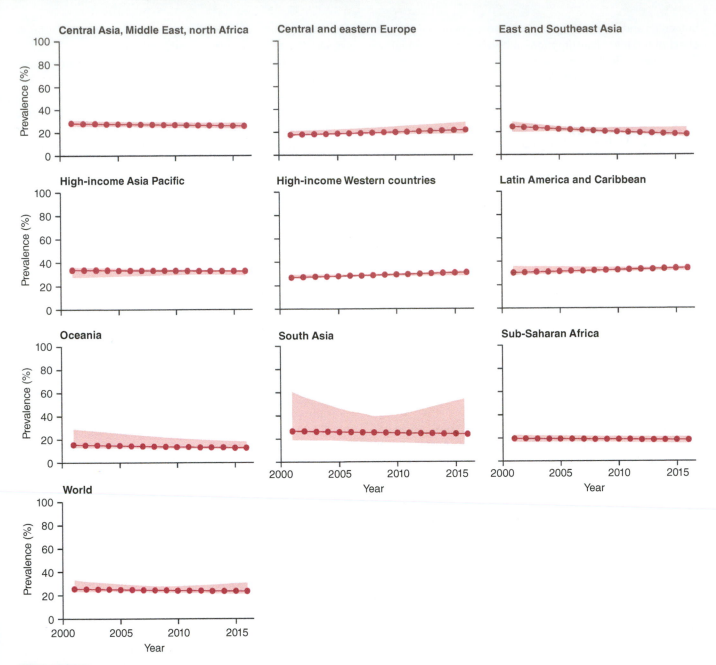

FIGURE 3.1   Trends in insufficient physical activity for three income groups from 2001 to 2016. The shaded areas show 95% uncertainty intervals. **Source:** Reprinted with permission from Guthold et al. (2018).

> **Key Point**
>
> Inactive adults have 20–30% increased risk of all-cause mortality.

decreased by 10% or 25%, more than 533,000 and 1.3 million deaths could be averted every year, respectively. Interestingly, using life-table analysis, Lee et al. also showed that the elimination of physical inactivity would increase the life expectancy of the world's population by 0.68 years (Figure 3.4).

Given the severe public health effects of physical inactivity, efficient multisectoral and multidisciplinary policies need to be implemented, in order to achieve an increase in PA in the population worldwide. Under this scope, in 2013, WHO member

states agreed to a target of reducing sedentariness by 10% by 2025 in the "Global Action Plan for the Prevention and Control of NCDs 2013–2020." The WHO suggested four policy actions for achieving this PA goal:

1. Adopt and implement national guidelines on PA for health.

2. Develop policy measures to promote PA through activities of daily living, including active transport, recreation, leisure, and sport.

3. Create and preserve built and natural environments that support PA in schools, universities, workplaces, clinics, and hospitals, and in the wider community.

(a)

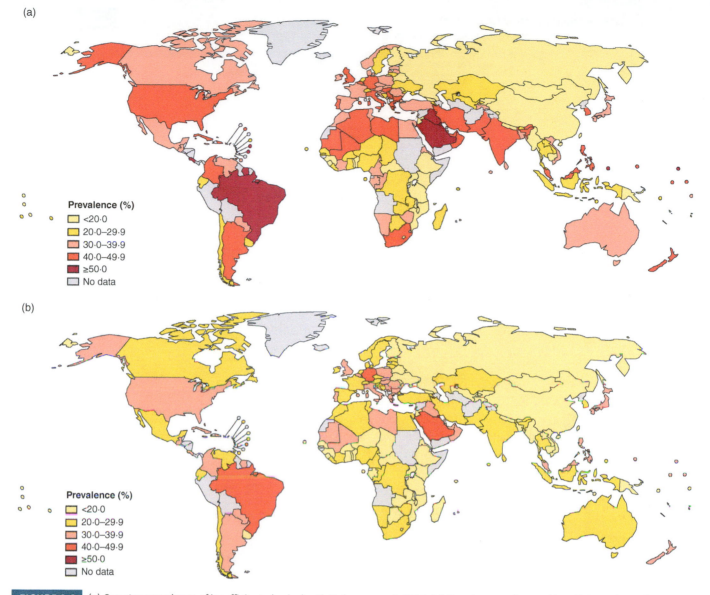

Prevalence (%)
- <20·0
- 20·0–29·9
- 30·0–39·9
- 40·0–49·9
- ≥50·0
- No data

(b)

Prevalence (%)
- <20·0
- 20·0–29·9
- 30·0–39·9
- 40·0–49·9
- ≥50·0
- No data

FIGURE 3.2   (a) Country prevalence of insufficient physical activity in women in 2016. (b) Country prevalence of insufficient physical activity in men in 2016. **Source:** Reprinted with permission from Guthold et al. (2018).

4. Implement evidence-informed public campaigns through mass media, social media, and at the community level to inform and motivate adults and young people to be more physically active.

The WHO has published guidelines to assist the member states and other stakeholders in the development and implementation of national PA plans and to provide guidance on policy options for effective promotion of PA at the national level. Most European and American countries have indeed integrated the promotion of PA at least to some extent in their national health and other policies. However, there is a need to continue updating the policies, both methodologically and substantially, in order to combat the current global sedentariness epidemic and promote the adoption of PA guidelines.

Key Point

Most European and American countries have integrated the promotion of PA at least to some extent in their national health and other policies.

Unhealthy Weight

Unhealthy weight is a well-documented risk factor for NCDs development, even in the absence of other major risk factors. Maintaining a healthy weight and refraining from smoking increases the years spent in good health, in both men and women. For obese men, the number of years spent in good health are decreased by 4.6 years, relative to men living a healthy life. For men who smoke, the number of years spent in good health are decreased by 7.8 years. The respective

Number of deaths by risk factor, world, 2017

Total annual number of deaths by risk factor, measured across all age groups and both sexes.

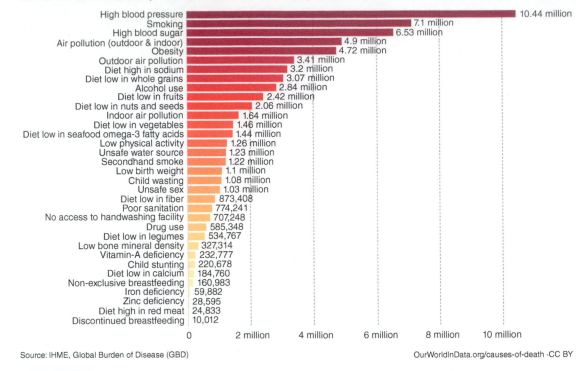

High blood pressure	10.44 million
Smoking	7.1 million
High blood sugar	6.53 million
Air pollution (outdoor & indoor)	4.9 million
Obesity	4.72 million
Outdoor air pollution	3.41 million
Diet high in sodium	3.2 million
Diet low in whole grains	3.07 million
Alcohol use	2.84 million
Diet low in fruits	2.42 million
Diet low in nuts and seeds	2.06 million
Indoor air pollution	1.64 million
Diet low in vegetables	1.46 million
Diet low in seafood omega-3 fatty acids	1.44 million
Low physical activity	1.26 million
Unsafe water source	1.23 million
Secondhand smoke	1.22 million
Low birth weight	1.1 million
Child wasting	1.08 million
Unsafe sex	1.03 million
Diet low in fiber	873,408
Poor sanitation	774,241
No access to handwashing facility	707,248
Drug use	585,348
Diet low in legumes	534,767
Low bone mineral density	327,314
Vitamin-A deficiency	232,777
Child stunting	220,678
Diet low in calcium	184,760
Non-exclusive breastfeeding	160,983
Iron deficiency	59,882
Zinc deficiency	28,595
Diet high in red meat	24,833
Discontinued breastfeeding	10,012

0   2 million   4 million   6 million   8 million   10 million

Source: IHME, Global Burden of Disease (GBD)   OurWorldInData.org/causes-of-death ·CC BY

FIGURE 3.3   Total annual number of deaths by risk factor. **Source:** Reprinted with permission from the Global Burden of Disease Collaborative Network. Global Burden of Disease Study 2017. Institute for Health Metrics and Evaluation (IHME) (2018).

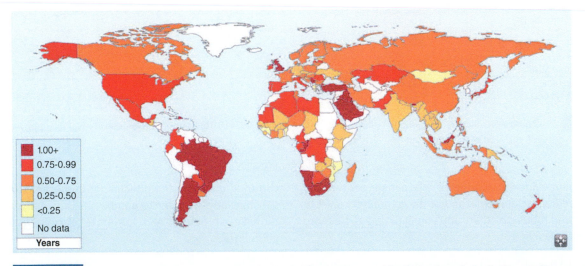

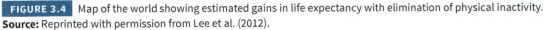

■	1.00+
■	0.75–0.99
■	0.50–0.75
■	0.25–0.50
■	<0.25
□	No data
Years	

FIGURE 3.4   Map of the world showing estimated gains in life expectancy with elimination of physical inactivity. **Source:** Reprinted with permission from Lee et al. (2012).

decreases for women are 4.5 and 6.0 years, for obese and smokers, respectively.

In addition, in a meta-analysis of 230 cohort studies (207 publications), overweight and obesity were associated with increased risk of all-cause mortality, with the lowest risk observed at BMI 23–24 kg/m² among never smokers, 22–23 kg/m² among healthy never smokers, and 20–22 kg/m² with longer durations of follow-up.

As is usually the case, not all studies agree; data from the Dutch Burden of Disease study suggest that elimination of smoking or obesity does not result in absolute compression of morbidity but slightly increases the part of life lived in good health (which, by the way, is very important!).

Regarding the risk for developing T2DM, findings from the Uppsala Longitudinal Study of Adult Men (ULSAM) cohort indicated that after 20 years of follow-up, those being overweight/

obese but free of MetS had approximately 3.5 times increased risk of developing T2DM; the risk was eight times higher for overweight/obese individuals with MetS, relative to those of normal weight and free of MetS.

Contrary to the above findings suggesting that overweight/obesity is a risk factor for NCDs, other studies have shown that overweight and even grade 1 obesity (BMI = 30–35 kg/m²) are related to decreased all-cause mortality by 6% and 5%, respectively, compared to those of normal BMI. Still, obesity grades 2 and 3 (BMI > 35 kg/m²) are associated with 18% and 29% increased risk of all-cause mortality, respectively, compared to those of normal BMI.

There are many studies on BMI and mortality without uniform results. This is because many factors have been shown to confound the relationship between BMI and longevity. Possible residual confounding factors might be age, disease-related weight loss, and individuals who smoked, had underlying diseases (e.g., cancer), or suffered early deaths.

In the elderly, mortality risk increases at BMIs lower than 22 kg/m², which is not seen in younger adults, while a lower risk is observed among those with overweight and mild obesity. This paradoxical finding, i.e., lower mortality at higher than "healthy" BMI levels, has been termed "the obesity paradox." There are many possible mechanisms to explain these findings. Excess fat may act as a metabolic reserve during illness or injury. In addition, because of lower noradrenaline-stimulated lipolytic activity in visceral fat as age increases (which leads to insulin resistance and morbidity), individuals may be less affected by excess adiposity. Moreover, physicians often prescribe more medications to those with overweight and obesity, which may indirectly contribute to the obesity paradox.

Frequent changes from normal to obese and back (yo-yo effect) have been linked to more than twofold increased risk of all-cause mortality, relative to stable normal BMI. However, changes from normal weight to overweight (not obesity) were not linked to elevated all-cause mortality risk, compared to stable normal weight. These findings were similar for CVD- and cancer-specific mortality.

Tobacco Use

According to the WHO, tobacco use is responsible for more than six million deaths annually. Smoking is responsible for more than five million of those fatal events, whereas secondhand smoking results in more than 600,000 deaths annually. More than 4000 chemical substances are present in tobacco smoke; more than 250 of those have been linked to negative effects for human health. Furthermore, more than 50 chemical substances in tobacco smoke have been robustly associated with increased incidence of oropharynx, esophagus,

> **Key Point**
> Smoking is the leading risk factor of cancer-specific deaths; it accounts for more than 20% of the global annual cancer-induced mortality.

stomach, liver, cervix, and colorectal cancer. Smoking is the leading risk factor of cancer-specific deaths; it accounts for more than 20% of the global annual cancer-induced mortality.

Tobacco use has been shown to have a causal relationship with the incidence of a variety of other chronic diseases, like stroke, CHD, T2DM, respiratory diseases, and impaired immune function. Smokers have 2–25 times higher risk for developing CHD and stroke when compared to nonsmokers. Smoking causes overall health deterioration, increases the number of days off from work, and increases healthcare utilization and cost. Quitting smoking can lead to important benefits in terms of longevity and mortality risk, especially for those who quit smoking early. Finally, it has been shown that heavy smokers live an unhealthier lifestyle compared to those who do not smoke, which usually includes sedentary lifestyle, excessive alcohol intake, and poor dietary habits.

> **Key Point**
> Quitting smoking can lead to important benefits in terms of longevity and mortality risk, especially for those who quit smoking early.

Excessive Alcohol Intake

Excessive alcohol intake has been recognized as a causal factor for more than 200 major types of diseases, injuries, and other health conditions – CVDs, T2DM, cancers, and gastrointestinal diseases, including liver cirrhosis and mental and behavioral disorders, as well as unintentional or intentional injuries. Figure 3.5 shows the distribution of alcohol-attributable deaths in 2012, by broad disease category.

According to the US dietary guidelines issued in 2015, excessive alcohol consumption may include binge drinking (i.e., 4 or more drinks for women and 5 or more drinks for men within 2 hours) or heavy drinking (i.e., 8 or more drinks a week for women and 15 or more drinks a week for men) with an alcoholic drink-equivalent defined as 14 g (0.6 fl oz) of pure alcohol. Examples of one alcoholic drink-equivalent include 12 fluid ounces (~355 ml) of regular beer (5% alcohol), 5 fluid ounces (~148 ml) of wine (12% alcohol), or 1.5 fluid ounces (~45 ml) of 80 proof distilled spirits (40% alcohol).

Alcohol-related health effects are associated with the volume of alcohol consumed and the pattern of drinking. For most alcohol-related diseases, there is a dose–response relationship, which means that the higher the consumption of alcohol the higher the risk for disease development. The drinking pattern, reflecting the way people consume alcohol, may be equally important as to the amount consumed. Heavy episodic drinking or binge drinking, i.e., 60 or more grams of pure alcohol on at least one single occasion at

> **Key Point**
> Alcohol-related health effects are associated with the volume of alcohol consumed and the pattern of drinking.

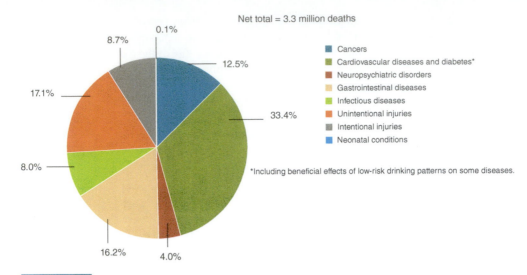

Net total = 3.3 million deaths

- Cancers
- Cardiovascular diseases and diabetes*
- Neuropsychiatric disorders
- Gastrointestinal diseases
- Infectious diseases
- Unintentional injuries
- Intentional injuries
- Neonatal conditions

*Including beneficial effects of low-risk drinking patterns on some diseases.

FIGURE 3.5   Distribution of alcohol-attributable deaths, as a percentage of all alcohol-attributable deaths by broad disease category, 2012. **Source:** Reprinted with permission from WHO Library Cataloguing-in-Publication Data Global status report on alcohol and health – 2014 ed.

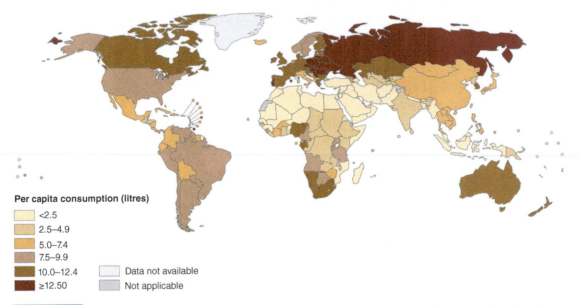

Per capita consumption (litres)

- <2.5
- 2.5–4.9
- 5.0–7.4
- 7.5–9.9
- 10.0–12.4
- ≥12.50
- Data not available
- Not applicable

FIGURE 3.6   Patterns of drinking score (15+ years), 2010. **Source:** Reprinted with permission from the WHO Library Cataloguing-in-Publication Data Global status report on alcohol and health – 2014 ed.

least monthly, is an indicator of the pattern of alcohol consumption associated with detrimental health consequences.

Countries with high per capita adult alcohol consumption, but with the least risky patterns of drinking, are in Southern and Western Europe, whereas the riskiest patterns of drinking are found in the Russian Federation, South Africa, Ukraine, Kazakhstan, and Mexico (Figure 3.6); half of all countries worldwide have a drinking pattern of intermediate risk.

Stress

People respond to life stresses in a variety of ways that may cause adverse health effects, especially when their reaction is fierce and violent. According to the American Psychological Association (APA), stressful circumstances hold the potential to affect several systems in the human body in a harmful way.

Under stressful conditions muscles are strained in an attempt to repel stress. However, chronic stress renders muscles constantly tensed, which in turn can lead to other abnormalities – neck and head muscle tension has been linked to tension-type experiences and migraine headaches. It has been suggested that

Key Point

Neck and head muscle tension has been linked to tension-type experiences and migraine headaches.

Key Point

Stressful circumstances hold the potential to affect several systems in the human body in a harmful way.

stress relaxation techniques can ease tensed muscles, reduce the occurrence of impairments linked to stress, and enhance the feeling of wellness and well-being.

Under stressful conditions, breathing becomes harder. This change can prove burdensome for people with chronic respiratory disorders, such as asthma. However, stress can also induce asthma attacks in people free of respiratory diseases and panic attacks among vulnerable people. Furthermore, psychological stress has been shown to increase heart rate, mainly due to increased secretion of stress hormones, such as adrenaline, noradrenaline, and cortisol. Thus, being under constant stress may result in aggravated heart function; in the long term, this condition may cause hypertension, CHD, or stroke.

> **Key Point**
>
> Being under constant stress may result in aggravated heart function.

Stressful experiences can trigger an inflammatory response, mainly in the coronary arteries, which is thought to be one of the mechanisms for the development of heart diseases. The way people cope with stress may affect blood cholesterol levels, which is also related to CVD events. Finally, stress hormones enhance hepatic glucose production and induce insulin resistance. Repeated stressful experiences can also cause disturbances in the gastrointestinal tract, the nervous system, and the male and female reproductive systems.

Lifestyle-Induced Epigenetic Alterations and NCD Risk

As mentioned in Chapter 2, the genetic background plays an important role in the development of several degenerative diseases. Nevertheless, the expression of genes that gives a variety of phenotypes linked to chronic diseases can be influenced by factors other than heritability. These factors and processes may be of developmental nature, occurring both in utero and during childhood, they may be chemicals found in the environment, drugs and/or pharmaceuticals, or caused by the aging progress and poor dietary habits (Figure 3.7). Provided that these parameters do not alter the DNA sequence but only the way genes act and are expressed, they are thought to exert an additional effect on the conventional genetic inheritance, thus characterized as epigenetic mechanisms – with the prefix *epi-* deriving from the Greek prefix επὶ- meaning over, outside of, around.

The term *epigenetic mechanisms* refers to the parameters involved in the modifications of gene regulation, including DNA methylation, histone modifications, and RNA-based mechanisms. Nutrigenomics is the epigenomics sector focusing on the effects of food and food constituents on gene expression. For example, adoption of a Mediterranean diet pattern rich in olive oil for 3 years can reduce the detrimental effects of the risk variant of the IL-6 gene, associated with weight gain, among middle-aged and older persons with high CVD risk. Compared

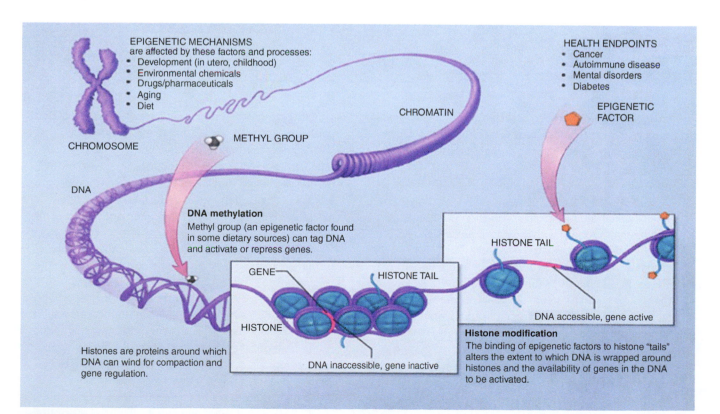

FIGURE 3.7   Epigenetic mechanisms. **Source:** National Institutes of Health (2018).

to the noncarriers and those heterozygous for the risk allele of the IL-6 gene, the homozygous ones had higher adiposity indexes pre-intervention, but after three years on the Mediterranean diet rich in olive oil, they appeared to have the most weight loss.

Moreover, variations in the gene-expressing adipokine (hormone) adiponectin have been implicated in weight gain in a cohort of middle-aged and elderly individuals at increased risk for CVD. Nevertheless, following a Mediterranean diet for three years proved to be advantageous in reversing weight gain among the carriers of the adiponectin gene SNPs, compared to noncarriers. Similarly, when the carriers of the fat-mass obesity (FTO) polymorphism, which is responsible for increased body weight, followed a Mediterranean diet pattern for three years, they appeared to have the lowest increase in weight after intervention, compared to the noncarriers.

The phytochemicals present in fruits and vegetables, herbs, and spices have been shown to be protective not only against oxidative stress but also chronic low-grade inflammatory responses, which constitute established risk factors of age-related brain impairments. Moreover, phytochemicals hold the potential to attenuate the oxidative damage of macromolecules, such as DNA. They can also protect against the deranged expression of genes, which can progressively lead to debilitating effects on brain function and the advent of brain disorders associated with aging.

The Effect of Maternal Health and Lifestyle Habits During Gestation

It is now widely accepted that maternal health and lifestyle habits, as well as infants' early nutrition and exposure to environmental factors, are involved in the development of metabolic diseases later in life. For instance, the presence of gestational diabetes mellitus (GDM) is related to reductions in methylation of the mesoderm-specific transcript (MEST) gene, a feature detected also among morbidly obese adults. When the fetus is exposed to GDM, the abnormal programming of the MEST gene increases the susceptibility of developing obesity later in life.

Another prenatal condition with future ramifications on the epigenome is that of famine exposure. Being exposed to famine prenatally can lead to alterations in the DNA methylation. Findings from a cohort study revealed that more young adults exposed to famine in gestation were underweight compared to young adults that were either exposed to famine postnatally or were never exposed. In contrast, more young adults exposed to famine postnatally were overweight compared to those gestationally exposed or unexposed. Underweight adults exposed to famine in gestation were hyperglycemic following a glucose tolerance test, and those exposed postnatally had elevated fasting glucose, compared to those unexposed.

Take-Home Messages

- An unhealthy diet has been associated with the development of a number of diseases, including CVD, cancer, diabetes, hypertension, liver and gallbladder diseases, and obesity.
- Excess caloric intake can adversely affect insulin sensitivity as well as plasma glucose, insulin, and triglyceride levels, which are all linked to obesity. Overeating has also been associated with increased aging rate and the development of age-related diseases.
- The effects of SFAs on CVD depend on what replaces them in the diet. Replacing saturated fat with PUFAs lowers the risk of coronary heart disease; on the other hand, replacing saturated fat with refined carbohydrates has no benefit on the prevention of coronary heart disease and may even increase the corresponding risk.
- Dairy products (e.g., yogurt and cheese) may have a neutral or even beneficial effect on CVD risk; in fact, it seems that CVD risk decreases from moderate dairy consumption.

- TFA intake has been positively and robustly associated with increased risk of CHD and related mortality.
- Dietary fiber has been associated with reduced all-cause and cardiovascular-related mortality, incidence of CHD, stroke incidence and mortality, T2DM, and colorectal cancer. The adequate daily intake of fiber is 14 g/1000 kcal, or 25 g/day for women and 38 g/day for men.
- Overconsumption of calories and unhealthy dietary patterns, such as the Western dietary pattern, might be the main contributing factors for chronic diseases.
- Western-type diets are positively associated with chronic diseases by increasing ROS production, insulin secretion, and insulin resistance; promoting low-grade inflammation and abnormal activation of the sympathetic nervous system and the renin-angiotensin system; and leading to gut microbiota alterations.
- Very-high and very-low carbohydrate diets have been associated with increased all-cause mortality,

with the lowest risk observed at 50–55% carbohydrate intake.

- Physical inactivity can explain 6–10% of the main NCDs and 9% of premature mortality, while physical activity may increase quality of life and possibly life expectancy.
- Obesity grades 2 and 3 (BMI > 35 kg/m²) may be a risk factor of NCD development, even in the absence of other major risk factors.
- Tobacco use increases the incidence of a variety of chronic diseases, such as stroke, CHD, diabetes, respiratory problems, impaired immune function, and several types of cancer.
- Excessive alcohol intake has been linked to the development of more than 200 major diseases.

- Stress can trigger the inflammatory response in the circulatory system, mainly in the coronary arteries, which is thought to be one of the mechanisms mediating the development of CVD.
- The term *epigenetic mechanisms* refers to the parameters involved in the modifications of gene regulation, including DNA methylation, histone modifications, and RNA-based mechanisms.
- Maternal health and lifestyle habits, as well as infants' early nutrition and exposure to environmental factors, are involved in the development of metabolic diseases later in life.

Self-Assessment Questions

1. Which of the following sentences is correct?
   a. Excess caloric intake has favorable effects on insulin sensitivity.
   b. Overeating has been associated with increased aging rate.
   c. One week of hypercaloric feeding does not affect fasting plasma insulin.
   d. a and b

2. Fill in the blanks:
   a. The substitution of _____ for SFAs might reduce CHD risk.
   b. Replacing SFA _____ reduces CVD risk.
   c. Results from prospective studies show _____ in CVD risk from full-fat dairy consumption.
   d. The highest degree of _____ is generated during the manufacturing process of hydrogenated vegetable and marine oils, such as margarines, confectionary fats, and fat spreads.
   e. Diets restricted in red meat may have _____ effect on cardiometabolic outcomes and cancer incidence and mortality.
   f. _____ smoking can lead to important benefits in terms of longevity and mortality risk.
   g. Very-high and very-low carbohydrate diets have been associated with increased all-cause mortality; the lowest risk is observed when _____ of daily energy comes from carbohydrate intake.

3. What is the recommended daily amount of fiber intake?

4. According to the World Cancer Research Fund, what is the recommendation of red meat consumption per week?

5. How much moderate- to vigorous-intensity physical activity should children engage in?
   a. 30 minutes or more per day
   b. 60 minutes or more per day
   c. 90 minutes or more per day
   d. 150 minutes or more per day

6. What are the recommendations for physical activity for adults?

7. Tobacco use has been shown to have a positive relationship with:
   a. stroke
   b. CHD
   c. T2DM
   d. respiratory problems
   e. impaired immune function
   f. all of the above

8. Define the terms *binge* and *heavy* drinking.

9. How can stress affect CVD development?

10. What does the term *epigenetic mechanisms* refer to?

11. Briefly describe the effects of SFAs on health.

12. How can TFAs increase CVD risk?

13. Which of the following statements about Western-type diets are correct?
    a. They are characterized by high intakes of meat, refined grains, fast food, eggs, high-sugar drinks and sweets, as well as low intake of fruits and vegetables.
    b. They represent a major risk factor for hypertension due to their high salt content.
    c. They can induce low-grade inflammation and oxidative stress and lead to an abnormal activation of the sympathetic nervous system.
    d. They seem to alter the structure of the microbiome even in the absence of obesity.
    e. All of the above

14. Fill in the blanks:
    a. Inactive adults have _____ increased risk of all-cause mortality, compared to those who engage in at least 150 minutes of moderate-intensity PA per week.
    b. _____ is the leading risk factor of cancer-specific deaths.
    c. _____ may be related to decreased all-cause mortality, compared to body weight values in the normal BMI range.

  d. _____but not_____TFAs are associated with increased risk of CHD.
  e. Changing our diet from_____-based foods to_____-based foods may result in better health outcomes.
15. Which of the following statements about TFAs are correct?
  a. TFA intake has been positively and robustly associated with increased risk of CHD and related mortality.
  b. TFAs are naturally present in foods, such as legumes and vegetable oils.
  c. Foods that commonly contain margarine, such as deep-fried foods, baked goods, and snacks, are therefore high in TFAs.
  d. Naturally occurring TFAs are associated with increased risk of CVD.
  e. TFAs are not dangerous as long as total fat intake is low.

Bibliography

Agorastos, A. and Chrousos, G.P. (2021). The neuroendocrinology of stress: the stress-related continuum of chronic disease development. *Mol. Psychiatry*. doi: 10.1038/s41380-021-01224-9.

American Psychological Association. (2017). Stress effects on the body. http://www.apa.org/helpcenter/stress-body.aspx.

Azadbakht, L., Haghighatdoost, F., Keshteli, A.H. et al. (2017). Consumption of energy-dense diets in relation to metabolic syndrome and inflammatory markers in Iranian female nurses. *Public Health Nutr.* 20 (5): 893–901.

Azais-Braesco, V., Sluik, D., Maillot, M. et al. (2017). A review of total & added sugar intakes and dietary sources in Europe. *Nutr. J.* 16 (1): 6.

Bielemann, R.M., Silva, B.G., Coll Cde, V. et al. (2015). Burden of physical inactivity and hospitalization costs due to chronic diseases. *Rev. Saude Publica* 49: 75.

Briggs, M.A., Petersen, K.S., and Kris-Etherton, P.M. (2017). Saturated fatty acids and cardiovascular disease: replacements for saturated fat to reduce cardiovascular risk. *Healthcare (Basel)* 5 (2): 29.

Cheng, F.W., Gao, X., Mitchell, D.C. et al. (2016). Body mass index and all-cause mortality among older adults. *Obesity (Silver Spring)* 10: 2232–2239.

Davinelli, S., Maes, M., Corbi, G. et al. (2016). Dietary phytochemicals and neuro-inflammaging: from mechanistic insights to translational challenges. *Immun. Ageing* 13: 16.

Davis, A., Liu, R., Kerr, J.A. et al. (2019). Inflammatory diet and preclinical cardiovascular phenotypes in 11–12 year-olds and mid-life adults: a cross-sectional population-based study. *Atherosclerosis* 285: 93–101. doi: 10.1016/j.atherosclerosis.2019.04.212.

de Souza, R.J., Mente, A., Maroleanu, A. et al. (2015). Intake of saturated and trans unsaturated fatty acids and risk of all cause mortality, cardiovascular disease, and type 2 diabetes: systematic review and meta-analysis of observational studies. *Br. Med. J.* 351: h3978.

Drouin-Chartier, J.P., Brassard, D., Tessier-Grenier, M. et al. (2016). Systematic review of the association between dairy product consumption and risk of cardiovascular-related clinical outcomes. *Adv. Nutr.* 7 (6): 1026–1040.

Finer, S., Iqbal, M.S., Lowe, R. et al. (2016). Is famine exposure during developmental life in rural Bangladesh associated with a metabolic and epigenetic signature in young adulthood? A historical cohort study. *BMJ Open* 6 (11): e011768.

Fransen, H.P., Boer, J.M.A., Beulens, J.W.J. et al. (2017). Associations between lifestyle factors and an unhealthy diet. *Eur. J. Public Health* 27 (2): 274–278.

Gassen, N.C., Chrousos, G.P., Binder, E.B. et al. (2017). Life stress, glucocorticoid signaling, and the aging epigenome: Implications for aging-related diseases. *Neurosci. Biobehav. Rev.* 74 (Pt B): 356–365. doi: 10.1016/j.neubiorev.2016.06.003.

GBD 2017 Diet Collaborators. (2019). Health effects of dietary risks in 195 countries, 1990–2017: a systematic analysis for the Global Burden of Disease Study 2017. *Lancet* 393 (10184): 1958–1972.

Gong, L., Cao, W., Chi, H. et al. (2018). Whole cereal grains and potential health effects: involvement of the gut microbiota. *Food Res. Int.* 103: 84–102.

Guthold, R., Stevens, G.A., Riley, L.M., and Bull, F.C. (2018). Worldwide trends in insufficient physical activity from 2001 to 2016: a pooled analysis of 358 population-based surveys with 1.9 million participants. *Lancet Glob. Health* 6 (10): e1077–e1086.

Institute for Health Metrics and Evaluation (IHME). (2018). *Findings from the Global Burden of Disease Study 2017*. Seattle, WA: IHME. http://ghdx.healthdata.org/gbd-results-tool.

Johnston, B.C., Zeraatkar, D., Han, M.A. et al. (2019). Unprocessed red meat and processed meat consumption: dietary guideline recommendations from the nutritional recommendations (NutriRECS) consortium. *Ann. Intern. Med.* 171 (10): 756–764.

Kleber, M.E., Delgado, G.E., Lorkowski, S., März, W., and von Schacky, C. (2016). Trans-fatty acids and mortality in patients referred for coronary angiography: the Ludwigshafen Risk and Cardiovascular Health Study. *Eur. Heart J.* 37 (13): 1072–1078. doi: 10.1093/eurheartj/ehv446.

Kokkinos, P., Faselis, C., Franklin, B. et al. (2019). Cardiorespiratory fitness, body mass index and heart failure incidence. *Eur. J. Heart Fail.* 21 (4): 436–444.

Kopp, W. (2019). How Western diet and lifestyle drive the pandemic of obesity and civilization diseases. *Diabetes Metab. Syndr. Obes.* 12: 2221–2236.

Krekoukia, M., Nassis, G.P., Psarra, G. et al. (2007). Elevated total and central adiposity and low physical activity are associated with insulin resistance in children. *Metabolism* 56 (2): 206–213.

Lee, I.M., Shiroma, E.J., Lobelo, F. et al. (2012). Effect of physical inactivity on major non-communicable diseases worldwide: an analysis of burden of disease and life expectancy. *Lancet* 380 (9838): 219–229. PMID: 22818936; PMCID: PMC3645500.

Li, Y., Hruby, A., Bernstein, A.M. et al. (2015). Saturated fats compared with unsaturated fats and sources of carbohydrates in relation to risk of coronary heart disease: a prospective cohort study. *J. Am. Coll. Cardiol.* 66 (14): 1538–1548.

Liska, D.J., Cook, C.M., Wang, D.D. et al. (2016). Trans fatty acids and cholesterol levels: an evidence map of the available science. *Food Chem. Toxicol.* 98 (Pt B): 269–281.

Livesey, G. and Livesey, H. (2019). Coronary heart disease and dietary carbohydrate, glycemic index, and glycemic load: dose-response meta-analyses of prospective cohort studies. *Mayo Clinic Proc. Innov. Qual. Outcomes* 3 (1): 52–69.

Livesey, G., Taylor, R., Livesey, H.F. et al. (2019). Dietary glycemic index and load and the risk of type 2 diabetes: assessment of causal relations. *Nutrients* 11 (6).

Lordan, R., Tsoupras, A., Mitra, B., and Zabetakis, I. (2018). Dairy fats and cardiovascular disease: do we really need to be concerned? *Foods* 7 (3): 29.

Ludwig, D.S., Willett, W.C., Volek, J.S. et al. (2018). Dietary fat: from foe to friend? *Science* 362 (6416): 764–770. doi: 10.1126/science.aau2096.

Magkos, F. and Sidossis, L.S. (2008). Exercise and insulin sensitivity – where do we stand? You'd better run! *Eur. J. Endocrinol.* 4 (1): 22–25.

Malek, A.M., Newman, J.C., Hunt, K.J. et al. (2019). Dietary sources of sugars and calories. *Nutr. Today* 54 (6): 296–304.

Medina-Remon, A., Kirwan, R., Lamuela-Raventos, R.M., and Estruch, R. (2018). Dietary patterns and the risk of obesity, type 2 diabetes mellitus, cardiovascular diseases, asthma, and neurodegenerative diseases. *Crit. Rev. Food Sci. Nutr.* 58 (2): 262–296.

Micha, R., Khatibzadeh, S., Shi, P. et al. (2014). Global, regional, and national consumption levels of dietary fats and oils in 1990 and 2010: a systematic analysis including 266 country-specific nutrition surveys. *Br. Med. J.* 348: g2272.

Mirmiran, P., Amirhamidi, Z., Ejtahed, H.S. et al. (2017). Relationship between diet and non-alcoholic fatty liver disease: a review article. *Iran. J. Public Health* 46 (8): 1007–1017.

Nassis, G.P., Papantakou, K., Skenderi, K. et al. (2005). Aerobic exercise training improves insulin sensitivity without changes in body weight, body fat, adiponectin, and inflammatory markers in overweight and obese girls. *Metabolism* 54 (11): 1472–1479.

Nassis, G.P., Psarra, G., and Sidossis, L.S. (2005). Central and total adiposity are lower in overweight and obese children with high cardiorespiratory fitness. *Eur. J. Clin. Nutr.* 59 (1): 137–141.

Oh, K., Hu, F.B., Manson, J.E. et al. (2005). Dietary fat intake and risk of coronary heart disease in women: 20 years of follow-up of the Nurses' Health Study. *Am. J. Epidemiol.* 161 (7): 672–679.

Panagiotakos, D., Pitsavos, C., Chrysohoou, C. et al. (2009). Dietary patterns and 5-year incidence of cardiovascular disease: a multivariate analysis of the ATTICA study. *Nutr. Metab. Cardiovasc. Dis.* 19 (4): 253–263.

Pervanidou, P. and Chrousos, G.P. (2018). Early-life stress: from neuroendocrine mechanisms to stress-related disorders. *Horm. Res. Paediatr.* 89 (5): 372–379. doi: 10.1159/000488468.

Pitsavos, C., Panagiotakos, D.B., Tambalis, K.D. et al. (2009). Resistance exercise plus to aerobic activities is associated with better lipids' profile among healthy individuals: the ATTICA study. *QJM* 102 (9): 609–616.

Prieto, M.S. and Kales, S.N. (2016). Dietary, lifestyle behaviors and obesity: towards modern science. *J. Obes. Eat. Disord.* 2 (2): 1–2.

Redman, L.M., Smith, S.R., Burton, J.H. et al. (2018). Metabolic slowing and reduced oxidative damage with sustained caloric restriction support the rate of living and oxidative damage theories of aging. *Cell Metab.* 27 (4): 805–815. e4.

Reynolds, A., Mann, J., Cummings, J. et al. (2019). Carbohydrate quality and human health: a series of systematic reviews and meta-analyses. *Lancet* 393 (10170): 434–445.

Romieu, I., Dossus, L., Barquera, S. et al. (2017). Energy balance and obesity: what are the main drivers? *Cancer Causes Control* 28 (3): 247–258.

Scientific Advisory Committee on Nutrition. (2019). Saturated fats and health. https://assets.publishing.service.gov.uk/government/uploads/system/uploads/attachment_data/file/814995/SACN_report_on_saturated_fat_and_health.pdf.

Seidelmann, S.B., Claggett, B., Cheng, S. et al. (2018). Dietary carbohydrate intake and mortality: a prospective cohort study and meta-analysis. *Lancet Public Health* 3 (9): e419–e428.

Stefanaki, C., Pervanidou, P., Boschiero, D. et al. (2018). Chronic stress and body composition disorders: implications for health and disease. *Hormones (Athens)* 17 (1): 33–43. doi: 10.1007/s42000-018-0023-7.

Tambalis, K., Panagiotakos, D.B., Kavouras, S.A., and Sidossis, L.S. (2009). Responses of blood lipids to aerobic, resistance, and combined aerobic with resistance exercise training: a systematic review of current evidence. *Angiology* 60 (5): 614–632.

Temple, N.J. (2018). Fat, sugar, whole grains and heart disease: 50 years of confusion. *Nutrients* 10 (1): 39.

Tobi, E.W., Lumey, L.H., Talens, R.P. et al. (2009). DNA methylation differences after exposure to prenatal famine are common and timing- and sex-specific. *Hum. Mol. Genet.* 18 (21): 4046–4053.

Tsekouras, Y.E., Magkos, F., Kellas, Y. et al. (2008). High-intensity interval aerobic training reduces hepatic very low-density lipoprotein-triglyceride secretion rate in men. *Am. J. Physiol. Endocrinol. Metab.* 295 (4): E851–E858.

Tsekouras, Y.E., Yanni, A.E., Bougatsas, D. et al. (2007). A single bout of brisk walking increases basal very low-density lipoprotein triacylglycerol clearance in young men. *Metabolism* 56 (8): 1037–1043.

Tsigos, C., Kyrou, I., Kassi, E., and Chrousos, G.P. (2000). Stress: endocrine physiology and pathophysiology. In K.R. Feingold, B. Anawalt, A. Boyce, G. Chrousos, W.W. de Herder, K. Dhatariya, K. Dungan, A. Grossman, J.M. Hershman, J. Hofland, S. Kalra, G. Kaltsas, C. Koch, P. Kopp, M. Korbonits, C.S. Kovacs, W. Kuohung, B. Laferrere, E.A. McGee, R. McLachlan, J.E. Morley, M. New, J. Purnell, R. Sahay, F. Singer, C.A. Stratakis, D.L. Trence & D.P. Wilson (Eds.), Endotext. South Dartmouth, MA: MDText. com, Inc.

World Cancer Research Fund/American Institute for Cancer Research. (2018). *Recommendations and public health and policy implications: continuous update project report*. World Cancer Research Fund. https://www.wcrf.org/sites/default/files/Recommendations. pdf.

World Health Organization. (2018). WHO plan to eliminate industrially produced trans-fatty acids from global food supply. https://www.who.int/news/item/14-05-2018-who-plan-to-eliminate-industrially-produced-trans-fatty-acids-from-global-food-supply.

Yang, Q., Zhang, Z., Gregg, E.W. et al. (2014). Added sugar intake and cardiovascular diseases mortality among US adults. *JAMA Intern. Med.* 174 (4): 516–524.

Yip, C.S.C., Lam, W., and Fielding, R. (2018). A summary of meat intakes and health burdens. *Eur. J. Clin. Nutr.* 72 (1): 18–29.

Zeraatkar, D., Johnston, B.C., Bartoszko, J. et al. (2019). Effect of lower versus higher red meat intake on cardiometabolic and cancer outcomes: a systematic review of randomized trials. *Ann. Intern. Med.* 171 (10): 721–731.

Zheng, Y., Li, Y., Satija, A. et al. (2019). Association of changes in red meat consumption with total and cause specific mortality among US women and men: two prospective cohort studies. *Br. Med. J.* 365: l2110.

CHAPTER 4

Characteristics and Principles of a Healthy Lifestyle

A strong body of evidence support that chronic diseases can be prevented if individuals adhere to healthy lifestyle behaviors. The term *healthy lifestyle* is used frequently in scientific literature, but its meaning may vary considerably. It may refer only to the avoidance of bad habits like smoking (preventive orientation), but it may also refer to behaviors that affect mostly the physical aspect of health (preventive and promotive orientation). It may also entail the broader meaning that includes behaviors that affect overall health (holistic, wellness-enhancing orientation). In the past, healthy lifestyle was associated more with the prevention of negative health consequences; today it is related to the promotion of positive health consequences. Adhering to a healthy lifestyle means practicing a way of living that builds, maintains, and promotes health and well-being through a cluster of positive health behaviors.

> **Key Point**
>
> Adhering to a healthy lifestyle means practicing a way of living that builds, maintains, and promotes health and well-being.

The main characteristics of a healthy lifestyle include following a healthy diet; being physically active; maintaining a healthy weight; avoiding tobacco use, excess alcohol use, and the use of other harmful substances; controlling stress; and resting adequately (Figure 4.1).

A healthy diet throughout our lifecycle starts from infancy through breastfeeding. Optimal nutrition through childhood and adolescence helps to foster healthy growth; adequate nutrition throughout the adult life preserves health and maintains a good quality of life. In general, a healthy diet may vary greatly, depending on the personal characteristics, age, gender, physical activity habits, dietary preferences, and cultural habits, but also on food availability and accessibility. Chapter 6 presents the various dietary patterns that are considered healthy, based on extensive research conducted over the past 50 years.

Regular physical activity reduces the risk of CVD, certain types of cancer, hypertension, and depression and contributes to weight control and prevention of overweight and obesity. To ensure good health, physical activity should be an essential component of everyday living. Physical activity may include sports or planned exercise; walking, biking, or running as transportation; leisure time physical activity (such as dancing); occupational (i.e., work) or household chores; play; games; and activities in the context of daily family and community life. Combining aerobic, muscle-strengthening, and bone-strengthening types of exercise provides optimal health benefits. Chapter 9 summarizes the various forms of physical activity and the benefits accrued from them.

> **Key Point**
>
> Regular physical activity reduces the risk of cardiovascular disease, certain types of cancer, hypertension, and depression and contributes to weight control and prevention of overweight and obesity.

Moderate alcohol intake may have some beneficial effects on CVD risk by lowering the risk of ischemic heart disease and ischemic stroke and associated mortality in some populations. When examining average alcohol consumption in comparison to lifetime abstainers, the relationship with ischemic heart disease risk follows a J-curve. The curve turns into a negative relationship at much lower average alcohol intake levels in women compared with men. However, average alcohol consumption alone is not sufficient to describe the relationship between alcohol and ischemic heart disease.

Drinking patterns play an important role in health; both episodic and chronic heavy drinking may counteract the beneficial association with ischemic heart disease risk and elevate other health risks substantially. There is some evidence to suggest that drinkers who have one to two drinks per day without episodic heavy drinking have a lower ischemic heart disease risk compared to lifetime abstainers. However, different drinking patterns are associated with very different health outcomes in diverse population groups with the same level of consumption.

Furthermore, large epidemiological studies suggest that any alcohol consumption may increase the risk for various

Textbook of Lifestyle Medicine, First Edition. Labros S. Sidossis and Stefanos N. Kales.
© 2022 John Wiley & Sons Ltd. Published 2022 by John Wiley & Sons Ltd.

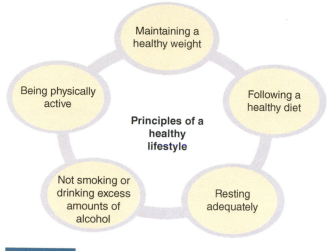

FIGURE 4.1 Basic principles of a healthy lifestyle.

> **Key Point**
>
> According to the WHO, there is no specific limit for alcohol consumption; drinking less is better.

types of cancers (Figure 4.2). Thus, recommendations for clinicians remain challenging because average low alcohol consumption may have both beneficial and detrimental health effects. According to the WHO, there is no specific limit for alcohol consumption; drinking less is better.

Refraining from smoking and all forms of tobacco use is a health-maintaining behavior. Quitting smoking at any age can greatly reduce the risk of developing smoking-related diseases.

> **Key Point**
>
> Although the health benefits are greater for people who quit smoking at earlier ages, benefits ensue at any age.

Although the health benefits are greater for people who quit smoking at earlier ages, benefits ensue at any age. Smoking cessation is associated with lower risk for lung cancer and many other types of cancer, heart disease, stroke, peripheral vascular disease, respiratory symptoms, and lung diseases.

Sleep is a basic element of everyday life, as people spend approximately one third of their lives sleeping; this topic has gained the interest of philosophers, physicians, and scientists since ancient and prehistoric times. The functions of sleep, the mechanisms that regulate sleep physiology, and its role in physical

> **Key Point**
>
> Sleep is not just a simple absence of wakefulness.

and mental health have been the subjects of debate since the fourth century BCE. Sleep is not just a simple absence of wakefulness. It is considered a physiologically active state in which specific processes and metabolic pathways occur that are essential for the regulation of daytime functioning and overall well-being.

The amount and quality of sleep may significantly affect the health of the person. For example, inadequate sleep is

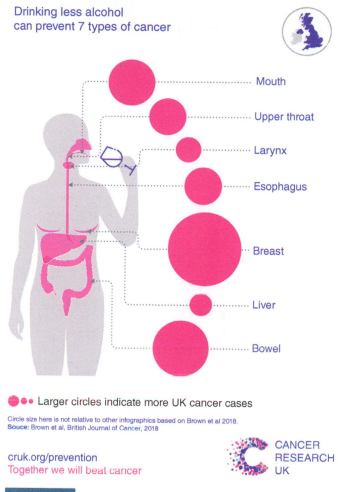

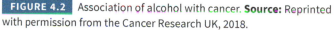

FIGURE 4.2 Association of alcohol with cancer. **Source:** Reprinted with permission from the Cancer Research UK, 2018.

detrimental to the process of learning and memory stabilization. Both insufficient and prolonged sleep are associated with increased risk for developing metabolic syndrome. The basic physiological determinants and the health effects of sleep will be presented in detail in Chapter 10.

Finally, the role of stress on human health has been studied extensively during the last three decades. Stress is caused by various life events; these events don't have to be negative to cause stress. For example, making wedding preparations is a good thing but nevertheless a source of stress. Routine daily activities can also induce stress. However, people's responses to stressors vary greatly and depend mainly on the perception of the specific event; i.e., an event that may cause stress to one person may have no effect on another person. It has been shown that even minor stressful events constitute a substantial source of stress, resulting in deterioration of both mental and physical health. When the adverse effects of daily difficulties and inconveniences congregate, they can aggravate susceptibility to several diseases and undermine overall well-being. Chapter 11 presents the effects of social life and stress on the prevention and treatment of major diseases.

Take-Home Messages

- Healthy lifestyle is a way of living that builds, maintains, and promotes health and well-being through a cluster of positive health behaviors.
- The main components of a healthy lifestyle are healthy diet, being physically active, maintaining a healthy weight, not smoking or drinking excess amounts of alcohol, controlling stress, and resting adequately.
- To maintain a healthy weight means to have a weight that does not cause illness or functional impairment and promotes a healthy self-esteem and a positive body image.

- Avoiding tobacco use is undoubtedly beneficial for health. Quitting smoking/tobacco use can also reduce the risk of developing smoking-related diseases.
- According to WHO, there is no specific limit for alcohol consumption; the less you drink the better it is for your health.
- Adequate sleep (i.e. 7 to 9 hours of sleep for adults) is associated with low mortality and morbidity.
- Stress-reduction approaches, such as mindfulness-based stress-reduction, yoga, and behavioral stress management programs, have all been proven effective in attenuating negative thoughts and feelings of anxiety.

Self-Assessment Questions

1. The term *healthy lifestyle*:
   a. refers to the avoidance of harmful habits, such as smoking
   b. includes behaviors that positively affect the physical aspect of health, such as physical activity and healthy diet
   c. encompasses behaviors that affect overall health and wellness
   d. is associated with the prevention of negative health consequences but also the promotion of positive ones
   e. all of the above
2. What are the main principles of a healthy lifestyle?
3. What are the factors that affect the quality of our diet?
4. Please define the term "physical activity" and give examples of a few types of physical activity.

5. How can alcohol cause cancer?
6. Describe the relationship between alcohol consumption and ischemic heart disease.
7. How is sleep related to health?
8. Which of the following statements about smoking are true?
   a. Smoking cessation is associated with increased risk for lung cancer ( ).
   b. Refraining from smoking is an important part of a heathy lifestyle ( ).
   c. Quitting smoking can reduce the risk of developing smoking-related diseases ( ).
   d. Passive smoking has no effect on health ( ).

Bibliography

Aljawarneh, Y.M., Al-Qaissi, N.M., and Ghunaim, H.Y. (2020). Psychological interventions for adherence, metabolic control, and coping with stress in adolescents with type 1 diabetes: a systematic review. *World J. Pediatr.* 16 (5): 456–470.

American Psychological Association. (2017). Stress effects on the body. http://www.apa.org/helpcenter/stress-body.aspx.

Antoni, M.H. and Dhabhar, F.S. (2019). The impact of psychosocial stress and stress management on immune responses in patients with cancer. *Cancer* 125 (9): 1417–1431.

Cancer Research UK. (2018). Alcohol and cancer. https://www.cancerresearchuk.org/about-cancer/causes-of-cancer/alcohol-and-cancer.

Ghazavi, Z., Rahimi, E., Yazdani, M., and Afshar, H. (2016). Effect of cognitive behavioral stress management program on psychosomatic patients' quality of life. *Iran J. Nurs. Midwifery Res.* 21 (5): 510–515.

Jimenez-Ruiz, C.A., Andreas, S., Lewis, K.E. et al. (2015). Statement on smoking cessation in COPD and other pulmonary diseases and in smokers with comorbidities who find it difficult to quit. *Eur. Respir. J.* 46 (1): 61–79.

Li, Y., Pan, A., Wang, D.D. et al. (2018). Impact of healthy lifestyle factors on life expectancies in the US population. *Circulation* 138 (4): 345–355.

Manigault, A.W., Shorey, R.C., Hamilton, K. et al. (2019). Cognitive behavioral therapy, mindfulness, and cortisol habituation: a randomized controlled trial. *Psychoneuroendocrinology* 104: 276–285.

Marteau, T.M. (2018). Changing minds about changing behaviour. *Lancet* 391 (10116): 116–117.

Roerecke, M. and Rehm, J. (2014). Alcohol consumption, drinking patterns, and ischemic heart disease: a narrative review of meta-analyses and a systematic review and meta-analysis of the impact of heavy drinking occasions on risk for moderate drinkers. *BMC Med.* 12: 182.

Sala-Vila, A., Estruch, R., and Ros, E. (2015). New insights into the role of nutrition in CVD prevention. *Curr. Cardiol. Rep.* 17 (5): 26. doi: 10.1007/s11886-015-0583-y.

Shield, K., Manthey, J., Rylett, M. et al. (2020). National, regional, and global burdens of disease from 2000 to 2016 attributable to alcohol use: a comparative risk assessment study. *Lancet Public Health* 5 (1): e51–e61.

Willett, W., Rockstrom, J., Loken, B. et al. (2019). Food in the Anthropocene: the EAT-Lancet Commission on healthy diets from sustainable food systems. *Lancet* 393 (10170): 447–492. doi: 10.1016/S0140-6736(18)31788-4.

Willett, W.C. and Stampfer, M.J. (2013). Current evidence on healthy eating. *Annu. Rev. Public Health* 34: 77–95. doi: 10.1146/annurev-publhealth-031811-124646.

World Health Organization. (2020). A healthy lifestyle. www.euro.who.int/en/health-topics/disease-prevention/nutrition/a-healthy-lifestyle.

Yu, E., Rimm, E., Qi, L. et al. (2016). Diet, lifestyle, biomarkers, genetic factors, and risk of cardiovascular disease in the Nurses' Health Studies. *Am. J. Public Health* 106 (9): 1616–1623. doi: 10.2105/AJPH.2016.303316.

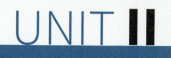

Healthy Diets

CHAPTER 5

Progression from Nutrients to Dietary Patterns

Nutrition epidemiology examines the correlations between dietary patterns, human health, and disease occurrence. In the past, the focus was on the effects of essential nutrient deficiency on health, since most diseases arose from malnutrition or "defective nourishment," e.g., ascorbic acid deficiency causing scurvy and deficiency of the B-complex vitamins causing pellagra and beriberi. However, nowadays most major diseases in the developed countries are lifestyle-related chronic diseases – heart disease, cancer, diabetes, etc. These diseases, unlike nutritional deficiencies, have a chronic development or result from a relatively short exposure to etiological factor(s) that may have occurred many years before diagnosis. Furthermore, they may not be reversible and they don't have single specific etiologic pathways.

Even though observational studies have suggested a link between specific nutrients and development of chronic diseases, clinical intervention studies do not confirm these associations. The reason may be that nutrients are ingredients of foods, and other aspects of the diet may confound the observed associations. Furthermore, it appears that examining the relationship between a single dietary factor and disease is not enough, since chronic diseases have multiple causes, including genetic makeup and occupational and other lifestyle factors. These factors act either independently or in sync with each other to affect our health. Therefore, examining whole food classes, whole diets or dietary patterns, and, lately, lifestyle patterns is more appropriate in order to investigate positive or negative effects on the development of specific chronic diseases.

In the following sections, we will review the progression from single nutrients to dietary and lifestyle patterns.

> **Key Point**
>
> Examining the relationship between a single dietary factor and disease is not enough.

Focus on Single Nutrient Deficiencies

The interest in the metabolic effect of food ingredients on the human body dates back to the nineteenth century. In his lecture "Disorders resulting from defective nutriment" given in 1842, George Budd noted, "There is no subject of more interest to the physiologist or of more practical importance to the physician . . . than the disorders resulting from defective nourishment."

In the first half of the twentieth century, scientists extensively studied the effects of single nutrients, mainly vitamins and minerals, on the development of various diseases. This perspective led into a new era in nutritional science and provided a myriad of scientifically based evidence on the effect of macro- or micronutrients deficiency or surplus on disease development. An example of a disease caused by a single nutrient deficiency is that of scurvy. Scurvy develops due to ascorbic acid deficiency, and it is accompanied by fatigue, lethargy, and malaise, in the early stages, and myalgia, anemia, depression, poor wound healing, and even death in late stages (Figure 5.1a and b). It is noteworthy that scurvy was the focus of what is considered to be the first controlled clinical trial. Specifically, in 1747, during his service as a physician at the British Royal Navy, James Lind studied the effect of citrus fruits (lemons and oranges) in the treatment of scurvy in British sailors. He noticed that the group allocated to including lemons and oranges in their diet showed significant improvement within a week, while those who didn't receive lemons and oranges did not recover even after 2 weeks.

Furthermore, back in the 1880s, the industrialization of milling was established and the refinement of grains became a common practice, as it increased the storage life

Textbook of Lifestyle Medicine, First Edition. Labros S. Sidossis and Stefanos N. Kales.
© 2022 John Wiley & Sons Ltd. Published 2022 by John Wiley & Sons Ltd.

(a)

(b)

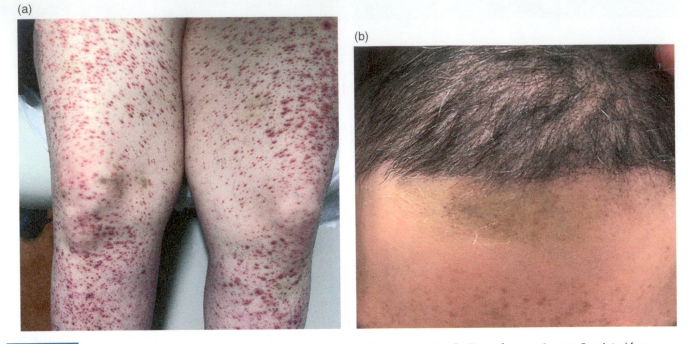

FIGURE 5.1 Perifollicular hemorrhages on both legs (a) and ecchymosis (b) are classic skin findings of scurvy. **Source:** Reprinted from Lipner (2018): 431.

of the grains. During the refinement process, the bran and the sperm are removed and hence, B-complex vitamins, fibers, and PUFAs are also removed. Soon, pellagra and beriberi epidemics appeared for the first time. In pellagra, the parts of the body exposed to sunlight suffer from dermatitis, but there are also mental and gastrointestinal implications. Using epidemiologic methods, scientists determined that pellagra was a disease of nutritional deficiency common in people who obtain most of their food energy from maize, notably rural South America, where maize is a staple food.

There are two types of beriberi – wet beriberi, which affects the cardiovascular system, and dry beriberi, which affects the nervous system. Around 1937, scientists detected that the lack of niacin (vitamin B$_3$) and thiamin (vitamin B$_1$) caused pellagra and beriberi, respectively.

In the last few decades, newly discovered food constituents have been shown to affect human health. For example, there is now considerable scientific evidence suggesting that plant polyphenols, which belong to the large group of phytochemicals, may account for some of the reported anti-carcinogenic and cardioprotective effects of plant foods. On the other hand, polyphenols, like flavonoids and lignans, have been associated with decreased risk for the development of CVDs. Two other polyphenolic classes, flavonols and flavones, have been shown to decrease mortality rate and prevent fatal and nonfatal coronary artery disease.

Even though it is now generally accepted that several nutrients have positive health effects, people do not consume single nutrients; they consume foods. And foods consist of many different nutrients in heterogeneous proportions.

Foods and Food Groups

Diseases caused by specific nutrient deficiencies usually manifest soon after initiating the nutrient-deficient diet and can be reversed within days or weeks after replacing the specific nutrient(s). However, the degenerative chronic diseases are not just a matter of nutrient deficiencies; their development is contingent on a constellation of risk factors, and they are characterized by heterogeneity and complexity. The interplay between human metabolism and all of the compounds found in foods of plant or animal origin create an intricate nexus of interactions, rendering the isolation of a single effect difficult and possibly misleading.

This notion triggered scientists to speculate that food components interact with the food matrix in which they are found, developing additive or even antagonistic effects on human metabolism and, by extension, on human health. This combined effect is defined as *food synergy* and *food antagonism,* respectively. Therefore, provided that the individual components of a food interact with each other and have a paired influence on health, questions began to emerge as to which is the best way to assess the overall impact of food consumption on health and disease. As a consequence, a new approach developed, that of the impact of whole foods and food groups on specific pathologies. For example, the increased consumption of whole-grain products has been shown to lower the risk for developing CVDs, T2DM, and some types of cancer. Whole-grain products are rich in several bioactive micronutrients and macronutrients with various health benefits; many of these beneficial micro- and macronutrients are lost during refining of the whole-grain product. Other food groups with high concentrations of nutrients and non-nutrients with advantageous influence on health are fruits, vegetables, and legumes.

Another important point to consider is that the health effects of foods depend on the biological properties that their nutrients maintain after digestion and not on the properties that they had before they were ingested. For example, although phytochemicals have been attributed advantageous effects against CVD, a study conducted in Welsh men, a population known for increased consumption of tea rich in flavonols, failed to detect such an effect. The researchers speculated that by adding milk to the tea, the flavonols could not be absorbed sufficiently, and therefore, this cohort of Welsh men did not benefit from the favorable effects of the tea flavanols. Another example of food antagonism is that of the inhibition of zinc absorption when iron is present. On the other hand, vitamin C enhances the absorption of plant-derived iron, i.e., nonheme iron.

> **Key Point**
>
> The health effects of foods depend on the biological properties that their nutrients maintain after digestion and not on the properties that they had before they were ingested.

Moreover, for many years, eggs were thought to increase the risk for the development of CVD, due to their high cholesterol content. However, the available evidence so far does not support the notion that dietary cholesterol increases the risk of heart disease in healthy individuals. Indeed, the effect of egg consumption, up to seven a week, on blood cholesterol is minimal, especially when compared with the effect of saturated fatty acids on blood cholesterol. Dietary cholesterol is common in foods that are high in saturated fatty acids, and this might have contributed to the notion that dietary cholesterol is atherogenic. Focusing only on the cholesterol content of eggs, without taking into consideration the fact that eggs are also a rich source of amino acids, vitamins, minerals, and other nutrients, may negatively influence the quality of our diet. It is obvious that our knowledge of the relationship between dietary cholesterol and cardiovascular disease in patients with diabetes is still incomplete. Therefore, further research is needed.

Holistic Approach to Diet; Dietary Patterns

Humans consume complex combinations of foods in the context of their meals, rather than individual foods or food groups. This is why it makes even more sense to assess dietary patterns rather than the effect of certain foods or even food groups. Dietary patterns can be described as the type, quantity, quality, frequency, and proportions of foods and drinks that are consumed by a particular population in a specific geographic region. Dietary patterns have developed over the centuries and have been influenced by environmental factors such as climate, terrain, and geography and cultural factors such as tradition and religion.

> **Key Point**
>
> Humans consume complex combinations of foods in the context of their meals, rather than individual foods or food groups.

There are many different dietary patterns around the world that reflect the dietary habits of the populations that have adopted them. The main dietary patterns that have been scientifically studied so far will be presented in the following chapters of the book. The various dietary patterns can be classified into the following categories: (i) those describing the dietary habits of whole populations residing in a specific geographic area (e.g., Mediterranean diet, Asian diet); (ii) those that have been shown to be healthy through epidemiological studies (e.g., the Prudent Dietary Pattern); (iii) those developed to serve certain health goals (e.g., the Dietary Approaches to Stop Hypertension [DASH] and the Therapeutic Lifestyle Changes [TLC] diet); and (iv) those created to be consistent with certain moral principles (e.g., vegetarian diet).

A dietary pattern is categorized as "healthy" by either (i) an a priori-defined healthy diet quality score/index based on the existing dietary guidelines; or (ii) a posteriori-derived healthy dietary pattern based on variations in food intake, developed using principal component analysis (PCA).

An example of a well-known dietary quality score/index is the Healthy Eating Index (HEI), originally published in 1995 to evaluate the extent to which Americans are following the dietary recommendations. Since then, the HEI index has been revised several times. The index has a number of questions, each of which receives a specific score as a reflection of an important aspect of diet quality. Higher scores indicate higher consumption and better adherence to a healthy dietary pattern. The DASH score and several Mediterranean diet scores (MedDietScore) are also well-established examples of such indexes, and they will be further discussed in later chapters of this book.

The second approach to define a healthy dietary pattern is to use PCA. PCA is a statistical method that is used to identify potential patterns from weighted food frequency questionnaires (FFQs) or 24-hour dietary recalls within a specific population. In other words, the method clusters variables that "behave in a similar way," forming new components instead of analyzing these variables independently. For example, someone eats a lot of vegetables but at the same time eats a lot of fruits and whole grains. Every new component can thereafter be associated with several characteristics of a study's sample.

Despite evidence of the efficacy of both approaches, major drawbacks exist. Scores are based on the current understanding of the relationship between diet and disease without taking into consideration possible unknown factors. Therefore, false-positive associations might be generated. A classic example is the one of serum cholesterol and eggs. While there is not a true relationship between the consumption of eggs with CHD and stroke, positive associations persist as eggs are high in cholesterol and saturated fat. Furthermore, an a posteriori-defined dietary pattern is derived from the population under consideration, but it is often not reproducible across populations.

According to the 2015–2020 Dietary Guidelines for Americans, a healthy dietary pattern should include consumption of a variety of vegetables, fruits, grains and especially whole grains, a variety of protein foods based on lean meats, poultry, eggs, low-fat dairy products, legumes, nuts, seafood, and soy products, while avoiding saturated and trans fats, as well as added sugars and sodium. It has been shown that people who adopt a healthy dietary pattern are also more likely to adopt other healthy lifestyle behaviors. For example, people who are more adherent to a prudent diet might also refrain from smoking and be more active compared to less-adherent individuals.

Scientific findings provide moderate-to-strong evidence that healthy dietary patterns are closely related to decreased prevalence of chronic diseases, such as CVDs, T2DM, and several types of cancer. Major dietary patterns that have been shown to have protective effects against diet-related diseases are the healthy Nordic dietary pattern, the healthy Asian dietary pattern, the healthy vegetarian pattern, and the healthy Mediterranean-style

> **Key Point**
>
> People who adopt a healthy dietary pattern are also more likely to adopt other healthy lifestyle behaviors.

dietary pattern. These dietary patterns share some typical features – increased consumption of fruits and vegetables, whole-grain cereals, legumes, and nuts, a modest alcohol intake, and moderate to low consumption of red and processed meats, refined grains, and sweets.

This is why in 2015 the US Dietary Guidelines Advisory Committee proposed the following:

A healthy dietary pattern is higher in vegetables, fruits, whole grains, low- or non-fat dairy, seafood, legumes, and nuts; moderate in alcohol (among adults); lower in red and processed meats; and low in sugar-sweetened foods and drinks and refined grains.

Even though most dietary patterns share common features, they differ significantly in the types of basic ingredients they use and the cooking methods. Hence, there is no one healthy dietary pattern for all, but people can adopt the one they prefer that satisfies not only their taste but also their sociocultural identity in an attempt to achieve long-term adherence to it and, eventually, better health.

> **Key Point**
>
> There is no one healthy dietary pattern for all, but people can adopt the one they prefer.

Take-Home Messages

- It appears that examining the relationship between a single dietary factor and disease is not enough, since chronic diseases have multiple causes.
- The interplay between human metabolism and all of the compounds found in foods of plant or animal origin create an intricate nexus of interactions, rendering the isolation of a single effect difficult and possibly misleading.
- Food compounds interact into the food matrix in which they are found, developing additive or even antagonistic effects. This combined effect is defined as *food synergy* and *food antagonism*.

- Nutrition epidemiology examines the correlations between dietary patterns and human health and disease occurrence.
- Two approaches exist for defining a prudent/healthy pattern: (i) an a priori-defined healthy diet quality score (or index) or (ii) an a posteriori-derived healthy dietary pattern based on variations in food intake, developed using PCA.
- There is no one healthy dietary pattern for all, but people can adopt the one they prefer that satisfies not only their taste but also their sociocultural identity in an attempt to achieve long-term adherence to it and, eventually, better health.

Self-Assessment Questions

1. Modern nutritional epidemiology examines:
   a. the prevalence of nutritional deficiencies, e.g., ascorbic acid deficiency and scurvy
   b. the health effects of acute viral and bacterial infections
   c. the impact of nutrition on chronic diseases, such as heart disease, cancer, and diabetes
   d. none of the above
2. Which of the following sentences is correct?
   a. Scurvy is caused by ascorbic acid deficiency.
   b. Oranges, but not lemons, are high sources of ascorbic acid.
   c. Scurvy is caused by lack of niacin (vitamin B$_3$).
   d. Scurvy is caused by lack of thiamin (vitamin B$_1$).

3. Describe the types of beri-beri disease.
4. Which of the following sentences is correct?
   a. Diseases caused by specific nutrient deficiencies usually manifest soon after initiating the nutrient-deficient diet.
   b. The degenerative chronic diseases are caused by specific nutrient deficiencies.
   c. The effects of a single nutrient deficiency are more important compared to the interaction of food components into the food matrix.
   d. "Food synergy" is a concept that can rarely explain how food and food groups affect health and disease.

5. Define the terms *food synergy* and *food antagonism*.
6. Why were eggs thought to be a risk factor for the development of CVD in the past?
7. The health effects of foods depend on:
   a. the time of their consumption during the day
   b. the biological properties that their nutrients maintain after digestion
   c. their energy content
   d. the combined effects of their nutrients, synergistic or antoagonistc
   e. all of the above
8. What are the available methods to categorize a dietary pattern as healthy?
9. Provide an example of a well-known dietary quality score/index.
10. What is principal component analysis (PCA)?
11. Which of the following dietary patterns was developed to achieve a specific health goal?
    a. the Mediterranean diet
    b. the Asian diet
    c. the Western-type diet
    d. the DASH diet
    e. all of the above
12. Which of the following dietary patterns is consistent with certain moral principles?
    a. the prudent diet
    b. the vegetarian diet
    c. the Asian diet
    d. the DASH diet
    e. none of the above
13. Complete the sentence: According to the 2015–2020 Dietary Guidelines for Americans, a healthy dietary pattern should include _____.
14. Report four dietary patterns that have been shown to have protective effects against diet-related diseases.
15. Do you agree with the statement, "There is no healthy dietary pattern for all"? Please justify your reply.

Bibliography

Budd, G. (1842). Lectures on the disorders resulting from defective nutriment. *Lond. Med. Gaz.* 2: 632–636. 712–716, 743–749, 906–915.

Burggraf, C., Teuber, R., Brosig, S., and Meier, T. (2018). Review of a priori dietary quality indices in relation to their construction criteria. *Nutr. Rev.* 76 (10): 747–764.

Carpenter, K.J. (2003). A short history of nutritional science: part 4 (1945–1985). *J. Nutr.* 133 (11): 3331–3342.

Dietary Guidelines for Americans. (2015–2020). https://health.gov/sites/default/files/2019-09/2015-2020_Dietary_Guidelines.pdf.

Dominguez, L.J., Barbagallo, M., Munoz-Garcia, M. et al. (2019). Dietary patterns and cognitive decline: key features for prevention. *Curr. Pharm. Des.* 25 (22): 2428–2442. doi: 10.2174/138161282566619072211 0458.

Grosso, G., Micek, A., Godos, J. et al. (2017). Dietary flavonoid and lignan intake and mortality in prospective cohort studies: systematic review and dose-response meta-analysis. *Am. J. Epidemiol.* 185 (12): 1304–1316.

Jayedi, A., Soltani, S., Abdolshahi, A., and Shab-Bidar, S. (2020). Healthy and unhealthy dietary patterns and the risk of chronic disease: an umbrella review of meta-analyses of prospective cohort studies. *Br. J. Nutr.* 124 (11): 1133–1144.

Krebs-Smith, S.M., Pannucci, T.E., Subar, A.F. et al. (2018). Update of the healthy eating index: HEI-2015. *J. Acad. Nutr. Diet.* 118 (9): 1591–1602.

Kritchevsky, S.B. and Kritchevsky, D. (2000). Egg consumption and coronary heart disease: an epidemiologic overview. *J. Am. Coll. Nutr.* 19 (5 Suppl): 549S–555S.

Lind, J. (1753). *A Treatise of the Scurvy*. Edinburgh: Sands, Murray and Cohran for A Kincaid and A Donaldson.

Lipner, S. (2018). A classic case of scurvy. *Lancet* 392 (10145): 431.

Martinez-Gonzalez, M.A. and Bes-Rastrollo, M. (2014). Dietary patterns, Mediterranean diet, and cardiovascular disease. *Curr. Opin. Lipidol.* 25 (1): 20–26. doi: 10.1097/MOL.0000000000000044.

Martinez-Gonzalez, M.A. and Martin-Calvo, N. (2013). The major European dietary patterns and metabolic syndrome. *Rev. Endocr. Metab. Disord.* 14 (3): 265–271. doi: 10.1007/s11154-013-9264-6.

Martinez-Gonzalez, M.A. and Sanchez-Villegas, A. (2016). Food patterns and the prevention of depression. *Proc. Nutr. Soc.* 75 (2): 139–146. doi: 10.1017/S0029665116000045.

Medina-Remon, A., Kirwan, R., Lamuela-Raventos, R.M. et al. (2018). Dietary patterns and the risk of obesity, type 2 diabetes mellitus, cardiovascular diseases, asthma, and neurodegenerative diseases. *Crit. Rev. Food Sci. Nutr.* 58 (2): 262–296. doi: 10.1080/10408398.2016.1158690.

Roman-Vinas, B., Ribas Barba, L., Ngo, J. et al. (2009). Validity of dietary patterns to assess nutrient intake adequacy. *Br. J. Nutr.* 101 (Suppl 2): S12–20. doi: 10.1017/S0007114509990547.

Ruiz-Canela, M., Bes-Rastrollo, M., and Martinez-Gonzalez, M.A. (2016). The role of dietary inflammatory index in cardiovascular disease, metabolic syndrome and mortality. *Int. J. Mol. Sci.* 17 (8): 1265. doi: 10.3390/ijms17081265.

Soliman, G.A. (2018). Dietary cholesterol and the lack of evidence in cardiovascular disease. *Nutrients* 10 (6): 780.

USDA. (2015–2020). Dietary guidelines for Americans, eighth edition. https://health.gov/our-work/food-nutrition/2015-2020-dietary-guidelines.

Wang, S., Meckling, K.A., Marcone, M.F. et al. (2011). Synergistic, additive, and antagonistic effects of food mixtures on total antioxidant capacities. *J. Agric. Food Chem.* 59 (3): 960–968.

CHAPTER 6

Popular Dietary Patterns Around the World

The Therapeutic Lifestyle Changes (TLC) Diet

The dietary management of dyslipidemia (defined as elevated total or LDL cholesterol or triglycerides levels, or low levels of HDL cholesterol) is a major goal in the management of CHD. According to the 2019 European Society of Cardiology/ European Atherosclerosis Society (ESC/EAS) guidelines for the management of dyslipidemias, the dietary strategy for lowering LDL cholesterol is to replace saturated and trans fatty acids with unsaturated and monosaturated fatty acids, as well as simple carbohydrates (e.g., sugars) with complex carbohydrates (e.g., whole grains, fruits, and vegetables).

In 2001, the National Cholesterol Education Program (NCEP) Expert Panel on Detection, Evaluation, and Treatment of High Blood Cholesterol in Adults (Adult Treatment Panel III, ATP III) published the dietary guidelines for lowering LDL cholesterol called the "Therapeutic Lifestyle Changes" (TLC) diet. These guidelines replaced what had been the most widely accepted dietary approaches for lowering LDL, the Step I and Step II diets. The basic principles of the TLC diet are shown in Table 6.1.

The first step of the TLC dietary approach is to reduce the intake of saturated fats, trans fatty acids, and cholesterol in order to lower LDL cholesterol. At this step, emphasis is also given to physical activity (at least 200 kcal/d of daily energy expenditure). After 6 weeks, if the LDL goal has not been achieved, other dietary choices for lowering LDL, such as plant stanols/sterols and soluble fiber, can be added. Sterols and stanols prevent the absorption of cholesterol in the human gastrointestinal tract, thereby decreasing cholesterol concentration in the bloodstream. When maximum LDL reduction is achieved with dietary therapy, emphasis is shifted to other metabolic abnormalities. Given that dyslipidemias are mostly prevalent among obese individuals who live a sedentary life, body weight loss plays an important role in further ameliorating not only LDL levels but also other risk factors associated with obesity. Physicians and other health professionals should

TABLE 6.1 **The basic principles of the TLC diet.**[a]

Saturated fat	Less than 7% of total calories
Polyunsaturated fat	Up to 10% of total calories
Monounsaturated fat	Up to 20% of total calories
Total fat	25–35% of total calories
Carbohydrates[b]	50–60% of total calories
Total fiber Soluble fiber	20–30 g/d 10–25 g/d
Proteins[c]	Approximately 15% of total calories
Cholesterol	Less than 200 mg/d
Plant stanols/sterols	2 g per day
Total calories (energy)	Balance energy intake and expenditure to maintain desirable body weight and prevent weight gain
Physical activity	Moderate physical activity to expend at least 200 kcal/day

[a] NCEP-ATPIII (2001).
[b] Carbohydrates should be derived predominantly from foods rich in complex carbohydrates, such as whole grains, fruits, and vegetables.
[c] Plant-based proteins can be used as a replacement for animal-based proteins.

Textbook of Lifestyle Medicine, First Edition. Labros S. Sidossis and Stefanos N. Kales.

advise their patients to visit a registered dietitian or other qualified nutritionist for expert advice and the development of appropriate/individualized nutritional plans.

The TLC diet reflects the recommendations included in the Dietary Guidelines for Americans 2000. Although in the TLC diet the total dietary fat is higher than in the aforementioned guidelines, this comes from unsaturated fat, which has been shown to favorably affect TAGs and HDL concentrations in individuals with MetS. As far as food components are concerned, the TLC diet promotes increased consumption of fruits and vegetables, whole-grain cereals, low-fat dairies, fish, and poultry.

Besides its dietary dimension, TLC is in accordance with the guidelines promoting physical activity and encouraging overweight/obese persons to maintain a healthy body weight. This dietary pattern has been shown to help improve several cardiovascular risk factors beyond dyslipidemias, like hypertension and diabetes mellitus.

A detailed description of the TLC dietary model and a sample menu plan can be found in Appendix B.1.

Take-Home Messages

- The TLC diet was developed for secondary prevention, for people at high risk or who have known CVD or other risk factors.
- The TLC dietary approach has several stages. The first step is to reduce the intakes of saturated fats and cholesterol in order to lower LDL cholesterol.

- Physicians should advise their patients to visit a registered dietitian or other qualified nutritionist for individualized nutritional intervention.

Self-Assessment Questions

1. What is the strategy for lowering LDL cholesterol according to the 2019 ESC/EAS guidelines?
2. Fill in the blanks:
   a. According to the TLC dietary approach, total fat should amount to _____ of total energy intake.
   b. The first step of the TLC dietary approach is to reduce _____ in order to lower LDL cholesterol.
   c. Plant stanols and sterols should be included in the TLC diet, if the _____ has not been accomplished.
   d. The TLC diet is in accordance with the guidelines recommending individuals to be _____ and encouraging obese persons to _____.

3. What is the recommended dietary fat intake in the TLC diet?
   a. Total fat intake is <20% of total energy.
   b. Total fat intake is 35–45% of total energy with emphasis on MUFA (up to 20%).
   c. Total fat intake is 25–35% of total energy with emphasis on SFA (<7%).
   d. Total fat intake is 20–30% of total energy, with emphasis on PUFA (>15%).
   e. None of the above.
4. Complete the sentence: Sterols and stanols _____ in the human gastrointestinal tract, thereby decreasing cholesterol concentration in the bloodstream.

The Dietary Approaches to Stop Hypertension (DASH) Diet

The **Dietary Approaches to Stop Hypertension (DASH)** dietary pattern originated in the 1990s as a dietary pattern to normalize BP in patients with hypertension. Since then, a large body of evidence has confirmed its beneficial effects on BP. This pattern advocates the consumption of fruits, vegetables, and low-fat dairy products. It incorporates whole grains, poultry, fish, and nuts, while discouraging the consumption of red and processed meat, sweets, and sugary soft drinks. As a result, it provides lower amounts of total and saturated fat and dietary cholesterol, while recommending the intake of dietary fiber, potassium (K), magnesium (Mg), and calcium (Ca). A typical serving guide of the DASH diet includes:

1. Vegetables: four to five servings/day
2. Fruits: four to five servings/day
3. Grain and grain products: seven to eight servings/day
4. Low-fat dairy products: two to three servings/day
5. Lean meat products: two or fewer servings/day
6. Nuts and seeds: four to five times/week
7. Fat and oils: two to three servings/day

The recommended sodium (Na) intake of the original DASH dietary pattern was 135 mmol/d (approximately 3100 mg/d). Since then, the effects of combining the DASH diet with lower dietary sodium intakes on BP have been investigated in individuals with hypertension. Further reducing sodium intake to 2000 mg/d reduces systolic BP more than the DASH diet alone. This effect has been shown in participants with or without hypertension, people from different races, and women and men. According to the WHO, the current recommendation for sodium intake is below 2000 mg/d (i.e., 5 g/d salt) to reduce BP and the risk of CVDs, stroke, and coronary heart disease.

Data from epidemiological prospective cohort studies suggest a synergistic effect when the DASH diet is combined with other healthy lifestyle measures. A healthy weight, half an hour or more of moderate- to high-intensity physical activity per day, alcohol intake less than 10 g/d, minimal use of nonnarcotic analgesics, and at least 400 μg/d supplemental intake of folic acid have been associated with lower risk for developing hypertension. In the Nurses' Health Study of 83,882 adult women aged 27–44 years, the adherence to the DASH diet, combined with improvements in several lifestyle parameters, was associated with lower risk for the development of hypertension.

Findings from the China Health and Nutrition Survey (CHNS) revealed that, after 11 years of follow-up, three factors were robustly linked to low hypertension prevalence: high adherence to the DASH diet, a healthy body weight, and at least half an hour of daily physical activity of moderate to high intensity. The combination of these lifestyle factors was associated with 38% reduced likelihood of developing hypertension among women and 43% among men.

Several alternatives to the original DASH dietary pattern have been developed to control BP and improve other health parameters. A similar reduction in BP is observed between a high-fat DASH diet (HF-DASH) and the original DASH diet; however, plasma triglyceride and very low-density lipoprotein (VLDL) concentrations decrease more in the HF-DASH diet, compared to the DASH diet, without any significant changes in LDL cholesterol. An alternative DASH diet, where the main protein source (55% of total proteins) is lean pork (DASH-P), instead of chicken and fish found in the typical DASH diet (DASH-CF), shows similar results.

Apart from its positive effect on hypertension, the DASH dietary pattern seems to also have positive effects on several other chronic diseases. This might be due to its high content in some bioactive compounds (such as fiber, vitamins, minerals, trace elements, and phytochemicals) found in whole grains, fruits, and vegetables, combined with its low content in harmful compounds found in processed meat and sugary beverages. The DASH diet has been suggested to have antioxidant, anti-atherogenic, anti-inflammatory, antiproliferative, and anti-

tumor properties. Indeed, it has been inversely associated with the risk of CVD, chronic kidney disease (CKD), and several types of cancer. There is also evidence for beneficial effects of the DASH diet on lipid profile, insulin sensitivity, inflammation, and oxidative stress. Most importantly, even modest adherence to the DASH diet has been associated with lower risk of all-cause mortality, while increasing the adherence to the diet also seems to strengthen this risk-reducing association.

Adherence to the DASH diet seems to reduce the incidence of CVDs, stroke, CHD, and heart failure (HF). According to a meta-analysis of six prospective observational studies with follow-up of 7–24 years, a DASH-like diet was found to be protective against CVDs, CHD, stroke, and HF risk by 20%, 21%, 19%, and 29%, respectively.

The DASH diet has been found to significantly reduce fasting insulin concentrations, independent of weight loss, compared with a control diet. Four weeks of the DASH diet were found to reduce fasting plasma glucose and serum insulin levels and Homeostatic Model Assessment of Insulin Resistance (HOMA-IR) compared to a control diet. Women diagnosed with gestational diabetes mellitus at 24–28 weeks of gestation showed significant improvements in plasma glucose and glycated hemoglobin (HbA1c) levels, compared to the control diet, after 4 weeks on the DASH diet.

The effectiveness of the DASH diet on insulin sensitivity and inflammation has also been investigated in obese women with established polycystic ovary syndrome (PCOS). After 8 weeks of intervention, the subjects assigned to the DASH diet had reduced insulin concentrations and HOMA-IR as well as high-sensitivity C-reactive protein (hs-CRP), compared to those assigned to the control diet.

Adherence to a DASH dietary pattern could also be beneficial for the prevention of CKD. Several meta-analyses have revealed a significant inverse correlation between adherence to the DASH diet and risk for the development of CKD. In addition, adherence to a DASH-style diet is inversely associated with a risk of rapid decline in estimated glomerular filtration rate (eGFR) and microalbuminuria, but not with low eGFR (<60 ml/min/1.73 m²).

The DASH dietary pattern may also decrease the risk of cancer. In a meta-analysis of 17 studies, of which 9 assessed the association between the DASH diet and risk of mortality from all cancer types, 4 assessed incidence of colorectal cancer, and 4 evaluated the association with the incidence of other types of cancers (i.e., breast, hepatic, endometrial, and lung cancer), it was found that high adherence to DASH was associated with decreased mortality from all cancer types; individuals with the highest adherence to the DASH diet had a lower risk of developing colorectal cancer compared to those with the lowest adherence.

A detailed description of the DASH dietary model and a sample menu plan can be found in Appendix B.2.

Take-Home Messages

- The DASH dietary pattern was developed to normalize BP in patients with hypertension. Many studies since then have confirmed the positive effects of this dietary modality on BP.
- The DASH dietary pattern advocates the consumption of fruits, vegetables, and low-fat dairy products. It incorporates whole grains, poultry, fish, and nuts, while discouraging the consumption of red and processed meat, sweets, and sugary soft drinks.
- The combination of the DASH diet with reduced dietary sodium intake holds the potential for further improvement of BP.
- The WHO recommends sodium intake below 2000 mg/d (i.e., 5 g/d salt) for management of BP and reduced risk of CVD, stroke, and CHD.
- Adherence to the DASH diet, combined with weight management and physical activity, is more beneficial for the risk of hypertension compared to the DASH diet alone.
- The DASH diet might also be a good choice for weight management in overweight and obese individuals.
- High levels of fiber, vitamins, minerals, trace elements, and phytochemicals found in whole grains, fruit, and vegetables combined with low levels in harmful compounds found in processed meat and sugary beverages may explain the antioxidant, anti-atherogenic, anti-inflammatory, antiproliferative, and anti-tumor properties of the DASH diet.
- The DASH dietary pattern has been inversely associated with the risk of CVD, CKD, and several types of cancer.
- The DASH dietary pattern has beneficial effects on lipid profile, insulin sensitivity, inflammation, and oxidative stress.
- Even modest adherence to the DASH diet has been associated with a lower risk of all-cause mortality, while higher adherence to the diet appears to strengthen this risk-reducing association.

Self-Assessment Questions

1. What is the main goal of the DASH dietary pattern?
2. Fill in the blanks:
   A typical serving guide of the DASH diet includes:
   a. Vegetables: _____
   b. Fruit: _____
   c. Grain and grain products: _____
   d. Low-fat dairy products: _____
   e. Lean meat products: _____
   f. Nuts and seeds: _____
   g. Fat and oils: _____
3. According to the WHO, what is the current recommendation for sodium intake?
4. Apart from the positive effects on hypertension, list other beneficial effects on health when following the DASH dietary pattern.

Vegetarian Diets

A vegetarian diet is a dietary pattern based predominantly on plant-origin products. Vegetarians exclude all kinds of meats (including fowl) and products containing meat from their diet. The most common types of vegetarian diets are: (i) vegan diets, devoid of all flesh foods (such as meat, poultry, seafood, and all animal products); (ii) ovovegetarian, vegan plus eggs; (iii) pesce-vegetarian, vegan plus fish and seafood; (iv) lacto-vegetarian, vegan plus dairy products; and (v) various combinations of the above (lacto-ovo-vegetarian, ovo-pescevegetarian). Cereals, vegetables, fruit, legumes, and seeds are common foods to the various types of vegetarian diets. In the recently defined flexitarian or semi-vegetarian diet, the person follows a primarily but not strictly vegetarian diet and occasionally eats meat or fish.

An individual chooses to adopt a vegetarian diet for several reasons, including the desire to protect the environment and animal welfare; ethical issues of world hunger and specific religious doctrines; and to prevent or mitigate chronic diseases. Results from several epidemiological studies suggest that vegetarian diets have a lower carbon footprint, meaning that they contribute less greenhouse gas emissions compared to diets including meat, making this dietary choice a more environmentally friendly type of a diet.

Key Point

Vegetarian diets have a lower carbon footprint.

Several national organizations and governments have published food guidelines for vegetarians. In 2013, a dietary pyramid illustrating the principles of the vegetarian diet was created by the Oldways Preservation Trust, which was a collaboration with scientists from several universities, including Harvard and Loma Linda University. In 2018, the VegPlate, a

(a)

(b)

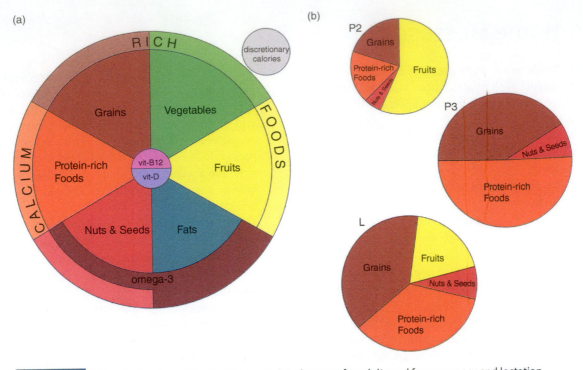

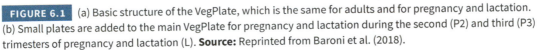

FIGURE 6.1 (a) Basic structure of the VegPlate, which is the same for adults and for pregnancy and lactation. (b) Small plates are added to the main VegPlate for pregnancy and lactation during the second (P2) and third (P3) trimesters of pregnancy and lactation (L). **Source:** Reprinted from Baroni et al. (2018).

new Mediterranean diet-based vegetarian food guide, was developed, based on the Italian Dietary Reference Intakes. The VegPlate contains six major food groups: grains, protein-rich foods, vegetables, fruits, nuts and seeds, and fats (Figure 6.1). Recommendations for specific populations, such as women in pregnancy or lactation, are also included in the VegPlate.

A well-planned vegetarian diet, containing a variety of foods and food groups such as vegetables, fruits, whole grains, legumes, nuts, and seeds, can provide adequate nutrition. In 2009, the American Dietetic Association (ADA) published a position statement regarding the nutrient adequacy and safety of a vegetarian diet:

It is the position of the American Dietetic Association that appropriately planned vegetarian diets, including total vegetarian or vegan diets, are healthful, nutritionally adequate, and may provide health benefits in the prevention and treatment of certain diseases. Well-planned vegetarian diets are appropriate for individuals during all stages of the lifecycle, including pregnancy, lactation, infancy, childhood, and adolescence, and for athletes.

> **Key Point**
>
> Vegans must regularly consume sources of vitamin B_{12} and D, omega-3 fatty acids, Ca, iodine, iron, and zinc.

However, more recent data support the notion that the risk of specific nutrient deficiencies is real, especially in those following a vegan diet. Therefore, vegans must regularly consume sources of vitamin B_{12} and D, omega-3 fatty acids, Ca, iodine, iron, and zinc, such as fortified foods or supplements –

otherwise they may become deficient in these nutrients. Recent data support that not only vegans but also lacto-ovo-vegetarians are at risk of developing B_{12} deficiency, and thus all vegetarians could benefit from B_{12} supplementation.

Many people consider vegetarian diets to be superior to nonvegetarian diets, in terms of quality. This is because the vegetarian food choices are high in dietary fibers, magnesium (Mg), potassium (K), vitamins C and E, folate, carotenoids, and other phytochemical substances, and they are low in saturated fat, cholesterol, and sodium content. Vegetarian dietary patterns have been shown to reduce cardiometabolic risk, including the risk of developing T2DM and hypertension. Results from large clinical trials suggest that vegetarian dietary patterns can improve HbA1c, fasting glucose levels, and other established cardiometabolic risk factors, such as high LDL-C and high systolic and diastolic BP compared to nonvegetarian dietary patterns.

Results from large cohort studies, with a follow-up period ranging from 4 to 21 years, show that the vegetarian dietary pattern is associated with reduced overall incidence of cancer, compared to nonvegetarians. The mechanism(s) mediating the effect of vegetarian diets on cancer risk is not known. It has been suggested that vegetarians have lower levels of hs-CRP compared to people who eat meat; the high antioxidant and anti-inflammatory effects of the food groups included in this pattern may also result in lower inflammation in the long term.

Adopting a vegetarian diet results in significantly lower CVD risk. The protective effect of vegetarian diets on cardiovascular risk seems to be mediated by the reduction of meat consumption and the increased consumption of fruits and vegetables. For each additional serving of fruits and vegetables consumed, the likelihood of all-cause mortality decreases by 5%, while eating more than five servings/day does not appear to further mitigate the

risk. Regarding CVD deaths, for each daily serving of fruits and vegetables per day, CVD mortality is reduced by 4%.

A detailed description of the vegeterian dietary model and a sample menu plan can be found in Appendix B.3.

Take-Home Messages

- A vegetarian diet is a dietary pattern based predominantly on plant-origin products. Vegetarians exclude most meat (including fowl) and products containing meat.
- Vegan diets are devoid of all flesh foods (such as meat, poultry, seafood, and their products). Other types of vegeterian diets are devoid of all flesh foods but may include egg (ovo-vegetarain), fish (pesce-vegetarian), dairy (lacto-vegetarian), or combinations.
- A well-planned vegetarian diet, containing a variety of foods and food groups such as vegetables, fruits, whole grains, legumes, nuts, and seeds, can provide adequate nutrition.
- However, the risk of specific nutrient deficiencies is real, especially in those who follow a vegan diet. The most common nutrient deficiencies are vitamins B_{12} and D, omega-3 fatty acids, calcium, iodine, iron, and zinc, as these micronutrients are derived mainly from animal products.
- Vegetarian diets are considered by some to be of higher diet quality compared to nonvegetarian diets due to their high content in dietary fibers, Mg, K, vitamin C and E, folate, carotenoids, and other phytochemical substances, and their low content in saturated fat, cholesterol, and sodium.
- Vegetarian dietary patterns have been shown to reduce cardiometabolic risk, including the risk of developing T2DM, hypertension, and obesity, as well as cancer incidence and mortality from CVD.

Self-Assessment Questions

1. What are the most common vegetarian diets?
2. Are there any risks of specific nutrient deficiencies when a person follows a vegan diet?
3. Why do people following a vegetarian diet have a lower risk of developing cancer?
4. How can a vegetarian diet contribute to sustainability?

The Religious/Fasting Diets

Disease prevalence and mortality rates differ between populations. Differences in genetic makeup, lifestyle habits, and other characteristics may explain these disparities. Religion is an important factor in shaping some people's beliefs; their lifestyle and dietary habits are often influenced by their religious traditions and practices. Many religious doctrines exist, each one having followers with varying degrees of devotion. It is common for these religious creeds to be related to specific religious food practices or customs; dietary restrictions may include the types of foods that are allowed in the diet, the foods that are allowed to be consumed on specific days of the week/month/year, the timing of food consumption, methods to prepare food, and when and how long to fast.

Fasting is common in most religions. It is considered a call to purification, holiness, and spirituality. The practice of fasting is acknowledged as the means by which the pious believers expiate for their sins, so as to be accepted by God, as well as to identify themselves with the anguish of the destitute.

Fasting signifies resistance to temptation, as a deed of expiation for committed sins but also as a means to prevent excessive eating and drinking. The duration of fasting may vary from a few hours during the day (e.g., from sunrise to sunset for Jews), to a fixed number of hours (e.g., 12-24 hours or more for Catholics, Greek Orthodox, and Mormons whose fasting is practiced on specific days), but also for several successive days, as happens during the Ramadan month for Muslims.

Detailed descriptions of the following religion-based dietary models and their corresponding sample menu plans can be found in Appendices B.4.- B.8.

Buddhism

"Do not kill or harm living things" is the first of five basic precepts of Buddhism. Thus, the majority of Buddhists abstain from meat consumption, and all of them exclude beef products from their diet. The major religious events for Buddhism are the birth, the enlightenment, and the death of Buddha; on these days devotees do not work but spend their time celebrating and fasting.

Buddhist monks undergo complete fast depending on the moon phase, and they refrain from solid food intake after noon.

The life of a Buddhist encompasses many other lifestyle factors that have been shown to improve health. For example, Buddhists practice meditation and yoga, activities that have been shown to cause favorable health effects. Meditation has positive effects on reducing stress and increasing mindfulness, as well as improving BP and vascular endothelial function. Numerous studies have demonstrated the role of mindfulness-based stress reduction in T2DM, showing modest improvements in body weight and glycemic control. Even short-term engagement in yoga practice has been found to improve obesity, CVD, and T2DM risk factors among high-risk populations.

> **Key Point**
>
> The life of a Buddhist encompasses many other lifestyle factors that have been shown to improve health status.

Hinduism

Fasting, known as *Vrat* or *Vratam,* is fundamental to the Hindu religion. It denotes the denial of the body's physical needs in favor of mental health. Each day in Hindu religion is devoted to a particular deity, and based on personal choice, believers can fast or not. *Tamasic* foods, such as fish and meat, are usually avoided for several days. During fasting, Hindus usually avoid solid foods and follow a liquid diet with vegetable or fruit juices. A stricter fasting ritual also exists, avoiding any solids and any form of liquid but water. Hindus follow fasting practices on each of the 18 major Hindu holidays but also on such days as birthdays, anniversaries, deaths, and marriages. Sunday is also a fasting day, as are certain days relative to the planetary scenery, i.e., the position of the moon and the planets.

> **Key Point**
>
> Fasting, known as *Vrat* or *Vratam,* is fundamental to the Hindu religion.

Although meat consumption is allowed in nonvegetarians, meat products such as those derived from pork, fowl, duck, snails, crabs, and camels are not preferred, as animals are considered part of the chain of life and should be treated with compassion. Because cows are considered sacred animals, beef intake is prohibited; however, the consumption of dairy products derived from cow, such as milk, yogurt, and butter, is allowed as they are considered to be pure and to contribute to the purity of body, spirit, and mind.

Judaism

In Judaism, believers consume only what is considered to be *kosher,* i.e., whatever has been prepared in agreement with the dietary regulations of *Kashrut.* Kashrut, which means "proper" or "correct," is a set of dietary laws determining the foods that Jews are permitted to eat and how they should be prepared. These laws are spelled out in detail in the written Torah, Leviticus 11. The dietary laws have the added benefit of preventing contamination and improving health. For example, Kashrut defines the proper handling of kitchenware, determines that the only types of meat that may be eaten are cattle and game that have "cloven hooves" and "chew the cud" (e.g., sheep, cattle, goats, and deer), notes that kosher and nonkosher foods cannot be served in the same plate, and states that meat and dairy products should be separated. After meat meals, one must wait several hours before eating dairy. However, after dairy consumption, no interval is required before meat may be eaten.

> **Key Point**
>
> Kashrut is a set of dietary laws determining the foods that Jews are permitted to eat and how they should be prepared.

The Jewish calendar has comparatively few days of fasting. Besides the Day of Atonement (Yom Kippur), which is the only fast day prescribed by the Mosaic law, there are only four regular fast days in commemoration of various historical events. Fasting lasts from sunrise to sunset, and the participants abstain from all food and drink, including water.

Islam

Halal (permissible) and *Haram* (forbidden) are the main concepts of Islamic dietary laws and are used to designate what is lawful to be eaten and what is prohibited for Muslims. Foods whose consumption is ambiguous are called *Mashbooh.* Muslims must follow these laws and never disobey irrespective of their age, sex, and caste.

The dietary laws of Islam have many similarities with dietary laws of Judaism. The followers of Islam eat foods that purify their body and spirit from all kinds of dirt and impurities, based on what Allah commands. For example, all kinds of birds are permitted expect for prey birds. In Islam, all kinds of vegetables, fruits, and crops that are not contaminated are allowed. Animal meat is lawful for consumption when it has been properly slaughtered, except for meat that is specifically forbidden (e.g., pork). The prescribed method of ritual slaughter of all lawful halal animals is called Dhabihah.

> **Key Point**
>
> The followers of Islam eat foods that purify their body and spirit from all kinds of dirt and impurities.

Islam discourages overconsumption of food and the intake of stimulants (such as coffee, tea, alcohol). Muslims fast on Mondays and Tuesdays and for a 6-day period during the 10th month of the Islamic year, named Shawwal. However, their most renowned fasting period is the holy month of *Ramadan,* the ninth month according to the Islamic calendar. During Ramadan, Muslims do not eat or drink anything from sunrise to sunset, approximately 13–18 hours/day.

Ramadan fasting has been associated with weight loss, attenuation of several metabolic markers (such as insulin resistance, high blood glucose, and high BP), improvements in lipid profile, prevention of chronic diseases (such as obesity, diabetes, CVDs, and cancer), and protection against neurodegeneration and inflammation. However, the results from the Epidemiology of Diabetes and Ramadan (EPIDIAR) study, which included patients with T1DM and T2DM, suggested that fasting during Ramadan can result in an increased number of hypoglycemic episodes. Education on diabetes management and medication adjustments prior to Ramadan has been shown to help overcome these problems.

In a systematic review and meta-analysis of 70 publications with a total of 2947 subjects, a significant reduction in body fat was found between the pre-Ramadan and post-Ramadan period, but only in overweight or obese individuals. However, a significant loss of fat-free mass (i.e., muscle and bone) was also found between pre-Ramadan and post-Ramadan. Nevertheless, 2–5 weeks after the end of Ramadan, weight and body composition returned to pre-Ramadan levels, as is the case when any kind of diet based on caloric restriction is discontinued.

Christianity

Fasting is a popular religious practice among many Christians. In many denominations, especially Protestant groups, there are no specific food restrictions or fasting days (although some groups prohibit alcohol or caffeine consumption). Prayer and fasting are often combined as preparation for important decisions or to seek God's blessing or guidance. However, other Christian denominations have more specific guidelines.

For example, the Greek Orthodox Church advises fasting for 180–200 days throughout the year, i.e., approximately 6.5 months/year. The diet during fasting resembles a vegetarian-style dietary pattern. Avoidance of meat, fish, milk, eggs, and cheese is recommended on Wednesdays and Fridays. The major fasting periods of the year are 40 days before Christmas, 48 days before Easter, and 15 days prior to the Assumption of Virgin Mary (August 15th). During the fasting before Christmas, devotees do not eat meat, eggs, and dairy, but they can eat fish and olive oil all days except Wednesdays and Fridays. Pre-Easter fasting has the same dietary restrictions as Christmas, but during this period fish consumption is permitted twice, on

March 25th (the Annunciation) and on Palm Sunday. Olive oil consumption is permitted only on weekends.

Orthodox fasting does not impose any restriction on the consumption of mollusks, shellfish, and snails, which are consumed freely during these periods. Animal-derived products are stored during this period in order to be consumed after the end of fasting. Similar to other religions, the dietary suggestions of the various Christian denominations are associated with low rates of chronic degenerative diseases, and they constitute a sustainable practice with positive financial implications.

Compliance with Orthodox Christianity not only offers a theological structure but also a flexible lifestyle pattern with health benefits. Orthodox fasting periods are characterized by a restriction in total energy and fat intake and an increase in the consumption of carbohydrate and fiber. Lipid profile seems to be optimal, while the reduction in total cholesterol and LDL-C levels is consistent across studies. However, the effect on HDL is still uncertain. Results regarding the impact on body weight and glucose homeostasis are conflicting, and a definite conclusion cannot be drawn. Further investigation is needed to evaluate the potentially negative effect of orthodox fasting on vitamins D and B_{12} and mineral (mainly calcium) intake.

According to Roman Catholicism, the pious believers must fast on the prescribed fasting days by reducing food intake (allowing one full meal and two smaller) and refraining from consuming meat or meat products on these holy days. Fasting is obligatory for all Catholics 18–60 years old on Ash Wednesday and Good Friday, unless they are exempt for health reasons. Abstinence from meat is obligatory for those more than 14 years of age. The dietary laws are not universal in the Catholic Church; episcopal conferences are able to propose adjustments on the fasting laws for their home countries.

> **Key Point**
> Compliance with Orthodox Christianity not only offers a theological structure but also a flexible lifestyle pattern with health benefits.

> **Key Point**
> The dietary laws are not universal in the Catholic Church; episcopal conferences are able to propose adjustments on the fasting laws for their home countries.

Take-Home Messages

- Religion is an important factor in shaping people's beliefs; their lifestyle and dietary habits may also be influenced by their religious traditions and practices.
- Fasting periods exist in almost all religions; they comprise a call to holiness and spirituality.
- Buddhist meditation has positive effects on reducing stress and increasing mindfulness, as well as improving BP and vascular endothelial function. Numerous studies have demonstrated the role of mindfulness-based stress reduction in T2DM showing modest improvements in body weight and glycemic control.

- A short-term engagement in yoga practice has been found to improve obesity, CVD, and T2DM risk factors among high-risk populations.
- Fasting, known as Vrat or Vratam, is fundamental to the Hindu religion; it shows the denial of the body's physical needs in favor of mental health.
- In Judaism, believers consume only what is considered to be kosher, i.e., whatever has been produced in agreement with the Jewish dietary laws.
- Islamic dietary laws dictate that Muslims can eat foods that purify their body and spirit from all kinds of dirt and impurities, based on what Allah commands. The most

renowned fasting period of Muslims is Ramadan.
- The health benefits associated with Ramadan fasting include weight loss, improvements in insulin resistance, blood glucose, BP, and lipid profile as well as the prevention of several chronic diseases.
- In Christianity, fasting is sometimes paired with prayer in seeking God's guidance. Some sects have specific dietary rituals. In the Greek Orthodox Church fasting is practiced throughout the year, about 6.5 months/year. The dietary rules of Orthodox Christianity offer a flexible lifestyle pattern with several, well-documented health benefits.

Self-Assessment Questions

1. Apart from diet, what other lifestyle factors improve health status in Buddhism?
2. What kinds of foods are usually avoided during fasting in Hinduism?
3. What does *Kashrut* mean in Judaism?
4. During Ramadan fasting, patients with T1DM should be aware of the possibility of:

   a. hyperglycemic episodes
   b. hypoglycemic episodes
   c. increase in body fat
   d. no changes in fat-free mass
5. Complete the sentence: Orthodox fasting periods are characterized by _____.

The Healthy Nordic Diet

The Nordic diet, also called the Baltic Sea diet, has been recently developed as a healthy dietary pattern. It is based on the principles of the traditional, plant-based Mediterranean diet using foods locally available in the Nordic regions of Scandinavian countries, such as Denmark, Finland, Norway, Sweden, and Iceland. This pattern is characterized by high consumption of fruits (e.g., berries, apples, and pears), vegetables (e.g., root vegetables, cabbage, potatoes, carrots), wild mushrooms, pulses (e.g., beans, peas), nuts, whole-grain foods (e.g., rye, barley, oats), rapeseed (canola) oil, oily fish (e.g., mackerel, salmon, herring), shellfish, and seaweed, while emphasis is given to low-fat choices of meat (such as poultry and game), low-fat dairy, salt restriction, and avoidance of sugar-sweetened products (Figure 6.2).

Compared to the Mediterranean and the DASH diets, the Nordic diet emphasizes the use of different types of oil and vegetables and fruit choices based on products indigenous to the Scandinavian region. In the Nordic diet the added culinary fat is the canola oil, a variety of rapeseed, instead of the olive oil that is used in the Mediterranean diet. Canola oil is rich in MUFAs and alpha-linolenic acid, a plant-based n-3 PUFA. Moreover, in

> **Key Point**
>
> The Nordic diet, also called the Baltic Sea diet, has been recently developed as a healthy dietary pattern.

the Nordic diet, berries constitute a common fruit choice with various potential health benefits. This group of fruits is rich in a class of polyphenols called *anthocyanins,* whose health effects on hypertension and CVD are well established.

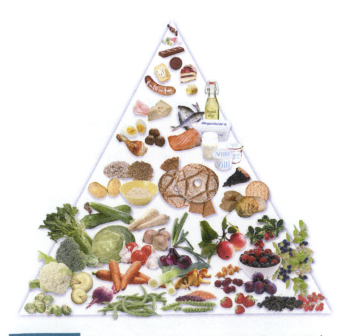

FIGURE 6.2   The Baltic Sea diet pyramid. **Source:** Kanerva et al. (2012).

Adherence to the Nordic diet could significantly decrease insulin levels and HOMA-IR and is associated with a significant reduction in systolic and diastolic BP. Total and LDL-cholesterol levels are also lower compared with a Western-type diet. In a model-based simulation study to find the number of deaths attributable to CVDs that could be prevented or delayed in the Nordic countries, it was found that the most lives could be saved by changes attributable to an increase in fruit and vegetable intakes.

In contrast, the Nordic diet is less effective in reducing inflammation, compared with other healthy dietary patterns such as the Mediterranean diet. The type of oil (canola oil vs. olive oil) consumed in the Nordic and the Mediterranean diets, respectively, may explain the different effects on inflammation. Overall, studies show that a higher degree of adherence to the Nordic diet is associated with a healthy lifestyle.

The Diet, Cancer, and Health cohort study, conducted in Danish people of both sexes, found that greater compliance with the Nordic dietary pattern was related to lower risk of developing colorectal cancer by 35% among women. It was further indicated that conformity to each component of this dietary pattern was associated with 9% lower risk of colorectal cancer occurrence in female participants. Furthermore, evidence derived from the Swedish Women's Lifestyle and Health cohort revealed that, after approximately two decades of follow-up, high compliance with the Nordic diet model decreased overall mortality by 18% compared to poor compliance. The studies demonstrated that lower overall mortality rates could be attributed solely to high intake of whole grains, apples, and pears.

Apart from the favorable health effects of the Nordic diet, this dietary pattern encompasses features of eco-friendliness. Like all plant-based diets, the Nordic diet employs a small number of natural resources in contrast to meat-based diets, which have been accused of increasing carbon dioxide production and, thus, carbon footprint. In order for a food to be characterized as "typical" of the Nordic diet, it has to fulfill a list of criteria, such as being produced within the Nordic countries without employing external energy sources, being related to Nordic dietary tradition (such as dark bread, root vegetables, and fish), being superior in terms of health effects compared to other foods of the same food group, and being consumed as food and not only in small amounts as dietary supplement, such as spices.

A detailed description of the Nordic dietary model and a sample menu plan can be found in Appendix B.9.

Take-Home Messages

- The Nordic diet is a plant-based diet and refers to the dietary pattern recently developed in the Nordic region.
- Compared to the Mediterranean and the DASH diets, the Nordic diet differs in the type of recommended oil and the vegetable and fruit choices.
- The Nordic diet has been proven to have favorable health effects in controlling weight status and blood glucose and in reducing cardio-metabolic and inflammatory markers.
- A food is characterized as "typical" of the Nordic diet if it fulfills a list of criteria, such as being produced within the Nordic countries, being related to Nordic dietary tradition, superior in terms of health effects compared to other foods of the same food group, and consumed as food and not as dietary supplement.

Self-Assessment Questions

1. What are the main characteristics of the Nordic diet?
2. What are the main differences of the Nordic diet compared to the Mediterranean and DASH diets?

3. When is a food characterized as typical of the Nordic diet?

The Healthy Asian Diet

Various aspects of the traditional Asian diet are followed by most Asian countries, including Bangladesh, Cambodia, China, India, Indonesian, Japan, Laos, Malaysia, Mongolia, Myanmar, Nepal, North Korea, South Korea, Philippines, Singapore, Sri Lanka, Taiwan, Thailand, and Vietnam. Although there are differences between countries, they all have many common food groups or items characteristic of the region.

The Asian diet is primarily characterized by high consumption of rice, foods of plant origin (e.g., soy products), fish and seafood, and fruits and vegetables. This dietary pattern includes fiber in amounts approximately threefold higher than a typical Western diet, whereas the consumption of red meat is usually very low. The majority of foods are boiled, steamed, or

Key Point

The Asian diet is primarily characterized by high consumption of rice, foods of plant origin (e.g., soy products), fish and seafood, and fruits and vegetables.

grilled without the addition of culinary fat, or fried with minimum quantities of seed oils, or they are consumed raw. Additionally, tea, a common drink among these populations, is drunk without sugar. Adherence to such a dietary pattern guarantees the intake of beneficial fatty acids, while limiting simple sugars and salt. The new Asian diet pyramid (Figure 6.3) was launched by the Oldways Preservation and Exchange Trust in 2018.

The Japanese and the Chinese dietary patterns represent two well-documented examples of the Asian diet. The "Dietary Guidelines for Japanese" were first published in 2000, and their latest version, namely, the "Japanese food guide spinning top" (Figure 6.4), was launched in 2010.

The illustration of these guidelines resembles the traditional Japanese spinning top toy, i.e., a turned-upside-down cone with separated layers displaying different foods. This illustration incorporates the number of servings for each food category.

Each food layer of the inverted cone reflects the frequency that each food should be consumed in a descending order. Cereal-based dishes, such as rice, noodles, bread, and pasta are on top (five to seven servings/day), followed by vegetable-based dishes (such as salads, cooked vegetables, and soups; five to six servings) and meat, fish, eggs, and soybean dishes

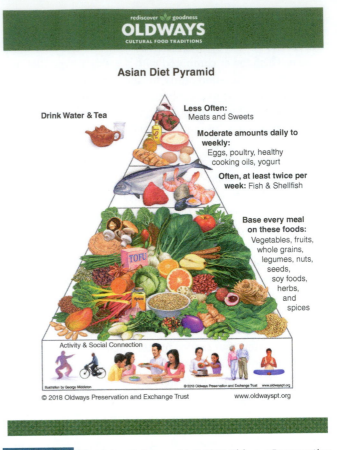

FIGURE 6.3   The Asian diet pyramid. © 2018 Oldways Preservation & Exchange Trust.

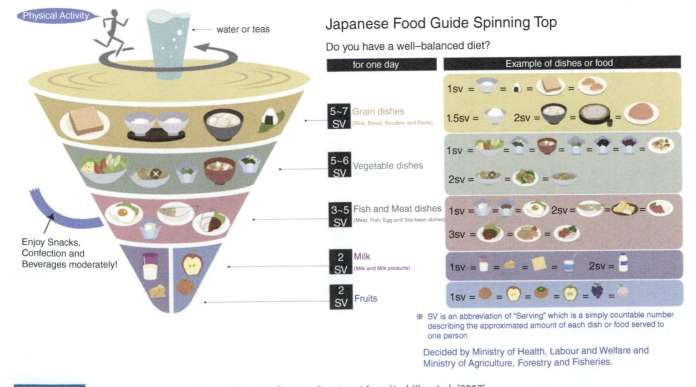

FIGURE 6.4   The Japanese food guide spinning top. **Source:** Reprinted from Yoshiike et al. (2007).

(three to five servings/day). At the bottom of the spinning top are foods that are consumed daily in two servings, namely, fruits and dairy products. Snacks, sweets, and beverages with added sugar should be consumed in moderate doses and not on a daily basis. In addition to nutrition advice, the Japanese health guidelines include hydration and exercise recommendations. A glass of water with the prompt to drink enough water is shown at the highest point of the spinning top, while a man is running around the spinning top to reflect the recommendation for physical activity.

The Japanese dietary guidelines emphasize the planning of a regular meal schedule for the establishment of a healthy rhythm, eating well-balanced meals, including staple foods, grains, vegetables and fruits, dairies, beans, and seafood, as well as enjoying both main meals and snacks. Furthermore, it highlights the avoidance of excessive amounts of salt and fat. Lifestyle recommendations are also included, such as managing body weight by controlling energy intake and being active and monitoring caloric intake. Finally, Japanese guidelines highlight the benefits of following the local dietary culture, avoiding food waste, and adopting suitable culinary practices and storage methods.

> **Key Point**
>
> Japanese guidelines highlight the benefits of following the local dietary culture, avoiding food waste, and adopting suitable culinary practices and storage methods.

Back in the 1950s, the Seven Countries Study, led by Ancel Keys, aiming to chart the incidence of CHD among seven countries (US, Japan, Italy, Greece, the Netherlands, Finland, Yugoslavia), underlined the effectiveness of the traditional Japanese diet in reducing CHD risk, as the Asian cohort demonstrated the lowest CHD incidence. The researchers from the Seven Countries Study concluded that the Asian diet was most effective in lowering CHD rates, although compared to the Greek cohort, Japanese showed more strokes due to the high sodium intake in Japan and higher stomach cancer rates due to traditional food preservation methods. Nevertheless, several studies have documented the beneficial role of specific dietary components of the Asian diet on various health outcomes.

> **Key Point**
>
> The researchers from the Seven Countries Study concluded that the Asian diet was most effective in lowering CHD rates.

Another example of dietary guidelines from Asia is that of China. The Chinese dietary guidelines were first launched in 1989 by the Chinese Nutrition Society. The Chinese dietary recommendations are illustrated by the "Chinese Food Guide Pagoda" (Figure 6.5), which consists of five gradually decreasing space levels, depicting the amount in which the foods of each level should be consumed.

The base of the pagoda is filled with cereals, such as rice, corn, bread, noodles, and crackers, as well as tubers. The next level includes fruits and vegetables, which should constitute the base of every meal, along with the cereals and tubers. Fish and shrimp, eggs, poultry, and meat should be eaten regularly, but in small amounts. The consumption of dairy products, beans, and bean-derived foods should be consumed in moderation, while at the top of the pagoda is the intake of fats, oils, and salt. Moreover, the Chinese dietary guidelines highlight the need for adequate hydration, suggesting 1500–1700 ml of water everyday as well as adequate physical activity equivalent to 6000 steps/day. Large prospective studies suggest that green tea consumption is significantly and inversely associated with CVD and all-cause mortality; black tea consumption is also significantly and inversely associated with cancer and all-cause mortality. Vegetables, fruits, legumes, fish, and eggs are the food groups associated with reduced risk of all-cause mortality.

The China-Cornell-Oxford Project, or simply the China Study, sought to explore the dietary habits along with the prevalence of age-related diseases in 10,200 Chinese of both genders. The study found that rural populations adhering to this traditional dietary pattern manifested very low prevalence of heart disease, breast and prostate cancer, obesity, and osteoporosis, compared to Western societies. However, urban Chinese adhering to a more Western-type diet with high intakes of animal-derived foods were more likely to be obese and suffer from heart disease, as well as breast and prostate cancer. When all the analyses were completed, Dr. Campbell, the principal investigator of the China Study, commented: "In the final analysis, we have strong evidence from this and other studies that nutrition becomes the controlling factor in the development of chronic degenerative diseases" Indeed, in a systematic review of 18 studies on the prevalence and trends for MetS in the Asia-Pacific region, more than 20% of the adult population had MetS.

> **Key Point**
>
> Nutrition becomes the controlling factor in the development of chronic degenerative diseases.

A detailed description of the Asian dietary model and a sample menu plan can be found in Appendix B.10.

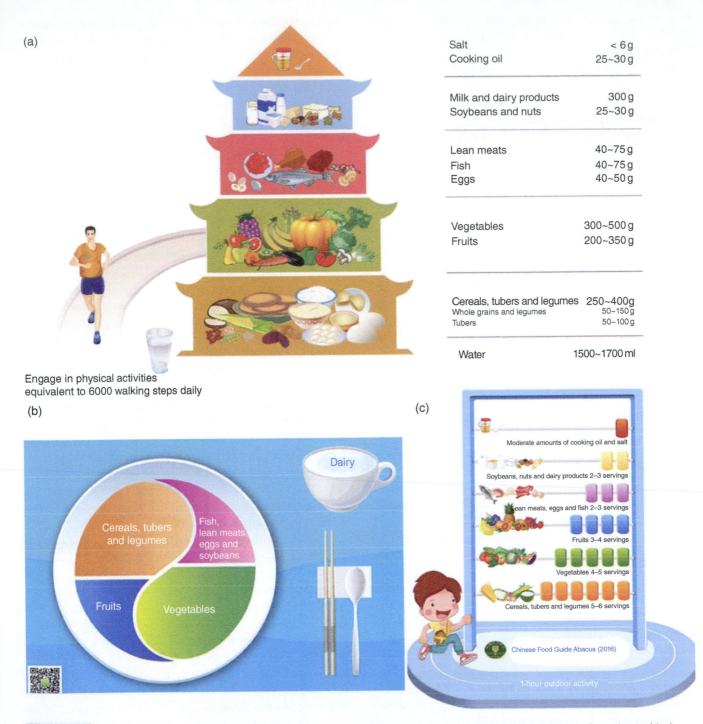

(a)

Salt	< 6 g
Cooking oil	25~30 g
Milk and dairy products	300 g
Soybeans and nuts	25~30 g
Lean meats	40~75 g
Fish	40~75 g
Eggs	40~50 g
Vegetables	300~500 g
Fruits	200~350 g
Cereals, tubers and legumes	250~400 g
Whole grains and legumes	50~150 g
Tubers	50~100 g
Water	1500~1700 ml

Engage in physical activities
equivalent to 6000 walking steps daily

(b)

Dairy

Cereals, tubers and legumes

Fish, lean meats, eggs and soybeans

Fruits

Vegetables

(c)

Moderate amounts of cooking oil and salt

Soybeans, nuts and dairy products 2–3 servings

Lean meats, eggs and fish 2–3 servings

Fruits 3–4 servings

Vegetables 4–5 servings

Cereals, tubers and legumes 5–6 servings

Chinese Food Guide Abacus (2016)

1-hour outdoor activity

FIGURE 6.5 Illustrations for the Chinese dietary guidelines launched in 2016: (a) Chinese Food Guide (CFG) G-Pagoda is the main graphical illustration; (b) CFG-Plate; and (c) CFG-Abacus function as supplementary illustrations for CFG-Pagoda. **Source:** Reprinted from Yang et al. (2018b).

Take-Home Messages

- The traditional Asian diet is followed in most Asian countries, and although it varies in many aspects between countries, it holds many similarities regarding the consumption of traditional Asian foods.
- The Asian diet is primarily characterized by high consumption of rice, foods of plant origin (e.g., soy products), fish and seafood, as well as fruits and vegetables.
- The Japanese and the Chinese dietary guidelines represent two well-documented examples of healthy Asian diets.
- The incidence of several chronic diseases, such as CVD and cancer, has been shown to be lower in most Asian societies compared to most Western countries.
- The recent shift from the traditional Asian diet to a more Western-like diet is characterized by an increase in meat consumption and a decrease in rice consumption.

Self-Assessment Questions

1. What are the main characteristics of the Asian diet?
2. State two well-documented examples of healthy Asian diets.

3. What kinds of foods are included at the base of the "Chinese Food Guide Pagoda"?

Bibliography

Abaidia, A.E., Daab, W., and Bouzid, M.A. (2020). Effects of Ramadan fasting on physical performance: a systematic review with meta-analysis. *Sports Med.* 50 (5): 1009–1026.

Akhlaghi, M. (2020). Dietary Approaches to Stop Hypertension (DASH): potential mechanisms of action against risk factors of the metabolic syndrome. *Nutr. Res. Rev.* 33 (1): 1–18.

Ali Mohsenpour, M., Fallah-Moshkani, R., Ghiasvand, R. et al. (2019). Adherence to Dietary Approaches to Stop Hypertension (DASH)-style diet and the risk of cancer: a systematic review and meta-analysis of cohort studies. *J. Am. Coll. Nutr.* 38 (6): 513–525.

Baroni, L., Goggi, S., and Battino, M. (2018). VegPlate: a Mediterranean-based food guide for Italian adult, pregnant, and lactating vegetarians. *J. Acad. Nutr. Diet.* 118 (12): 2235–2243.

Chen, J., Campbell, T.C., Li, J., and Peto, R. (1990). *Diet, Lifestyle and Mortality in China. A Study of the Characteristics of 65 Chinese Counties.* A joint publication of: Oxford University Press, Cornell University Press, and the People's Medical Publishing House.

Coronary heart disease in seven countries. XVII. The diet. (1970). *Circulation* 41 (4 Suppl): I162–I183.

Derbyshire, E.J. (2016). Flexitarian diets and health: a review of the evidence-based literature. *Front. Nutr.* 3: 55.

Eliasi, J.R. and Dwyer, J.T. (2002). Kosher and halal: religious observances affecting dietary intakes. *J. Am. Diet. Assoc.* 102 (7): 911–913.

Eveleigh, E.R., Coneyworth, L.J., Avery, A., and Welham, S.J.M. (2020). Vegans, vegetarians, and omnivores: how does dietary choice influence iodine intake? A systematic review. *Nutrients* 12 (6): 1606.

FAO. (2010). Food-based dietary guidelines for Japanese. www.fao.org/nutrition/education/food-dietary-guidelines/regions/countries/Japan/en.

Fernando, H.A., Zibellini, J., Harris, R.A. et al. (2019). Effect of Ramadan fasting on weight and body composition in healthy non-athlete adults: a systematic review and meta-analysis. *Nutrients* 11 (2): 478.

Gonzalez-Garcia, S., Esteve-Llorens, X., Moreira, M.T., and Feijoo, G. (2018). Carbon footprint and nutritional quality of different human dietary choices. *Sci. Total Environ.* 644: 77–94.

Haghighatdoost, F., Bellissimo, N., Totosy, de Zepetnek, J.O., and Rouhani, M.H. (2017). Association of vegetarian diet with inflammatory biomarkers: a systematic review and meta-analysis of observational studies. *Public Health Nutr.* 20 (15): 2713–2721.

Haider, L.M., Schwingshackl, L., Hoffmann, G., and Ekmekcioglu, C. (2018). The effect of vegetarian diets on iron status in adults: a systematic review and meta-analysis. *Crit. Rev. Food Sci. Nutr.* 58 (8): 1359–1374.

Iguacel, I., Huybrechts, I., Moreno, L.A., and Michels, N. (2021). Vegetarianism and veganism compared with mental health and cognitive outcomes: a systematic review and meta-analysis. *Nutr. Rev.* 79 (4): 361–381.

Kanerva, N., Kaartinen, N.E., Schwab, U., Lahti-Koski, M., and Männistö, S. (2014). The Baltic Sea Diet Score: a tool for assessing healthy eating in Nordic countries. *Public Health Nutr.* 17 (8): 1697–1705. doi: 10.1017/S1368980013002395.

Koufakis, T., Karras, S.N., Zebekakis, P., and Kotsa, K. (2018). Orthodox religious fasting as a medical nutrition therapy for dyslipidemia: where do we stand and how far can we go? *Eur. J. Clin. Nutr.* 72 (4): 474–479.

Landberg, R. and Hanhineva, K. (2019). Biomarkers of a healthy Nordic diet: from dietary exposure biomarkers to microbiota signatures in the metabolome. *Nutrients* 12 (1): 27.

Lankinen, M., Uusitupa, M., and Schwab, U. (2019). Nordic diet and inflammation – a review of observational and intervention studies. *Nutrients* 11 (6): 1369.

Lee, I.M., Shiroma, E.J., Lobelo, F. et al. (2012). Effect of physical inactivity on major non-communicable diseases worldwide: an analysis of burden of disease and life expectancy. *Lancet* 380 (9838): 219–229.

Li, Y., Hruby, A., Bernstein, A.M. et al. (2015). Saturated fats compared with unsaturated fats and sources of carbohydrates in relation to risk of coronary heart disease: a prospective cohort study. *J. Am. Coll. Cardiol.* 66 (14): 1538–1548.

Mach, F., Baigent, C., Catapano, A.L. et al. (2020). 2019 ESC/EAS guidelines for the management of dyslipidemias: lipid modification to reduce cardiovascular risk. *Eur. Heart J.* 41 (1): 111–188.

Makarem, N., Bandera, E.V., Lin, Y. et al. (2018). Consumption of sugars, sugary foods, and sugary beverages in relation to adiposity-related cancer risk in the Framingham offspring cohort (1991–2013). *Cancer Prev. Res. (Phila).* 11 (6): 347–358.

Martin, C.A., Gowda, U., Smith, B.J., and Renzaho, A.M.N. (2018). Systematic review of the effect of lifestyle interventions on the components of the metabolic syndrome in South Asian migrants. *J. Immigr. Minor. Health.* 20 (1): 231–244.

Melina, V., Craig, W., and Levin, S. (2016). Position of the Academy of Nutrition and Dietetics: vegetarian diets. *J. Acad. Nutr. Diet.* 116 (12): 1970–1980.

Meltzer, H.M., Brantsaeter, A.L., Trolle, E. et al. (2019). Environmental sustainability perspectives of the Nordic diet. *Nutrients* 11 (9): 2248.

Mihrshahi, S., Ding, D., Gale, J. et al. (2017). Vegetarian diet and all-cause mortality: evidence from a large population-based Australian cohort – the 45 and up study. *Prev. Med.* 97: 1–7.

NCEP-ATPIII. (2001). Executive summary of the third report (NCEP) expert panel on detection, evaluation, and treatment of high blood cholesterol in adults (adult treatment panel III). *JAMA* 285 (19): 2486–2497.

Nishimura, T., Murakami, K., Livingstone, M.B. et al. (2015). Adherence to the food-based Japanese dietary guidelines in relation to metabolic risk factors in young Japanese women. *Br. J. Nutr.* 114 (4): 645–653.

Oba, S., Nagata, C., Nakamura, K. et al. (2009). Diet based on the Japanese food guide spinning top and subsequent mortality among men and women in a general Japanese population. *J. Am. Diet. Assoc.* 109 (9): 1540–1547.

OLDWAYS. (2018). Asian Heritage Diet. https://oldwayspt.org/traditional-diets/asian-heritage-diet.

Pakeeza, M. and Munir, M. (2010). Dietary laws of Islam and Judaism: a comparative study. *AL-ADWA* 45: 1–14.

Pakkir Maideen, N.M., Jumale, A., Alatrash, J.I., and Abdul Sukkur, A.A. (2017). Health benefits of Islamic intermittent fasting. *J. Nutr. Fasting Health* 5: 162–171.

Parker, H.W. and Vadiveloo, M.K. (2019). Diet quality of vegetarian diets compared with nonvegetarian diets: a systematic review. *Nutr. Rev.* 77 (3): 144–160.

Picasso, M.C., Lo-Tayraco, J.A., Ramos-Villanueva, J.M. et al. (2019). Effect of vegetarian diets on the presentation of metabolic syndrome or its components: a systematic review and meta-analysis. *Clin. Nutr.* 38 (3): 1117–1132.

Ramezani-Jolfaie, N., Mohammadi, M., and Salehi-Abargouei, A. (2019). The effect of healthy Nordic diet on cardio-metabolic markers: a systematic review and meta-analysis of randomized controlled clinical trials. *Eur. J. Nutr.* 58 (6): 2159–2174.

Ranasinghe, P., Mathangasinghe, Y., Jayawardena, R. et al. (2017). Prevalence and trends of metabolic syndrome among adults in the Asia-Pacific region: a systematic review. *BMC Public Health* 17 (1): 101.

Rogerson, D. (2017). Vegan diets: practical advice for athletes and exercisers. *J. Int. Soc. Sports Nutr.* 14: 36.

Sacks, F.M., Obarzanek, E., Windhauser, M.M. et al. (1995). Rationale and design of the Dietary Approaches to Stop Hypertension trial (DASH). A multicenter controlled-feeding study of dietary patterns to lower blood pressure. *Ann. Epidemiol.* 5 (2): 108–118.

Saha, S., Nordstrom, J., Mattisson, I. et al. (2019). Modelling the effect of compliance with Nordic nutrition recommendations on cardiovascular disease and cancer mortality in the Nordic countries. *Nutrients* 11 (6): 1434.

Sakhaei, R., Ramezani-Jolfaie, N., Mohammadi, M., and Salehi-Abargouei, A. (2019). The healthy Nordic dietary pattern has no effect on inflammatory markers: a systematic review and meta-analysis of randomized controlled clinical trials. *Nutrition* 58: 140–148.

Schaefer, E.J., Lichtenstein, A.H., Lamon-Fava, S. et al. (1995). Efficacy of a National Cholesterol Education Program Step 2 diet in normolipidemic and hypercholesterolemic middle-aged and elderly men and women. *Arterioscler. Thromb. Vasc. Biol.* 15 (8): 1079–1085.

Schurmann, S., Kersting, M., and Alexy, U. (2017). Vegetarian diets in children: a systematic review. *Eur. J. Nutr.* 56 (5): 1797–1817.

Shah, M. and Garg, A. (2019). The relationships between macronutrient and micronutrient intakes and type 2 diabetes mellitus in South Asians: a review. *J. Diabetes Complications* 33 (7): 500–507.

Soeters, P.B. (2020). Editorial: vegan diets: what is the benefit? *Curr. Opin. Clin. Nutr. Metab. Care* 23 (2): 151–153.

Soltani, S., Arablou, T., Jayedi, A., and Salehi-Abargouei, A. (2020). Adherence to the Dietary Approaches to Stop Hypertension (DASH) diet in relation to all-cause and cause-specific mortality: a systematic review and dose-response meta-analysis of prospective cohort studies. *Nutr. J.* 19 (1): 37.

Stewart, O., Yamarat, K., Neeser, K.J. et al. (2014). Buddhist religious practices and blood pressure among elderly in rural Uttaradit Province, northern Thailand. *Nurs. Health Sci.* 16 (1): 119–125.

Taghavi, M., Sadeghi, A., Maleki, V. et al. (2019). Adherence to the dietary approaches to stop hypertension-style diet is inversely associated with chronic kidney disease: a systematic review and meta-analysis of prospective cohort studies. *Nutr. Res.* 72: 46–56.

Tomova, A., Bukovsky, I., Rembert, E. et al. (2019). The effects of vegetarian and vegan diets on gut microbiota. *Front. Nutr.* 6: 47.

Unger, T., Borghi, C., Charchar, F. et al. (2020). 2020 International Society of Hypertension global hypertension practice guidelines. *Hypertension* 75 (6): 1334–1357.

United States Conference of Catholic Bishops. (2020). Fast & abstinence. www.usccb.org/prayer-and-worship/liturgical-year-and-calendar/lent/catholic-information-on-lenten-fast-and-abstinence.

van den Brink, A.C., Brouwer-Brolsma, E.M., Berendsen, A.A.M., and van de Rest, O. (2019). The Mediterranean Dietary Approaches to Stop Hypertension (DASH), and Mediterranean-DASH Intervention for Neurodegenerative Delay (MIND) diets are associated with less cognitive decline and a lower risk of Alzheimer's disease: a review. *Adv. Nutr.* 10 (6): 1040–1065.

Viguiliouk, E., Kendall, C.W., Kahleova, H. et al. (2019). Effect of vegetarian dietary patterns on cardiometabolic risk factors in diabetes: a systematic review and meta-analysis of randomized controlled trials. *Clin. Nutr.* 38 (3): 1133–1145.

Wang, X., Ouyang, Y., Liu, J. et al. (2014). Fruit and vegetable consumption and mortality from all causes, cardiovascular disease, and cancer: systematic review and dose-response meta-analysis of prospective cohort studies. *BMJ* 349: g4490.

Williams, B., Mancia, G., Spiering, W. et al. (2018a). 2018 practice guidelines for the management of arterial hypertension of the European Society of Hypertension and the European Society of Cardiology: ESH/ESC Task Force for the Management of Arterial Hypertension. *J. Hypertens.* 36 (12): 2284–2309.

Williams, B., Mancia, G., Spiering, W. et al. (2018b). 2018 ESC/ESH guidelines for the management of arterial hypertension. The Task Force for the Management of Arterial Hypertension of the European Society of Cardiology (ESC) and the European Society of Hypertension (ESH). *G. Ital. Cardiol. (Rome)* 19 (11 Suppl 1): 3S–73S.

World Health Organization. (2012). Guideline: sodium intake for adults and children. Geneva: WHO www.who.int/publications/i/item/9789241504836.

Yang, J., Siri, J.G., Remais, J.V. et al. (2018a). The Tsinghua-Lancet commission on healthy cities in China: unlocking the power of cities for a healthy China. *Lancet* 391 (10135): 2140–2184.

Yang, Y.X., Wang, X.L., Leong, P.M. et al. (2018b). New Chinese dietary guidelines: healthy eating patterns and food-based dietary recommendations. *Asia Pac. J. Clin. Nutr.* 27 (4): 908–913.

Yoshiike, N., Hayashi, F., Takemi, Y et al. (2007). A new food guide in Japan: the Japanese food guide spinning top. *Nutr. Rev.* 65 (4): 149–154.

Yu, D., Zhang, X., Xiang, Y.B. et al. (2014). Adherence to dietary guidelines and mortality: a report from prospective cohort studies of 134,000 Chinese adults in urban Shanghai. *Am. J. Clin. Nutr.* 100 (2): 693–700.

Zagożdżon, P. and Wrotkowska, M. (2017). Religious beliefs and their relevance for treatment adherence in mental illness: a review. *Religions* 8: 150.

Zimorovat, A., Mohammadi, M., Ramezani-Jolfaie, N., and Salehi-Abargouei, A. (2020). The healthy Nordic diet for blood glucose control: a systematic review and meta-analysis of randomized controlled clinical trials. *Acta Diabetol.* 57 (1): 1–12.

CHAPTER 7

The Mediterranean Diet

A Dietary Pattern That Has Stood the Test of Time

The Mediterranean Diet

The term *Mediterranean diet* (MedD) (Figure 7.1) is commonly used to describe the dietary pattern followed by the populations in the Mediterranean region.

However, the term "diet" does not refer only to food and eating. The word *diet* originated from the Greek word $\delta\acute{\iota}\alpha\iota\tau\alpha$ (*diaita*), which means "way of living," "lifestyle." Therefore, MedD does not refer only to nutrition but to a way of living, our lifestyle. This way of living incorporates an assortment of knowledge, expertise, and competences that have been gained empirically, as well as customs and rituals, synthesizing inherited traditions conveyed from previous generations to the next.

> **Key Point**
>
> The word *diet* originated from the Greek word $\delta\acute{\iota}\alpha\iota\tau\alpha$ (*diaita*), which means "way of living." Therefore, MedD does not refer only to nutrition but to a way of living, our lifestyle.

> **Key Point**
>
> Today there are several versions of the Mediterranean diet.

The MedD concept dates back to the 1960s. It is characterized by food patterns typical of the Greek island of Crete, much of the rest of Greece, and Southern Italy in the early 1960s. This is when Ancel Keys, an American physiologist, based on the results of the Seven Countries Study (SCS; discussed below), demonstrated that these populations (Italy and Greece) had a reduced incidence of cardiovascular disease and cancer compared to the other populations of the study.

Based on the results of this epidemiological study, MedD is now considered the outcome of the interactions between the natural Mediterranean environment and major civilizations, different cultures, and religions of people living in the Mediterranean basin. Consequently, today there are several versions of the Mediterranean diet, reflecting knowledge, traditions, and customs of the different Mediterranean populations, in the subjects of cooking, sharing, and consumption of foods, that are conveyed from previous generations to the next. In 2013, Cyprus, Croatia, Spain, Greece, Italy, Morocco, and Portugal proposed the inclusion of the Mediterranean diet in the list of Intangible Cultural Heritage of Humanity; the proposal was approved by the United Nations Educational, Scientific and Cultural Organization (UNESCO) with the following description:

The Mediterranean diet constitutes a set of skills, knowledge, practices and traditions ranging from the landscape to the table, including the crops, harvesting, fishing, conservation, processing, preparation and consumption of food. A nutritional model which remained constant over time and space, consisting mainly of olive oil, cereals, fresh or dried fruits and vegetables, a moderate amount of fish and dairy products, low amount of meat, condiments, spices, accompanied by wine, according to the beliefs of each community. It is more than food, it promotes social interaction and communal events, since communal meals are the cornerstone of social customs and festivities. It has enriched knowledge, generated songs and music, tales and legends over centuries in the Mediterranean. The Mediterranean diet is rooted in respect to the territory, biodiversity and is closely related to traditional activities and crafts linked to farming and fishing. Women played a vital role in the transmission from generation to generation of expertise, as well as knowledge of gestures, celebration practices and the culture of the table. (UNESCO, 17 November 2013)

Textbook of Lifestyle Medicine, First Edition. Labros S. Sidossis and Stefanos N. Kales.

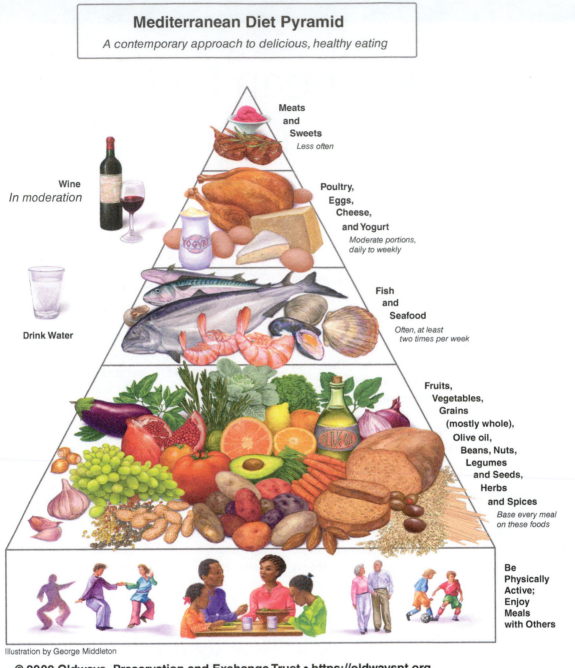

Mediterranean Diet Pyramid
A contemporary approach to delicious, healthy eating

Illustration by George Middleton

© 2009 Oldways Preservation and Exchange Trust • https://oldwayspt.org

FIGURE 7.1 The Mediterranean Diet Pyramid. © 2009 OLDWAYS Preservation & Exchange Trust.

The Emergence of the Mediterranean Diet

The MedD belongs to what one would call "ancient diets." Its adoption goes back to the mists of times, starting in Ancient Crete with the Minoans, and subsequently the other Greeks exporting olive oil and wine and expanding olive cultivation. Several archeological findings and literature apothegms, such as those found in Homer's epics, denote the way Mediterranean people used to eat. Obviously, the traditional MedD has

undergone significant changes over time. During the Middle Ages, eating habits of the populations of the Mediterranean region such as Romans fused, at least partly, with those of other populations, such as the German nomads who were more into hunting, farming, and gathering food resources. Although the Roman culture kept most of the "Mediterranean" style of dieting, the Arabic food culture, which had developed on the southern shores of the Mediterranean, was slowly incorporated into the Roman cuisine. The Arabs facilitated the introduction of yet unknown agricultural products, such as various spices and fruits, contributing greatly to the formation of several new cooking habits.

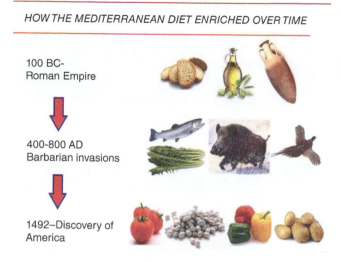

HOW THE MEDITERRANEAN DIET ENRICHED OVER TIME

100 BC-
Roman Empire

400-800 AD
Barbarian invasions

1492–Discovery of
America

FIGURE 7.2 The development of the Mediterranean diet over the centuries. **Source:** Reprinted from Capurso et al. (2018).

The discovery of the Americas also affected the European food culture. The newly discovered land provided new kinds of foods, such as potatoes and tomatoes. Interestingly, tomatoes were erroneously thought to be poisonous, up until the mid-1800s; later they became one of the flagships of the MedD. Consequently, the MedD reflects a collection of dietary habits and food-handling practices adopted in the countries bordering the Mediterranean Sea (Figure 7.2).

The MedD has a strong societal dimension. For instance, shared meals in the context of traditional festivities or during the breaks of rural manual labor are the essence of the social character that food consumption holds in the Mediterranean lifestyle (MedL). This further suggests that the MedD describes a holistic way of eating that incorporates relevant social and cultural aspects of everyday life, rather than the simple consumption of nutrients, foods, or food groups. That is exactly what the Greek word *diaita* denotes, i.e., the holistic character of lifestyle.

Scientific interest for the role of the MedD in the health of the populations flourished in the middle of the twentieth century. Contrary to the popular belief that the Seven Countries Study (SCS) is the first study to examine the dietary habits of the people living in the Mediterranean region, the first systematic attempt was carried out in the late 1940s in the Greek island of Crete by a scientific team headed by Leland C. Allbaugh, an American epidemiologist commissioned by the Rockefeller Foundation. His team, consisting mainly of trained nurses from the Greek Red Cross, collected weighed food records from 128 households, obtained seven-day dietary intake records from more than 500 individuals from those households, and administered food-frequency questionnaires to 765 households. The results were published as a case study: *Crete: A Case Study of an Underdeveloped Area.*

> **Key Point**
>
> MedD describes a holistic way of eating that incorporates relevant social and cultural aspects of everyday life, rather than the simple consumption of nutrients, foods, or food groups.

The main findings were that the foundation of the Cretan diet was plant-based foods (~61%). It included few animal products (7%), but fat intake was relatively high (~29%). The survey showed that olives, cereal grains, pulses, wild greens and herbs, and fruits, together with limited quantities of goat meat and milk, game, and fish, had remained the basic Cretan foods for 40 centuries. Olives and olive oil contributed significantly to energy intake. Olive oil was freely used as a cooking fat and was also added to salads, soups, and cooked vegetables. Moreover, no meal was complete without bread. Bread had a symbolic meaning, as it was an important component in church ceremonies and in family gatherings, in joy or in grief. Furthermore, it was observed that wine consumption accompanied all meals in the MedD except breakfast. Table 7.1 shows the percent contribution of the main food groups to the Cretan diet, compared to the rest of Greece and the USA during the period 1948–1949.

However, again contrary to popular belief, the dietary practices of Crete in the 1950s were not out of choice but more out of necessity, i.e., people were eating whatever was available; they didn't have the luxury to choose. Only one out of six surveyed households judged their diet to be satisfactory. Many complained of hunger and stated that they would like to have more meat, rice, fish, pasta, butter, and cheese in their diet. Indeed, when life conditions improved, the Cretans started consuming more meat, butter, and carbohydrates. As a result, the contemporary diet in Crete scarcely resembles the model diet described by Leland Allbaugh in 1953.

Despite the plethora of information presented in the Rockefeller report, the interest in the health effects of the MedD peaked with the publication of the results from the SCS. Ancel Keys and his team collected data on lifestyle, biomarkers, and heart disease prevalence from cohorts in the USA, Finland, former Yugoslavia, Japan, the Netherlands, Italy, and Greece. The primary finding of the study was that men from the USA and northern Europe experienced a much higher incidence of CHD and mortality rate from CHD than did men of the same age in southern and central Europe. Based on these results, Keys proposed the notion that the fat content of the diet correlates positively with the number of deaths from CHD (Figure 7.3). However, after 5, 10, and 15 years of follow-up, it became evident that the various types of fats have different effects on CHD mortality and morbidity; all-cause mortality and CHD deaths are positively associated with SFA intake and negatively with MUFA intake and high MUFAs to SFAs ratio.

The risk of CHD mortality was also evaluated in the SCS in relation to the total cholesterol (TC) measurements. It was found that for a cholesterol concentration of ~210 mg/dl, the risk of CHD mortality was 4–5% in the Mediterranean cohorts of southern Europe and Japan, but it reached 15% for northern Europe. This observation led to the speculation that other factors had contributed

> **Key Point**
>
> Different types of fats have very different health effects.

TABLE 7.1   **Contribution of the main food groups to the Cretan diet (%) compared with accessibility in Greece and in the USA, 1948–1949.**

Food group	Crete 7-d weighed food records	Greece Respective food accessibility	USA: Respective food accessibility
Energy			
(Mj/d)	10.6	10.4	13.1
(kcal/d)	2547	2477	3129
Foods (% of total)			
Cereals	39	61	25
Pulses, nuts, and potatoes	11	8	6
Vegetables and fruits	11	5	6
Meat, fish, and eggs	4	3	19
Dairy products	3	4	14
Table oils and fats	29	15	15
Sugar and honey	2	4	15
Wine, beer, and spirits	1	NA	NA

Source: Allbaugh, L.C. (1953). *Crete: A Case Study of an Underdeveloped Area*. Princeton, NJ: Princeton University Press.

to the different CHD mortality rates in countries of the Mediterranean region, northern Europe, and the United States. This is when the term "Mediterranean diet" emerged to describe not only nutrient intake but also a way of living. It is obvious that the appropriate term to describe "way of living in the

Mediterranean region" is Mediterranean lifestyle and not Mediterranean diet. Since Cretans had the lowest CHD rates, the Cretan diet is considered the archetype of the Mediterranean diet.

In 1963, Ancel Keys and his wife, Margaret, settled in the village Pioppi in Southern Italy and lived and worked there

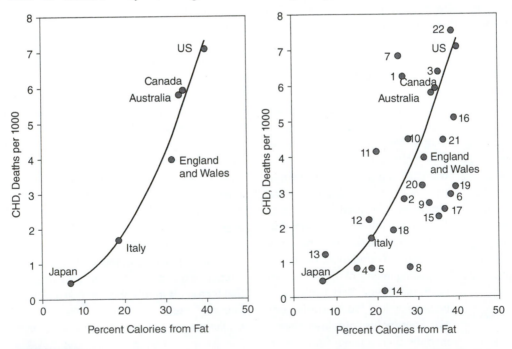

FIGURE 7.3   Data from Keys et al. depicting the correlation between percent calories from fat in the diet and CHD deaths (left panel). Keys was criticized that he "cherry-picked" six of 22 countries to present in the left panel. When data from the other 16 countries studied by Keys' group were included in the graph (right panel), the association is obviously not as strong (the line in the right panel was drawn for comparison purposes).

until 1998. He died at the age of 101 years in Minneapolis in 2004. He described the experience of tasting the MedD in his writings with intense enthusiasm:

We liked so much to taste that simple food – homemade vegetable soup, thousands of kinds of pasta always freshly cooked, dressed with tomato sauce and some minced cheese, rarely enriched with meat or local fish; a nice dish of pasta and beans; a great plenty of fresh bread, never served with sauces or butter; abundant fresh vegetables, a little portion of meat or fish, maximum once or twice a week; some local wine; and for dessert some fresh fruit.

According to Keys, the consumption of olive oil, bread, and wine constituted the pillars of the MedD, at least for the Mediterranean populations of the 1960s.

In the years that followed, a considerable volume of research focused on determining the individual components of the MedD that exert beneficial effects on human health. To date,

there is accumulating evidence stemming from numerous studies confirming many of these health benefits, as will be discussed in detail below. The MedD has proven to be effective in primary and secondary noncommunicable disease prevention, without side effects. Therefore, well-orchestrated efforts are needed to reinvent, reevaluate, and preserve the MedD as a palatable tool of disease prevention and as an element of cultural identity. Unfortunately, globalization has changed the diet of the Mediterranean region toward a Western-type diet; therefore, from this point on, the use of the term MedD in this book refers to the diet that the populations in the Mediterranean basin used to follow up to 30–40 years ago.

Deconstructing the Mediterranean Diet Pyramid into Its Primary Characteristics

As was the case with the Asian diet, it seems that there is more than one version of the MedD, even though the basic characteristics are common. For example, total daily lipid intake is ~40% of total energy intake in Greece and ~30% in Italy; however, in both cases the main source of dietary lipids is olive oil. The MedD is primarily a plant-based dietary pattern, including a high consumption of whole grains, bread, fruits, vegetables, legumes, nuts, and seeds. It is characterized by the low consumption of red meat and meat products, whole-fat dairy products (mainly in the form of cheese and yogurt), processed foods, and simple and refined cereals. Egg yolks are consumed less than four times per week. Fish and seafood (traditionally varied based on the population's proximity to the sea) is consumed in moderation. Olive oil is the main source of dietary fat, while a moderate amount of red wine is consumed with every meal (except breakfast).

The MedD is considered high in MUFAs (approximately 15–25% of daily energy intake), mainly deriving from olive oil, and PUFAs, deriving from fish and plant foods. Due to the low consumption of animal origin foods, this pattern has a low saturated fat content (less than 8% of daily energy intake). The omega-6 to omega-3 ratio varies from 2:1 to 1:1, denoting a very favorable balance of essential fatty acids. The high content of dietary fibers results in low glycemic index and glycemic load. Moreover, the MedD contains a wide variety of bioactive non-nutrients, such as phenolic and antioxidant compounds, with well-established benefits for human health.

In 1992, the United States Department of Agriculture presented the Food Guide Pyramid, based on the characteristics of the MedD (Figure 7.4). It was designed to highlight graphically the frequency of the food groups meant to be consumed by Americans, incorporating foods and food groups that were part of the MedD pattern. Later versions of the pyramid and the nutritional guidelines introduced other lifestyle aspects, such as physical activity, adequate hydration, and moderate wine intake, highlighting the contribution of these factors to health promotion.

The first "Mediterranean Diet pyramid" was presented in 1993 at the "International Conference on the Diets of the Mediterranean" in Cambridge, Massachusetts. It was the product of an initiative by the OLDWAYS Preservation & Exchange Trust, in collaboration with the Harvard School of Public Health and the European Office of the WHO. Figure 7.5 depicts this pyramid, which was composed based primarily on the dietary habits of people living in Crete and Corfu islands, but also in Southern Italy in the 1960s. The pyramid also included two basic habitual elements of those people: the engagement with physical activity, which was fundamental in everyday life, and moderate wine consumption, which was drunk mainly during meals (except breakfast).

The updates of the MedD pyramid that followed gave emphasis to adequate water intake, wine intake in moderation, and adequate hydration (Figure 7.6). The revised version of the MedD pyramid was published in 2009 (Figure 7.1). The major changes included: (i) the merging of all the plant-derived foods in the same section at the base of the pyramid, highlighting the basic role of these foods in every meal; (ii) the increased frequency of fish and shellfish consumption to at least twice per week, because of their beneficial effects on brain function and reproduction; and (iii) the introduction of herbs and spices in the structure of the pyramid; they enhance the flavor of meals and contribute to health promotion.

In the 2009 MedD pyramid, other aspects of lifestyle, such as sharing meals and regular exercise, covered the base of the

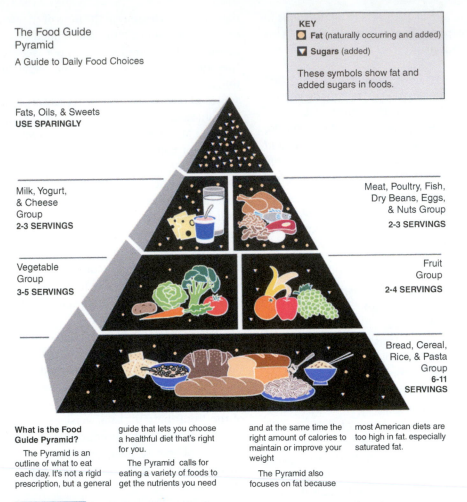

The Food Guide
Pyramid
A Guide to Daily Food Choices

KEY
◻ **Fat** (naturally occurring and added)
▽ **Sugars** (added)

These symbols show fat and
added sugars in foods.

Fats, Oils, & Sweets
USE SPARINGLY

Milk, Yogurt,
& Cheese
Group
2-3 SERVINGS

Meat, Poultry, Fish,
Dry Beans, Eggs,
& Nuts Group
2-3 SERVINGS

Vegetable
Group
3-5 SERVINGS

Fruit
Group
2-4 SERVINGS

Bread, Cereal,
Rice, & Pasta
Group
**6-11
SERVINGS**

What is the Food Guide Pyramid?

The Pyramid is an outline of what to eat each day. It's not a rigid prescription, but a general guide that lets you choose a healthful diet that's right for you.

The Pyramid calls for eating a variety of foods to get the nutrients you need and at the same time the right amount of calories to maintain or improve your weight

The Pyramid also focuses on fat because most American diets are too high in fat. especially saturated fat.

FIGURE 7.4   The Food Guide Pyramid – a guide to daily food choices (1992). **Source:** Reprinted from United States Department of Agriculture (USDA).

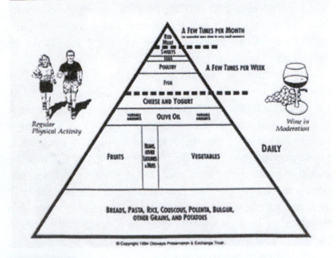

FIGURE 7.5   The traditional healthy Mediterranean Diet Pyramid; first version presented in 1993. **Source:** Reprinted from Callaway (1997).

pyramid, forming gradually the transition from dietary patterns to lifestyle patterns.

In 1999, the Health Ministry of Greece created a Mediterranean Diet Pyramid to visually describe the recommendations included in the "Dietary Guidelines for Greek Adults" (Figure 7.7). One serving was defined as half of the serving size that was designated in the Greek market regulations. For instance, one serving of cereals was defined as one slice of bread (25 g) or half a cup of cooked rice or pasta (about 50–60 g). Apart from specific servings, recommendations for daily physical activity and moderate wine intake during meals were also present in this pyramid. Specific recommendations were given about water intake and the substitution of salt with herbs and spices in order to enhance the palatability of cooked dishes.

In 2011, the Mediterranean Diet Foundation published a new pyramid. An important change in this MedD pyramid (Figure 7.8) was the food group at the top of the pyramid; sweets and sugary foods (such as candies, pastries, and sweetened beverages, e.g., soft drinks) had replaced red meats. Together with recommendations for portions and frequency of food consumption, healthy lifestyle recommendations and cultural elements were also added. Socialization, cooking with friends and family, and sharing

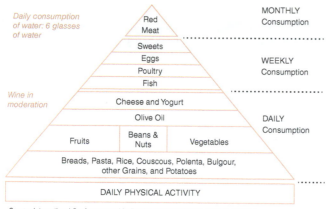

FIGURE 7.6 The Traditional Healthy Mediterranean Diet with updated graphics, published in 2000. © 2000 OLDWAYS Preservation & Exchange Trust.

foods, as well as seasonality, biodiversity, and the eco-friendliness characteristics of the MedD pattern were presented at the bottom of the pyramid to highlight aspects such as relaxation, community togetherness, and sustainability. Regular physical activity (such as walking, taking the stairs versus an elevator or escalator, and housework for at least 30 minutes throughout the day) is also represented for

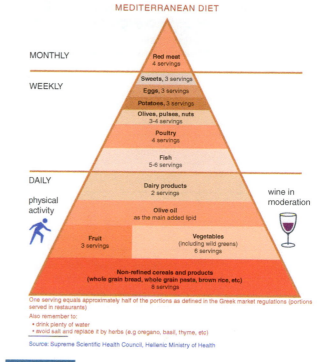

FIGURE 7.7 The MedD pyramid as depicted in the "Dietary Guidelines for Greek Adults." **Source:** Reprinted from Ministry of Health and Welfare Supreme Scientific Health Council (1999).

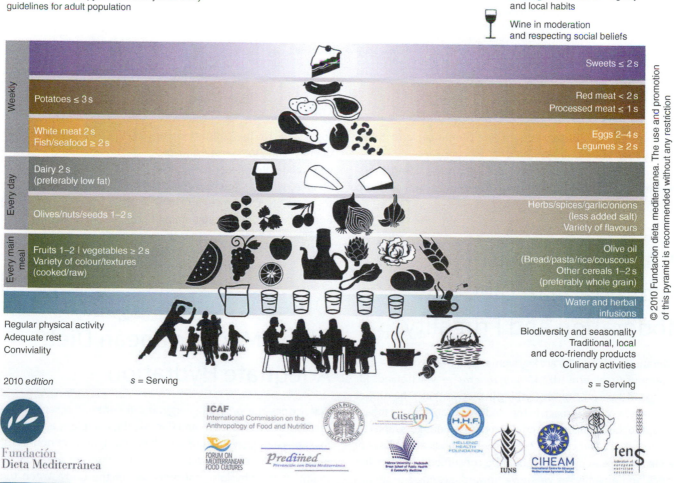

FIGURE 7.8 The Mediterranean pyramid today. **Source:** Reprinted from Bach-Faig et al. (2011).

TABLE 7.2 Comparison of the MedD pyramids, published 1993–2011.

Foods	OLDWAYS Preservation and Exchange Trust (2009)[b]	Mediterranean Diet Foundation (2011)[c]	1999 Greek Dietary Guidelines (1999)[a,d]
Olive oil	Every meal	Every meal	Main added lipid
Vegetables	Every meal	≥2 servings every meal	6 servings daily
Fruits	Every meal	1–2 servings every meal	3 servings daily
Breads and cereals	Every meal	1–2 servings every meal	8 servings daily
Legumes	Every meal	≥2 servings weekly	3–4 servings weekly
Nuts	Every meal	1–2 servings daily	3–4 servings weekly
Fish/Seafood	Often, at least two times per week	≥2 servings weekly	5–6 servings weekly
Eggs	Moderate portions, daily to weekly	2–4 servings weekly	3 servings weekly
Poultry	Moderate portions, daily to weekly	2 servings weekly	4 servings weekly
Dairy foods	Moderate portions, daily to weekly	2 servings daily	2 servings daily
Red meat	Less often	<2 servings/week	4 servings monthly
Sweets	Less often	<2 servings/week	3 servings weekly
Red wine	In moderation	In moderation and respecting social beliefs	Daily in moderation

[a] Dietary Guidelines for Greek Adults, Ministry of Health and Welfare Supreme Scientific Health Council (1999).
[b] 2008 Mediterranean Diet Pyramid, OLDWAYS Preservation and Exchange Trust (2009).
[c] Mediterranean Diet Foundation (2011); Bach-Faig et al. (2011).
[d] Serving sizes specified as: 25 g bread, 100 g potato, 50–60 g cooked pasta, 100 g vegetables, 80 g apple, 60 g banana, 100 g orange, 200 g melon, 30 g grapes, 1 cup milk or yogurt, 1 egg, 60 g meat, 100 g cooked dry beans.
Source: Reprinted with permission from C. Davis, J. Bryan, J. Hodgson, and K. Murphy. (2015). Definition of the Mediterranean diet: A literature review. *Nutrients* 7 (11): 9139–9153.

balancing energy intake, weight maintenance, and other health benefits.

In a published review, Davis et al. provide a comprehensive table of the similarities and differences between the published dietary pyramids (Table 7.2).

Other Aspects of the Mediterranean Diet: Moderation and Frugality

Moderation and frugality are key elements of the MedD, based on the famous Greek proverb "*Μέτρον άριστον*" – which stands for "all in good measure," or "everything in moderation." There is not "a one size fits all" approach in the MedD; portion sizes are meant to adapt to the population needs related to various geographical, socioeconomic, and cultural contexts. The foods at the base of the Mediterranean pyramid should be consumed in greater frequency and quantity; as we move upward, serving size shrinks and consumption frequency declines. The notion is that the foods

suggested to be consumed frequently enhance satiety and provide moderate energy for a given volume, whereas foods suggested to be rarely consumed are more energy-dense per unit volume and usually have higher glycemic index and glycemic load.

> **Key Point**
> Moderation and frugality are key elements of the MedD, based on the famous Greek proverb "*Μέτρον άριστον*" – which stands for "all in good measure," or "everything in moderation."

Other Aspects of the Mediterranean Diet: Adequate Hydration

Water does not provide energy, but it contains essential elements, such as iodine (I) and fluoride (F), and plays a vital role in all physiological functions, making it a significant non-nutrient source. Adequate water intake is therefore essential to maintain the physiological functions of the body. When the climate is hot and dry, as in the Mediterranean region for

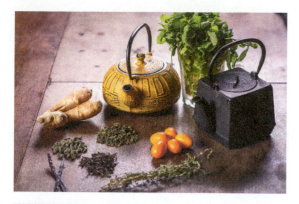

FIGURE 7.9 Herbal infusions can also contribute to adequate daily hydration.

several months during the year, it is essential to maintain *euhydration* (normal water content in the body). Under normal environmental and physical activity conditions, water intake is effectively governed by the feeling of thirstiness.

Key Point

Adequate water intake is essential to maintain the physiological functions of the body.

When temperature and humidity rise and physical activity levels increase, the need for water intake also increases. In the MedD, adequate daily hydration is achieved not only by drinking water but also by drinking herbal teas, low-fat broths, and other nonalcoholic beverages with low concentrations in sugar and sodium (Figure 7.8). Weather conditions, age, activity level, and pathological conditions should be taken into account in order to estimate daily water needs. The easiest and safest way to assess hydration is by comparing urine color to a urine color chart.

Key Point

The easiest and safest way to assess hydration is by simply comparing urine color to a urine color chart.

Pale yellow, or "straw-colored," urine, means hydration is optimal. On the other hand, darker urine means one may not be drinking enough liquids. The darker the urine, the more risk there is to be dehydrated!

A detailed description of the Mediterranean dietary model and a sample menu plan can be found in Appendix B.11.

The Health Effects of the Mediterranean Diet

Noncommunicable diseases (NCDs) are nontransmittable, chronic, lifestyle-related diseases that evolve gradually over time. As a component of the Mediterranean lifestyle, the MedD is an effective nutritional strategy against NCDs. The term *NCDs* primarily encompasses CVD, diabetes, cancer, and CRDs. These four groups of diseases account for more than 80% of all premature NCD deaths. According to the WHO, 41 million people died from NCDs in 2017; this number is projected to increase to 52 million by 2030; about 35% of them

are people less than 70 years old, mostly from a lower socioeconomic status. Lower socioeconomic status has been associated with approximately 75% of total deaths attributed to NCDs.

The main risk factors associated with NCDs are elevated blood pressure (hypertension), increased blood glucose (hyperglycemia), increased blood lipid levels (hyperlipidemia), and increased body weight (obesity). Prevention and management of

Key Point

As a component of the Mediterranean lifestyle, the MedD is an effective nutritional strategy against NCDs.

these cardiometabolic disorders can be achieved through the adoption of a healthy lifestyle, characterized by an adequate level of physical activity, a prudent dietary pattern, modest alcohol consumption, control of stress, and abstinence from smoking. The term *cardiodiabesity* has been used to describe the close inter-relationship between chronic metabolic abnormalities caused by a less than optimal lifestyle pattern, namely CVD, T2DM, MetS, and obesity.

A plethora of scientific studies have shown the effectiveness of the MedD in preventing and treating NCDs linked to dietary factors. In the following sections, we will review some of the main evidence associating long-term adherence to the MedD to better health.

Quality of Life and Wellness

Quality of life (QoL) is a broad, multidimensional concept that includes subjective evaluations of positive and negative aspects of life. Although health is one of the fundamental domains of overall QoL, there are several other important determining factors, such as the person's job, housing, school, and neighborhood. Aspects of culture, values, and spirituality are also key domains of overall QoL that add to the complexity of its nature. The concept of health-related quality of life (HRQoL) evolved in the 1980s to encompass the aspects of overall QoL that have been clearly shown to affect health – physical and mental. On the individual level, HRQoL includes physical and mental health perceptions (e.g., energy level and mood) and their correlates, including health risks and conditions, functional status, social support, and socioeconomic status. As mentioned previously, wellness connotes to a constellation of interdependent and interacting features that embody not only the components of adequate physical activity and sound dietary habits but also the aspects of harmonic socialization, coex-

Key Point

QoL is strongly connected with wellness.

istence with natural and personal environment, and balance between work and personal life, as well as emotional, spiritual, and intellectual well-being. Thus, QoL is strongly connected with wellness.

Long-term adherence to the MedD has been linked to a better quality of life. The SUN (Seguimiento Universidad de Navarra) Project found that high adherence to the MedD was strongly associated with better QoL, in terms of mental and physical health. These health-related parameters encompassed primarily vitality, general health, somatic pain, and physical and body function. Data from the Dutch cohort of the European Prospective Investigation into Cancer and Nutrition (EPIC-NL) study revealed that greater compliance to the MedD was related with two more months of living without health problems. Moreover, the same cohort highlighted that a higher adherence to the MedD was related to reduced disease burden, as assessed by the Disability-Adjusted Life Years (DALY) questionnaire. The Wellbeing, Eating and Exercise for a Long Life (WELL) study was conducted in a sample of men and women aged 55–65 years residing in Victoria, Australia. Adults with better-quality diets, resembling the MedD, reported better quality of life, whereas additional associations with emotional well-being and enhanced self-reported energy were observed in women. In addition, in the frame of the InCHIANTI study involving men and women >65 years old observed for 9 years, greater MedD scores resulted in 29% lower mobility deterioration of the lower limbs.

> **Key Point**
>
> Long-term adherence to the MedD has been linked to a better quality of life.

The relationship between high adherence to the MedD and wellness can be, at least in part, attributed to the ability of some components of the MedD to mitigate oxidative stress inflammation, which is inversely associated with longevity and healthy aging. Non-nutrient components belonging to the polyphenols family, such as resveratrol (found in grapes, wine, dried fruits, and nuts), quercetin (found in red wine and red onions), and oleuropein and oleacein (found in extra-virgin olive oil), induce the activity of a protein called sirtuin 1, which may prolong lifespan and promote healthy aging.

Mortality

The MedD offers protection against overall and disease-specific mortality. As early as 1995, Trichopoulou et al. suggested that even small increases in adherence to the MedD reduce all-cause mortality in the elderly by 17%. Almost a decade later, the same research team showed that, after 3.6 years of follow-up, an increase in the level of adherence to the MedD was related to an even lower risk of total, CHD, and cancer mortality, in the Greek cohort of the EPIC study. However, in the same study, no benefit was found for cerebrovascular mortality.

> **Key Point**
>
> The relationship between high adherence to the MedD and wellness can be attributed to the ability of some components of the MedD to mitigate oxidative stress and inflammation.

Many other prospective cohorts have demonstrated a negative correlation between the relative risk of all-cause mortality and adherence to the MedD. The Survey in Europe on Nutrition and the Elderly Concerted Action (SENECA) showed a 21% reduced likelihood of overall mortality in a Danish population when adherence to the MedD was increased. Moreover, women from the Nurses' Health Study diagnosed with breast cancer who reported a high adherence to a Mediterranean-like dietary pattern had a 61% reduced risk of mortality not caused by breast cancer. In a more recent meta-analysis of longitudinal studies, Sofi et al. confirmed the finding that a moderate increase in the level of adherence to the MedD leads to an 8% decrease in overall mortality, a 10% decrease in CVD-related mortality, and a 4% decrease in malignancies-associated mortality.

The effect of the MedD on mortality could be attributed to the beneficial effects of some of its individual components and their possible combinations and interactions. For instance, the high fruit and vegetable content of the MedD has been accredited for the 20–30% decrease in overall mortality among CVD patients. Additionally, daily consumption of olive oil (~30 g) has been found to attenuate all-cause mortality by 26%, when compared with a daily consumption of less than 15 g. Data on the association between red and white meat consumption and mortality are less consistent, since some studies have reported a negative association with overall and cancer-related mortality in both genders, while others have linked red and white meat consumption with a higher CVD mortality only in men.

Chronic Inflammation

Inflammatory response is a physiological function to guard the body from pathogens, stress, and diseases. However, when the inflammatory response is prolonged (e.g., low-grade inflammation), metabolic abnormalities ensue. Subclinical low-grade inflammation is omnipresent in obesity and has been associated with chronic abnormalities that often accompany obesity. It has been demonstrated that the production of inflammatory markers – such as C-reactive protein (CRP); tumor necrosis factor-α (TNF-α); interleukins-1β (IL-1β), -6 (IL-6), and -18 (IL-18); fibrinogen; and adhesion molecules – induce and aggravate inflammation in NCDs. On the other hand, adiponectin levels, a well-documented anti-inflammatory biomarker, are usually reduced in these chronic diseases.

The MedD, with foods naturally rich in bioactive compounds with antioxidant and anti-inflammatory properties, constitute a dietary pattern able to attenuate inflammatory state and endothelial dysfunction. In the PREDIMED (Prevención con Dieta Mediterránea) trial, a primary prevention interventional trial, the relationship between MedD and CVD incidence was assessed in a sample of 7447 individuals at high risk for CVD, randomly assigned to one of three arms: a low-fat control diet, a Mediterranean diet supplemented with extra-virgin olive oil, or a Mediterranean diet supplemented with a mixture of nuts. The MedD groups supplemented with virgin olive oil or nuts showed an anti-inflammatory effect, with reductions in serum CRP, IL-6, and endothelial and monocyte adhesion molecules and chemokines, whereas these parameters increased after the low-fat diet intervention. A relevant meta-analysis revealed that, in obese adults at increased CVD risk, the adoption of a Mediterranean-style diet can attenuate inflammation through high-sensitivity CRP reduction within two years.

> ### Key Point
> Subclinical low-grade inflammation is omnipresent in obesity and has been associated with chronic abnormalities that often accompany obesity.

> ### Key Point
> The MedD, with foods naturally rich in bioactive compounds with antioxidant and anti-inflammatory properties, constitutes a dietary pattern able to attenuate inflammation and endothelial dysfunction

The underlying mechanisms for the inverse association between the MedD and chronic inflammation are not yet fully elucidated. Available data suggest that they may relate to the bioactive micronutrients present in typical Mediterranean foods, such as vegetables and fruits, cereals, and red wine. These foods may decrease inflammation through the anti-inflammatory and antioxidant properties they exert. Likewise, fish consumption has been linked to improved inflammatory status due to its high content in PUFA. Phenolic compounds present in extra-virgin olive oil have also been reported to lower inflammation through modulation of the expression of inflammatory genes. For example, oleocanthal has been found to decrease the cyclooxynase-induced inflammation and thus protect against chronic degenerative diseases. Furthermore, other findings suggest that consuming extra-virgin olive oil in breakfast blunts the expression of some inflammatory genes.

Cardiovascular Diseases

Cardiovascular diseases, such as CHD, cerebrovascular disease, peripheral arterial disease, rheumatic and congenital heart disease, as well as deep vein thrombosis and pulmonary embolism, are leading causes of death. Large prospective epidemiological studies have shown a lower risk of developing CVD when compliance with the MedD or Mediterranean-like dietary patterns is high. Of note, even a marginal increase in adherence to the MedD produces a significant decrease in CVD risk. The first interventional trial highlighting the role of the MedD in the secondary prevention of CVDs was the Lyon Diet Heart Study. Its findings were impressive; they showed that adherence to a MedD rich in alpha-linolenic acid decreased the risk of recurrent CVD events by 47–72% for four years in patients with a previous myocardial infarction, compared with a prudent Western-type

diet. Most importantly, the adoption of the MedD has been shown to prevent the onset of CVDs, even in the presence of well-documented CVD risk factors. In the PREDIMED trial, after 4.8 years of follow-up, the magnitude of protection that the MedD conferred

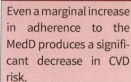

> ### Key Point
> Even a marginal increase in adherence to the MedD produces a significant decrease in CVD risk.

against CVD was 30% for the MedD enhanced with olive oil and 28% for the MedD supplemented with nuts, compared to the control low-fat diet.

Furthermore, the beneficial effects of the MedD have been evaluated in atherosclerosis and arterial stiffness, well-established predictors for stroke. Adherence to the MedD reduced carotid intima-media thickness (IMT) and the presence of unstable atheroma and was found to correlate with reduced arterial stiffness in later adulthood. Furthermore, a meta-analysis concluded that high adherence to the MedD positively modifies several CVD risk factors, such as body weight, systolic (SBP) and diastolic blood pressure (DBP), fasting glucose, CRP, and TC levels.

Genetic predisposition is a well-established determinant of CVD morbidity. Greater compliance with the MedD blunts the unfavorable impact of homozygosity for the risk alleles of certain genes, closely related to T2DM, in terms of glucose, triglycerides (TG), and TC and LDL levels, and it reduces new stroke events. Evidence from a nutrigenomic trial also underscores the modulatory effect of the MedD on the expression of genes implicated in several molecular mechanisms contributing to CVD risk.

The CLOCK (circadian locomotor output cycles kaput) gene is involved in the regulation of the circadian rhythm and human metabolism. The PREDIMED trial concluded that, as far as the CLOCK-rs4580704 C > G single nucleotide polymorphism is concerned, T2DM patients who are homozygous for the polymorphism of CLOCK-rs4580704 C > G are less vulnerable to experience stroke by 52%, compared to those lacking the polymorphism. Patients who adhered to the MedD presented a protection against stroke incidence, albeit not statistically significant.

With regard to individual foods and nutrients of the MedD, pooled analyses of 17 prospective studies, with 730,994 participants and 17,134 cumulative incident cases of CVD (including deaths), revealed that the protective effects of the diet were mostly attributable to olive oil, vegetables, and legumes.

Eating whole-grain-rich meals results in a 20–30% decrease in CVD incidence. Additionally, regular consumption of certain vegetables (especially dark green leafy, cruciferous, and deep yellow-orange) and fruits (especially citrus and deep yellow-orange) has been linked to the prevention of heart disease and stroke. Possible mechanisms mediating the health benefits of these foods may involve fiber, folic acid, and flavonoids intake, for which an effect at lowering risk of stroke and CHD has been well documented. Folic acid, present in high concentrations in fruits and vegetables, further enhances CVD health, as it decreases homocysteine, a well-established CVD risk factor. Ω-3 PUFA, found in fish, walnuts, and flax seeds, has also been shown to prevent CVD and ameliorate a host of CVD functions. Furthermore, daily intake of garlic attenuates cholesterol levels and thrombosis, offering additional protection against atherosclerosis.

Polyphenols exert antioxidant and anti-inflammatory properties, thus combating the common denominator of chronic metabolic disturbances, the combination of oxidative stress and chronic low-grade inflammation. Red wine, a typical component of the MedD, is thought to play a significant role in CVD prevention, due to its high concentration in polyphenols and its stress-reducing effects. A suggested mechanism for its health benefits against atherosclerosis involves the decrease in oxidized LDL levels, obstruction of platelet aggregation, better function of the endothelium, a strong antihypertensive and anti-inflammatory effect, and the prevention of cell deterioration. The same inhibitory effect on LDL oxidation seems to apply for herbs and spices; their broad usage in Mediterranean cuisine may also contribute to atherosclerosis prevention.

Olive oil, another key element of the MedD, also shows beneficial effects against atherosclerosis and CVD. Owing to its phenolic compounds, olive oil consumption has been found to reduce oxidized LDL concentrations. Indeed, a number of mechanistic studies have demonstrated that olive oil renders LDL resistant to oxidation via the coupling of its phenolic compounds to LDL molecules. Higher olive oil intake was associated with a lower risk of CHD and total CVD in two large prospective cohorts of US men and women. The authors of these studies concluded that substitution of margarine, butter, mayonnaise, and dairy fat with olive oil could lead to significantly lower risk of CHD and CVD.

Metabolic Syndrome

Metabolic syndrome is a cluster of metabolic abnormalities including central body fat adiposity, decreased HDL, increased TG levels, elevated blood pressure, and high fasting glucose concentration, and it is a well-established risk factor of CVD and T2DM. This risk is further increased by the co-presence of increased inflammatory and oxidative stress biomarkers, creating a pro-inflammatory and pro-thrombotic state.

Adherence to the MedD has been shown to ameliorate the risk of MetS as well as several features of the MetS, i.e., abdominal adiposity, fasting glucose concentrations, DBP, insulin resistance, and inflammation. The positive health effects of the MedD on MetS cannot be ascribed to any single nutrient, food, or food component, but they have to be extended to the entire meal pattern and lifestyle. In the following sections, we will discuss the effects of the MedD on specific components of MetS.

Dyslipidemias

The MedD lowers total, medium–small, and very small LDL particles, large VLDL fractions, and TC concentration. In addition, its adoption augments the total number of HDL fractions and large LDL particles and improves TG to HDL cholesterol ratio. When individuals at moderate risk for CVD followed a Mediterranean-style diet for three months, they managed to ameliorate post-prandial lipemia (TG-rich lipoprotein levels in the circulation after a meal ingestion) and hypercholesterolemia. The MedD in healthy adults improved TC and apolipoprotein B (ApoB) but not HDL, LDL or TG levels.

Epidemiological studies have demonstrated that people who consume high quantities of whole-grain cereals, as is the case in the MedD, have reduced risk of CHD and stroke. A possible mechanism explaining this observation is the clinically significant decreases in TC and LDL levels, attributed to the soluble fiber contained in whole grains. Furthermore, fruits and vegetables have been proposed to decrease the magnitude of arterial cholesterol oxidation, probably mediated by the presence of the antioxidant agents found naturally in them. A similar preventive effect against oxidized LDL concentrations is exerted by red wine, herbs, and spices.

Nonalcoholic Fatty Liver Disease

Nonalcoholic fatty liver disease (NAFLD) covers a spectrum of liver injury in the absence of excessive alcohol consuption, ranging from simple steatosis to nonalcoholic steatohepatitis (NASH) that may lead to advanced fibrosis and cirrhosis. It is one of the most common complications of obesity and T2DM in Western populations, affecting approximately 50% of diabetics and more than 70% of obese patients. NAFLD is the hepatic dimension of the MetS and constitutes a critical CVD risk factor. The Mediterranean diet has been shown to benefit NAFLD patients. In an RCT performed by Katsagoni et al., overweight/obese individuals with NAFLD were randomized to (i) control group (CG), (ii) Mediterranean diet group (MDG), or (iii) Mediterranean lifestyle group (MLG). Participants of the MDG and MLG groups attended seven 60-minute group sessions for 6 months, aiming at weight loss and increasing adherence to MedD, whereas in the MLG, additional guidance for increasing physical activity and improving sleep habits was given. Patients in CG received only written information for a healthy lifestyle. At the end of the intervention, MLG showed significant improvements in alanine transaminase (ALT) levels and liver stiffness compared with CG. MDG improved only liver stiffness compared with CG, suggesting that the Mediterranean lifestyle as a

> **Key Point**
>
> NAFLD is the hepatic dimension of the MetS and constitutes a critical CVD risk factor.

pattern may be superior to the MedD in improving liver outcomes in NAFLD patients.

Moreover, better adherence to the MedD has been associated with reduced SBP and serum TG levels and improvements in insulin resistance in NAFLD patients.

Hypertension

High blood pressure is a well-documented risk factor of CVDs and renal disease. Adherence to the MedD, for at least one year, ameliorates SBP and DBP, but whether the extent of the improvement holds clinical significance remains controversial. Nevertheless, it has been suggested that whole-grain products (primarily fruits and vegetables) and dairy products, all main components of the MedD, significantly improve blood pressure. Several randomized controlled clinical trials have highlighted a favorable impact of dietary fibers on blood pressure, to such extent that at least some patients can decrease or even terminate their antihypertensive treatment regimen. However, more studies are needed to further elucidate the underlying mechanisms for this effect. With respect to herbs and spices, it has been suggested that daily consumption of garlic has the potential to improve SBP. Furthermore, olive oil consumption is positively associated with favorable SBP and DBP responses. The mechanistic pathways explaining this effect possibly involve amelioration of endothelial function, through the reduction of ROS, mediated by the oleic acid and the phenolic compounds contained in olive oil. Again, more well-designed studies are needed to shed light on the mechanisms mediating the beneficial effect of the MedD on the regulation of blood pressure in humans.

Type 2 Diabetes Mellitus

Diabetes mellitus is a group of metabolic diseases characterized by hyperglycemia resulting from defects in insulin production, insulin action, or both. There is consistent evidence suggesting an inverse association between the adherence to a Mediterranean diet and incidence of T2D. A high score on the Mediterranean Diet Adherence Questionnaire has been associated with a reduction of approximately 20% in T2D risk. A meta-analysis of eight cohort studies with >120,000 subjects found that higher adherence to the Mediterranean diet was associated with a 19% lower risk of T2DM.

In summary, it appears that the MedD that includes whole-grain cereals, plant-based products (fruits, vegetables, legumes, nuts), prudent wine ingestion, and limited intake of red and processed meat and sweets may improve glycemic control and lipid profile in T2DM.

Cross-sectional studies are not able to detect causal effects; well-designed and executed RCTs are needed to describe the effect of an intervention or treatment on the outcome variable, e.g., the effect of the MedD on the prevention and treatment of T2DM. RCTs are scientific studies that aim to reduce certain

sources of bias when testing the effectiveness of new treatments. This is accomplished by randomly assigning subjects to two or more groups, treating them differently, and then comparing the groups prospectively with respect to a measured response. The multicenter PREDIMED trial enrolled 418 nondiabetic individuals with high risk of CVD and randomly assigned them on either a low-fat diet or a MedD supplemented with extra-virgin olive oil (1 l/wk) or nuts (30 g/d). After approximately four years of follow-up, it was found that the groups following the MedD supplemented with olive oil or nuts exhibited 50% lower risk of developing T2DM, compared to the participants who received the low-fat diet. Approximately five years after the end of the study, nondiabetic patients who had received the MedD supplemented with olive oil had 40% reduced risk to develop T2DM, whereas those who received the nut-enhanced MedD had 20% lower risk to experience T2DM, compared with the control group.

High compliance with the MedD may also protect from development of gestational diabetes mellitus. The health benefits that the MedD offers are also substantial for CVD patients and women who had previously experienced gestational diabetes.

> **Key Point**
> High compliance with the MedD may also protect from development of gestational diabetes mellitus.

Cancer

Cancers are responsible for a large number of annual deaths. Up to 30% of overall cancer mortality is attributed to increased body weight, inadequate ingestion of fibers, physical inactivity, elevated ethanol intake, and smoking. Cancer prevalence constitutes a crucial health burden and is expected to further increase by 70% over the next 20 years.

The traditional MedD has been associated with decreased risk for the development of several types of cancer, such as colorectal, epithelial, breast, prostate, pancreas, endometrial, and cancers of the upper aerodigestive tract. Intake of whole-grain cereals, fruits, and vegetables may lower the risk of cancers of the gastrointestinal tract but also those of the breast, female genital tract, and epithelium. According to the American Institute for Cancer Research, "a diet high in vegetables and fruits (more than 400 g/d) could possibly prevent at least 20% of all cancer incidence" No single substance has been identified as responsible for the alleged protection against cancer development; the cancer preventive effect is likely the result of a synergistic effect of multiple components in foods that are common in the MedD. Evidence also exists that olive oil intake has the potential to reduce oncogenesis, due to reduction in DNA oxidation (about 30%), possibly mediated by its phenolic compounds. Additionally, it has been

> **Key Point**
> The cancer preventive effect is likely the result of a synergistic effect of multiple components in foods that are common in the MedD.

postulated that consumption of oleic acid, the basic MUFA found in olive oil, may exert a preventive effect against breast, colon, and prostate cancers. The suggested effects of oleic acid may be via gene-diet interaction, meaning that oleic acid intervenes in the genome and subdues the expression of carcinogenic genes.

Neurodegenerative Diseases

Long-term adherence to the MedD decreases the risk for the development of neurodegenerative diseases and may even delay their onset. Relevant studies cover a range from intact cognitive ability to mild cognitive impairment (MCI) and dementia. The latter form of cognitive deterioration is present in ~4% of the elderly population worldwide. Alzheimer's disease (AD) constitutes the most prominent cause of dementia and accounts for 60–70% of all dementia events. Previous experience of depression, CVD, traumatic head injury, high blood pressure, unfavorable gut microflora composition, and the presence of T2DM have all been characterized as risk factors for the development of AD. The brain is an organ characterized by complexity and high energy demand; therefore, continuous delivery of nutrients and intense metabolic processes are required to maintain its physiological role. High metabolic rate increases reactive oxygen species and other oxidative stress biomarkers. Reactive oxygen species are free radicals, also called *oxygen radicals*. Their accumulation in brain cells may cause damage to DNA, RNA, and proteins and may cause brain abnormalities.

Lifestyle modification may play a critical role in the development and progression of these brain pathologies. Several nutrients, such as PUFAs and MUFAs, B-complex vitamins, as well as bioactive nutrients (polyphenols and antioxidant vitamins) may mitigate oxidative stress and inflammation. For example, the oleocanthal contained in olive oil hinders the deteriorating effect of a set of proteins on brain nerve cell function. Moreover, fish PUFAs seem to have a beneficial effect on patients with mild AD in terms of cognitive function. Even alcohol may exert some beneficial effects, assuming it is consumed in small to moderate doses.

The mechanisms underlying the protective effects of these nutrients against the age-related brain abnormalities are probably inextricably linked and intertwined. Therefore, the investigation of a dietary pattern containing all these nutrients is more appropriate compared to studying these nutrients separately. Indeed, prospective cohort studies have demonstrated that long-term adherence to the MedD can limit the occurrence of AD by 40%. In addition, after 4.4 years of follow-up, AD patients on a MedD presented 73% lower risk of disease-related mortality, and they had lower risk of developing mild cognitive decline. When the MedD was accompanied by physical activity, the preventive effect on mild cognitive decline was even more robust. The Australian Imaging, Biomarkers and Lifestyle Study of Aging demonstrated that individuals with a greater conformity to the MedD were less likely to develop AD. A more recent systematic review and meta-analysis reported that the MedD was associated with 33% decreased likelihood of developing MCI and AD. With respect to Parkinson's disease (PD), a 16-year prospective epidemiological study combining participants from the Health Professionals Follow-Up Study and the Nurses' Health Study revealed that a greater compliance to the MedD led to a 25% reduced risk of incident PD. Moreover, the MIND trial (a combination of MedD and DASH) seems to substantially slow cognitive decline with age. In the PREDIMED study, the MedD supplemented with olive oil or nuts was associated with improved composite measures of cognitive function.

> **Key Point**
>
> Reactive oxygen species accumulation in brain cells may cause damage to DNA, RNA, and proteins and may cause brain abnormalities.

> **Key Point**
>
> When the MedD was accompanied by physical activity, the preventive effect on mild cognitive decline was even more robust.

Chronic Respiratory Diseases

CRDs are diseases of the respiratory system that encompass impairments of the air passages and the lungs. The most prevalent CRDs are chronic obstructive pulmonary disease (COPD), asthma, obstructive sleep apnea (OSA) syndrome, occupational lung diseases, and pulmonary hypertension. The predominant risk factors for the development of CRDs are smoking, followed by indoor and outdoor pollution, occupational chemicals and dusts, and repetitive infections of the respiratory tract during childhood. WHO projections show that by 2030, COPD may be the third most prevalent cause of death. OSA syndrome is positively correlated with BMI and other obesity-related comorbidities, such as CVD, possibly because of the dysfunction of the endothelium triggered by inflammatory and oxidative biomarkers.

Findings from RCTs suggest that when people with OSA syndrome adopt MedD-like nutrition, they have fewer apnea episodes during the rapid eye movement (REM) stage of sleep, which usually accounts for approximately 25% of total sleep during the night. Moreover, physical activity has been shown to improve the apnea-hypopnea index (AHI) and several anthropometric measurements. Weight loss has been shown to further decrease oxidative stress and other obesity-related risks in patients with OSA syndrome.

Mental Disorders

Depression is a common mental disorder, characterized by sadness, loss of interest or pleasure, feelings of guilt or low self-worth, disturbed sleep or appetite, feelings of tiredness, and poor concentration. The disease often first appears at a young age. It affects women more often than men; unemployed people are also at high risk. Depression is significantly associated with decreased mental and physical ability but also increased disease burden.

Scientific evidence is mounting to support a positive association between the adoption of healthy dietary patterns and the prevention of depression. Data from the SUN cohort suggested that high compliance to the MedD exerts a protective effect against depression incidence. Of note, this association was not linear, indicating that the MedD can prevent depression development only to a certain degree. Clinical trials assessing the effect of MD on mental health show promising results; depressive symptoms decrease and remission rates increase substantially under this healthy diet regimen. Furthermore, a review of 37 studies highlighted the beneficial role of polyphenols consumption on depression risk, as well as in the reduction of depressive symptom severity.

Adherence to a diet composed of vegetables, fruits, whole grains, fish, and legumes, i.e., similar to the MedD, may protect against the development of depressive symptoms in older adults. Furthermore, sufficient intakes of B-complex vitamins and omega-3 PUFA have been related to preserved mental health. Folate intake lowers the risk of depression in men, especially in smokers. Additionally, adequate B_{12} vitamin intake is related to decreased depression rates in women, mainly in smokers and those performing physical activity.

> **Key Point**
>
> People who follow a MedD regimen may, to a certain degree, be protected from depression.

Sufficient intake of omega-3 PUFA appears beneficial in depression prevention only for women. MedD contains foods high in these nutrients, and therefore it is expected that people who follow a MedD regimen may, to a certain degree, be protected from depression.

Autoimmune Diseases

In autoimmune disorders, the immune system attacks healthy cells, tissues, and organs of its own organism, resulting in aberrant or total loss of function of these sites. It has been suggested that adherence to the MedD may have beneficial effects on the management or the relief of symptoms of the autoimmune disorders. Rheumatoid arthritis (RA) is an autoimmune disorder affecting the joints and accompanied by inflammation, pain, and malformations. Three months on the MedD resulted in a decrease in several RA symptoms and inflammation, improved physical function, and increased vitality and patients' self-evaluation of health condition compared to the previous year. In addition, a dietary pattern featuring fish, olive oil, and cooked vegetables – typical characteristics of the MedD – has been related to decreased risk for RA, possibly due to the omega-3 PUFA content of these foods. Of interest, a synergistic effect has been proposed to exist between olive oil and fish oils on RA symptom alleviation. Furthermore, olive oil may lower the incidence of RA. These findings are in accordance with the lower RA rates and its milder variants recorded in south European populations, where the MedD constitutes the traditional dietary pattern.

> **Key Point**
>
> In autoimmune disorders, the immune system attacks healthy cells, tissues, and organs of its own organism, resulting in aberrant or loss of function of these sites.

Inflammatory bowel diseases, e.g., Crohn's disease and ulcerative colitis, constitute another form of autoimmune diseases in which the predominant characteristic is the chronic inflammation of the gastrointestinal tract. Adoption of a Mediterranean-like dietary pattern has been shown to attenuate inflammation, restore gut microbiota colonization, and favorably affect gene expression in Crohn's disease patients.

Last but not least, evidence suggests that the adoption of a diet high in fibers may lower blood glucose and HbA1c measurements and produce fewer hypoglycemic episodes in T1DM patients.

Allergic Diseases

Allergic diseases include asthma, allergic rhinitis (or hay fever), atopic dermatitis (eczema), anaphylaxis, and food allergies. Their prevalence increased significantly during the last 50 years; it is estimated that currently they affect more than 40% of the childhood population. This trend has been ascribed to lifestyle changes, e.g., dietary, environmental, hygiene, and socioeconomic changes. It is speculated that these changes intervene in the immune system and cause epigenetic modifications (postnatal genome alterations). With respect to dietary habits, there is a shift from traditional and healthy dietary patterns to the adoption of a Western-style diet. The adoption of this dietary pattern contributes to obesity and asthma development; obesity itself constitutes a risk factor for asthma.

The exact mechanisms connecting obesity with asthma have not been fully elucidated; it has been suggested that they incorporate airway smooth cell dysfunction due to airway obstruction, inflammation, oxidative stress, and obesity-related disturbances, which, in turn, exacerbate asthma symptoms. Nonetheless, the Western-style diet features energy-dense foods rich in saturated fats and simple sugars, increased intake of red meat and its products, full-fat dairy products, and decreased vegetable and fruit intake. Hence, this dietary pattern leads to high risk for both age-related and allergic diseases.

Studies evaluating a possible connection between nutrition and allergies have examined the effects of antioxidants, long-chain PUFAs, nuts, vitamin D, fish, fruits, and vegetables on the development of several allergic diseases. The findings suggest beneficial effects, attributed mostly to the antioxidant properties and the immune-protective potential of these nutrients and foods. Furthermore, it has been proposed that any nutritional intervention aiming to prevent the onset of allergies should focus on maternal nutrition during pregnancy and on the infant's nutrition during the first months after delivery. The notion behind this suggestion is that the human immune, respiratory, and digestive systems affected by allergies have not been totally shaped until several months after birth. Thus, benefits mediated via nutrition may affect their function and reinforce prevention.

Omega-3 PUFAs have received broad attention in the context of immune modulation and allergy prevention, due to their strong anti-inflammatory and antioxidant potential. Enhanced maternal consumption of omega-3 PUFAs appears to moderate the prevalence of prenatal atopic dermatitis. However, findings from postnatal dietary modifications with omega-3 PUFAs are inconclusive. Following the MedD rich in omega-3 PUFAs decreased atopic dermatitis symptoms and wheezing recurrence in children at high risk for allergies, though not all patients with established asthma and atopic dermatitis can benefit from an increase in omega-3 PUFA intake.

The International Study on Allergies and Asthma in Childhood (ISAAC) has shown an inverse association between fruit consumption and current wheezing in developed (14%) and developing countries (29%). Current wheezing was also decreased when fish consumption and cooked green vegetable consumption was high in developed and developing countries. Finally, the consumption of olive oil during pregnancy has been shown to significantly decrease infants' wheezing during the first year of life.

Antonogeorgos et al. attempted to determine the contribution of the MedD to the association between living in cities compared to rural areas and the development of asthma in children aged 10–12 years old. These investigators suggested that urban environment is positively correlated with asthma. Nevertheless, conformity to the MedD was negatively associated with asthma, and its adoption could act protectively against asthma for those children living in urban centers.

Take-Home Messages

- The term *Mediterranean diet (MedD)* is commonly used to refer to the dietary pattern followed by populations living in the Mediterranean region but is most closely related to the traditional dietary patterns followed in rural Greece and Southern Italy in the 1950s and 1960s. The word *diet* originates from the Greek word *diaita*, which means "way of life" rather than food-eating pattern, as we know it today.
- MedD is characterized by high intakes of plant-derived foods, such as whole grains, fruits, and vegetables, and low intake of foods of animal origin. Legumes, poultry, and eggs, fish, and seafood are consumed on a weekly basis. Olive oil is the primary source of fat in this diet. Herbs and spices are also used in cooking in order to enhance taste and to avoid the overuse of salt.
- The MedD reflects a blend of dietary habits and food-handling practices adopted in the countries bordering the Mediterranean Sea.
- The first systematic attempt to investigate the diet of the people in the Mediterranean region was carried out in the Greek island of Crete by a scientific team headed by Leland Allbaugh, an American epidemiologist commissioned by the Rockefeller Foundation.
- The Seven Countries Study was the first to systematically examine the effect of diet and lifestyle on health. The most impressive finding of this study was the significantly lower incidence of CHD and mortality rate from CHD of men from Italy, Greece, and Japan compared to men of the same age in Finland and the United States.
- Another important finding of the Seven Countries Study is something that is now widely accepted: different types of fats exert different health effects.

- Globalization has changed the diet of the Mediterranean region toward a Western-type diet. This change may, at least in part, explain the increased prevalence of metabolic diseases observed over the last decades in all the Mediterranean countries.
- The most recent MedD pyramid was published in 2011 by the Mediterranean Diet Foundation food group; healthy lifestyle and cultural elements were added to the dietary recommendations.
- The MedD, albeit rich in total fat (30–40% of total daily energy intake coming mainly from monounsaturated fat from extra-virgin olive oil), is widely recognized as an effective nutritional strategy against NCDs, i.e., diseases that are the leading cause of death globally, killing 38 million people each year.
- A large amount of scientific evidence suggests that high adherence to the MedD is inversely associated with the risk of developing cancer, cardiometabolic, neurodegenerative, mental, autoimmune, and allergic diseases. This protection is largely attributed to the synergistic effect of its components, such as fruits, vegetables, whole grains, olive oil, and wine, which are rich in numerous bioactive nutrients.
- Even small increases in the level of adherence to the MedD can produce clinically significant reductions in all-cause mortality and promote longevity.
- Besides physical health, adherence to the MedD is positively associated with QoL and wellness; this relationship can be attributed to the ability of some components of the MedD to mitigate oxidative stress and inflammation and therefore promote healthy aging.

Self-Assessment Questions

1. Describe the main characteristics of the MedD.
2. Is there only one version of the MedD? Please justify your answer.
3. Characterize the following statements as true (T) or false (F).
   a. The MedD is considered high in MUFAs (approximately 15–25% of daily energy intake), mainly deriving from olive oil ( ).
   b. Foods in the base of the MedD pyramid should be consumed in lower frequency and quantity; moving up the pyramid, the recommended serving size and consumption frequency increases ( ).
   c. Total daily lipid intake is ~40% of total energy intake in the Greek version of the MedD and ~30% in the Italian version of the MedD; however, in both cases, the main source of dietary fat is butter ( ).
   d. The Seven Countries Study (SCS) was the first study to examine dietary intake in the Mediterranean region ( ).
   e. The traditional dietary practices of the Cretans were not out of choice but more out of necessity, i.e., they consumed whatever was available without having the luxury of choosing ( ).
4. How has the MedD evolved through the years?
5. What is the main source of fat in the MedD?
   a. canola oil
   b. margarine
   c. butter
   d. olive oil
   e. coconut oil
6. What are the primary findings of the Seven Countries Study?
7. Choose the correct statement:
   a. The MedD is characterized by high intakes of whole grains, fruits, and vegetables.
   b. The MedD is characterized by high intake of animal origin foods.
   c. Eggs are not allowed in the MedD.
   d. Seafood is part of the Asian diet but not the MedD.
   e. 30% of total energy intake in the MedD is attributed to protein intake.
8. Describe the most recent MedD pyramid published in 2011.
9. What is the meaning of the term frugality in the MedD?
10. Which of the following statements about hydration are true?
    a. Water contains essential elements but also provides large amounts of energy.
    b. Adequate water intake is essential to maintain the physiological functions of the body.
    c. Under normal environmental and physical activity conditions, water intake is effectively governed by the feeling of thirst.
    d. When temperature and humidity rise and physical activity levels increase, the need for water intake decreases.
    e. The darker your urine, the more dehydrated you are.
11. What are the major health effects of the MedD?
12. The relationship between high adherence to the MedD and wellness can be attributed to which of the following?
    a. The MedD has low-energy content, which contributes to a healthy body weight.
    b. The MedD has a high simple carbohydrate content.
    c. Some components of the MedD can mitigate oxidative stress and inflammation.
    d. The MedD has a beneficial effect on blood lipids.
    e. There is an inverse association between the MedD and T2DM.
13. Which of the components of the MedD have anti-inflammatory properties?
    a. the bioactive micronutrients present in fruits, vegetables, cereals, and red wine
    b. the polyunsaturated fatty acids found in fish
    c. the phenolic compounds present in extra-virgin olive oil
    d. all of the above
14. Characterize the following statements as true (T) or false (F).
    a. The MedD offers protection against overall and disease-specific mortality ( ).
    b. The MedD increases total, medium–small, and very small LDL particles and large VLDL fractions ( ).
    c. Adoption of the MedD can benefit NAFLD patients; it can lead to reductions in blood pressure and lipids and improvements in insulin sensitivity ( ).
    d. The MedD is not recommended for diabetic patients, given that it contains high amounts of fat that can aggravate insulin resistance ( ).
    e. The MedD reduces apneas-hypopneas, attenuates oxidative stress, and improves obesity-related indexes in patients with OSA ( ).

Bibliography

Allbaugh, L.C. (1953). *Crete: A Case Study of an Underdeveloped Area*. Princeton, NJ: Princeton University Press.

Antonogeorgos, G., Panagiotakos, D.B., Grigoropoulou, D., Yfanti, K., Papoutsakis, C., Papadimitriou, A., Anthracopoulos, M.B., Bakoula, C., and Priftis, K.N. (2014). Investigating the associations between Mediterranean diet, physical activity and living environment with childhood asthma using path analysis. *Endocr. Metab. Immune Disord. Drug Targets* 14 (3): 226–233. doi: 10.2174/1871530314666140826102514.

Bach-Faig, A., Berry, E.M., Lairon, D. et al. (2011). Mediterranean Diet Pyramid today. Science and cultural updates. *Public Health Nutr.* 14 (12A): 2274–2284. https://doi.org/10.1017/S1368980011002515. PMID: 22166184.

Becerra-Tomas, N., Blanco Mejia, S., Viguiliouk, E. et al. (2020). Mediterranean diet, cardiovascular disease and mortality in diabetes: a systematic review and meta-analysis of prospective cohort studies and randomized clinical trials. *Crit. Rev. Food Sci. Nutr.* 60 (7): 1207–1227.

Callaway, C.W. (1997). Dietary guidelines for Americans: an historical perspective. *J. Am. Coll. Nutr.* 16 (6): 510–516.

Capurso, A., Crepaldi, G., and Capurso, C. (2018). The historical origins and composition of Mediterranean diet. In: *Benefits of the Mediterranean Diet in the Elderly Patient*, 1–9. Berlin: Springer.

Casas, R., Sacanella, E., and Estruch, R. (2014). The immune protective effect of the Mediterranean diet against chronic low-grade inflammatory diseases. *Endocr. Metab. Immune Disord. Drug Targets* 14 (4): 245–254. doi: 10.2174/1871530314666140922153350.

Chiva-Blanch, G., Badimon, L., and Estruch, R. (2014). Latest evidence of the effects of the Mediterranean diet in prevention of cardiovascular disease. *Curr. Atheroscler. Rep.* 16 (10): 446. doi: 10.1007/s11883-014-0446-9.

Dernini, S. and Berry, E.M. (2015). Mediterranean diet: from a healthy diet to a sustainable dietary pattern. *Front. Nutr.* 2: 15.

Estruch, R. and Bach-Faig, A. (2019). Mediterranean diet as a lifestyle and dynamic food pattern. *Eur. J. Clin. Nutr.* 72 (Suppl 1): 1–3.

Estruch, R. and Ros, E. (2020). The role of the Mediterranean diet on weight loss and obesity-related diseases. *Rev. Endocr. Metab. Disord.* 21 (3): 315–327. doi: 10.1007/s11154-020-09579-0.

Food Guide Pyramid. (1992). U.S. Department of Agriculture and U.S. Department of Health and Human Services. https://www.fns.usda.gov/FGP.

Foscolou, A., D'Cunha, N.M., Naumovski, N. et al. (2020). The association between the level of adherence to the Mediterranean diet and successful aging: an analysis of the ATTICA and MEDIS (MEDiterranean Islands Study) epidemiological studies. *Arch. Gerontol. Geriatr.* 89: 104044.

Franquesa, M., Pujol-Busquets, G., Garcia-Fernandez, E. et al. (2019). Mediterranean diet and cardiodiabesity: a systematic review through evidence-based answers to key clinical questions. *Nutrients* 11 (3): 655.

Garcia-Fernandez, E., Rico-Cabanas, L., Rosgaard, N. et al. (2014). Mediterranean diet and cardiodiabesity: a review. *Nutrients* 6 (9): 3474–3500. doi: 10.3390/nu6093474.

George, E.S., Kucianski, T., Mayr, H. L. et al. (2018). A Mediterranean diet model in Australia: strategies for translating the traditional Mediterranean diet into a multicultural setting. *Nutrients* 10 (4). doi: 10.3390/nu10040465.

Georgousopoulou, E.N., Naumovski, N., Mellor, D.D. et al. (2017). Association between siesta (daytime sleep), dietary patterns and the presence of metabolic syndrome in elderly living in Mediterranean area (MEDIS study): the moderating effect of gender. *J. Nutr. Health Aging* 21 (10): 1118–1124.

Grammatikopoulou, M.G., Maraki, M.I., Giannopoulou, D. et al. (2018). Similar Mediterranean diet adherence but greater central adiposity is observed among Greek diaspora adolescents living in Istanbul, compared to Athens. *Ethn. Health.* 23 (2): 221–232.

Itsiopoulos, C., Hodge, A. and Kaimakamis, M. (2009). Can the Mediterranean diet prevent prostate cancer? *Mol. Nutr. Food Res.* 53 (2): 227–239. doi: 10.1002/mnfr.200800207.

Katsagoni, C.N., Papatheodoridis, G.V., Ioannidou, P., Deutsch, M., Alexopoulou, A., Papadopoulos, N., Papageorgiou, M.V., Fragopoulou, E., and Kontogianni, M.D. (2018). Improvements in clinical characteristics of patients with non-alcoholic fatty liver disease, after an intervention based on the Mediterranean lifestyle: a randomised controlled clinical trial. *Br. J. Nutr.* 120 (2): 164–175. doi: 10.1017/S000711451800137X.

Keys, A., Anderson, J.T., and Grande, F. (1965). Serum cholesterol response to changes in the diet: II. The effect of cholesterol in the diet. *Metabolism* 14 (7): 759–765.

Keys, A. and Keys, M. (1959). *Eat Well and Stay Well.* New York: Doubleday & Company.

Keys, A., Menotti, A., Karvonen, M.J. et al. (1986). The diet and 15-year death rate in the Seven Countries Study. *Am. J. Epidemiol.* 124 (6): 903–915.

Martinez-Gonzalez, M.A., Bes-Rastrollo, M., Serra-Majem, L., et al. (2009). Mediterranean food pattern and the primary prevention of chronic disease: recent developments. *Nutr. Rev.* 67 (Suppl 1): S111–116. doi: 10.1111/j.1753-4887.2009.00172.x.

Martinez-Gonzalez, M.A., Gea, A., and Ruiz-Canela, M. (2019). The Mediterranean diet and cardiovascular health. *Circ. Res.* 124 (5): 779–798. doi: 10.1161/CIRCRESAHA.118.313348.

Martinez-Gonzalez, M.A., Guillen-Grima, F., De Irala, J. et al. (2012). The Mediterranean diet is associated with a reduction in premature mortality among middle-aged adults. *J. Nutr.* 142 (9): 1672–1678. doi: 10.3945/jn.112.162891.

Martinez-Gonzalez, M.A., Hershey, M.S., Zazpe, I., and Trichopoulou, A. (2017). Transferability of the Mediterranean diet to non-Mediterranean countries. What is and what is not the Mediterranean diet. *Nutrients* 9 (11): 1226.

Martinez-Gonzalez, M.A. and Martin-Calvo, N. (2016). Mediterranean diet and life expectancy; beyond olive oil, fruits, and vegetables. *Curr. Opin. Clin. Nutr. Metab. Care* 19 (6): 401–407. doi: 10.1097/MCO.0000000000000316.

Martinez-Gonzalez, M.A., Salas-Salvado, J., Estruch, R. et al. (2015). Benefits of the Mediterranean diet: insights from the PREDIMED Study. *Prog. Cardiovasc. Dis.* 58 (1): 50–60. doi: 10.1016/j.pcad.2015.04.003.

Martín-Peláez, S., Fito, M., and Castaner, O. (2020). Mediterranean diet effects on type 2 diabetes prevention, disease progression, and related mechanisms. A review. *Nutrients* 12 (8): 2236.

Menotti, A. and Puddu, P.E. (2015). How the Seven Countries Study contributed to the definition and development of the Mediterranean diet concept: a 50-year journey. *Nutr. Metab. Cardiovasc. Dis.* 25 (3): 245–252.

Mentella, M.C., Scaldaferri, F., Ricci, C., Gasbarrini, A., and Miggiano, G. (2019). Cancer and Mediterranean diet: a review. *Nutrients* 11 (9): 2059. https://doi.org/10.3390/nu11092059.

Minelli, P. and Montinari, M.R. (2019). The Mediterranean diet and cardioprotection: historical overview and current research. *J. Multidiscip. Healthc.* 12: 805–815.

Ministry of Health and Welfare Supreme Scientific Health Council. (1999). Dietary guidelines for Greek adults. *Arch. Hellen Med.* 16 (5): 516–524.

OLDWAYS. (2009). The Mediterranean diet. www.oldwayspt.org/traditional-diets/mediterranean-diet.

OLDWAYS. (2020). History of the Mediterranean Diet Pyramid. http://www.oldwayspt.org/history-mediterranean-diet-pyramid.

OLDWAYS Preservation & Exchange Trust. (2000). https://oldwayspt.org/traditional-diets/mediterranean-diet.

Papamichael, M.M., Itsiopoulos, C., Susanto, N.H. et al. (2017). Does adherence to the Mediterranean dietary pattern reduce asthma symptoms in children? A systematic review of observational studies. *Public Health Nutr.* 20 (15): 2722–2734. doi: 10.1017/S1368980017001823.

Parletta, N., Zarnowiecki, D., Cho, J., Wilson, A. et al. (2019). A Mediterranean-style dietary intervention supplemented with fish oil improves diet quality and mental health in people with depression: a randomized controlled trial (HELFIMED). *Nutr. Neurosci.* 22 (7): 474–487. doi: 10.1080/1028415X.2017.1411320.

Ryan, M.C., Itsiopoulos, C., Thodis, T. et al. (2013). The Mediterranean diet improves hepatic steatosis and insulin sensitivity in individuals with non-alcoholic fatty liver disease. *J. Hepatol.* 59 (1): 138–143. doi: 10.1016/j.jhep.2013.02.012.

Simopoulos, A.P. (2006). Evolutionary aspects of diet, the omega-6/omega-3 ratio and genetic variation: nutritional implications for chronic diseases. *Biomed. Pharmacother.* 60 (9): 502–507.

Sofi, F., Macchi, C., Abbate, R., Gensini, G.F., and Casini, A. (2014). Mediterranean diet and health status: an updated meta-analysis and a proposal for a literature-based adherence score. *Public Health Nutr.* 17 (12): 2769–2782. doi: 10.1017/S1368980013003169.

Soltani, S., Jayedi, A., Shab-Bidar, S. et al. (2019). Adherence to the Mediterranean diet in relation to all-cause mortality: a systematic review and dose-response meta-analysis of prospective cohort studies. *Adv. Nutr.* 10 (6): 1029–1039.

Trichopoulou, A., Kouris-Blazos, A., Wahlqvist, M.L., Gnardellis, C., Lagiou, P., Polychronopoulos, E., Vassilakou, T., Lipworth, L., and Trichopoulos, D. (1995). Diet and overall survival in elderly people. *BMJ* 311 (7018): 1457–1460. doi: 10.1136/bmj.311.7018.1457.

UNESCO. (2020). The Mediterranean Diet. https://www.unesco.org/archives/multimedia/?s=films_details&pg=33&vl=&id=1680&vo=2.

Zaragoza-Marti, A., Cabanero-Martinez, M.J., Hurtado-Sanchez, J.A. et al. (2018). Evaluation of Mediterranean diet adherence scores: a systematic review. *BMJ Open* 8 (2): e019033.

Zhong, Y., Zhu, Y., Li, Q. et al. (2020). Association between Mediterranean diet adherence and colorectal cancer: a dose-response meta-analysis. *Am. J. Clin. Nutr.* 111 (6): 1214–1225.

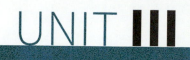

From Mediterranean Diet to Mediterranean Lifestyle

CHAPTER 8

The Mediterranean Lifestyle Paradigm

Snowflakes were beginning to fly as we left Strasbourg in the 4th of February. All the way to Switzerland we drove in a snowstorm. . . On the Italian side the air was mild, flowers were gay, birds were singing, and we basked at an outdoor table drinking our first espresso coffee at Domodos-sola. We felt warm all over. . . .

Ancel & Margaret Keys

The 2015–2020 Dietary Guidelines for Americans promotes the healthy Mediterranean-style diet (MedD) pattern as a healthy eating paradigm, since it has long been associated with positive health outcomes. Compliance with these recommendations entails the adoption of several healthy eating behaviors, which can maintain and improve health but also prevent the development of degenerative diseases.

However, what makes the MedD so special is that it was not constructed to improve health but was based on the availability of local food sources and was inextricably intertwined with other aspects of traditional life and culture: the conviviality of meals, the agricultural practices (*seasonality, biodiversity, eco-friendliness, traditional,* and *local food products*), the deeply rooted religious consciousness, the local cooking practices, the daily engagement in physical activity, the sleeping, rest, and stress management practices.

Consequently, the combination of all these unique idiosyncratic features synthesizes a complex and multifaceted entity – *the Mediterranean lifestyle (MedL)*. Therefore, MedL is defined as the lifestyle paradigm encompassing the various traditional components of the daily life of the people residing in the Mediterranean basin – a plant-based diet characterized by moderation, seasonality, participation in culinary activities and conviviality, daily engagement in physical activity as an inherent feature of everyday life, healthy sleeping practices, stress management practices, adequate rest, engagement in spiritual activities, active social life, and the rich cultural heritage (Figure 8.1).

In the following paragraphs and chapters we will discuss in detail the various components of the Mediterranean lifestyle, starting with the diet-related features that make the Mediterranean diet unique among other local diets.

> **Key Point**
>
> Mediterranean lifestyle is defined as the lifestyle paradigm encompassing the various traditional components of the daily life of the people residing in the Mediterranean basin.

Conviviality and Socialization

A very significant aspect of the MedL pattern is the conviviality of meals, i.e., the practice of eating your meals together with others, in a pleasant environment. The word *companion* comes from the Latin *a cum panis*, i.e., someone with whom we are sharing bread. Likewise, "companion" in Greek is σύντροφος, literally meaning "someone with whom we are eating together." The social aspect of eating and drinking was a prominent feature of many civilizations that existed in the Mediterranean region. For example, ancient Greeks had established specific rules during meals, including the proper way to serve wine, the order of the various food groups, the combination of wine with meals, etc. Eating was not to satisfy physical needs but was a social event: *"We do not sit at the table to eat. . . but to eat together"* (Plutarch, ancient Greek historian).

Even today, people in the Mediterranean countries spend more time eating than people anywhere else in the world. This

> **Key Point**
>
> "Companion" in Greek is σύντροφος, literally meaning "someone with whom we are eating together."

> **Key Point**
>
> *"We do not sit at the table to eat. . . but to eat together."* (Plutarch, ancient Greek historian)

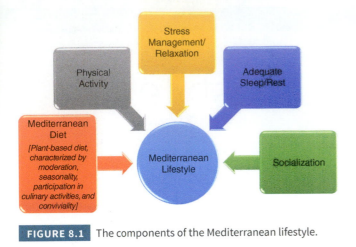

FIGURE 8.1   The components of the Mediterranean lifestyle.

difference demonstrates the social character of meals in this area of the world. Interestingly, it has been suggested that people who pay more attention to satisfaction during eating (by eating foods that they like, with friends and loved ones) tend to adopt more health-conscious eating habits compared to people who focus more on health recommendations. For example, the project EAT (Eating Among Teens)–II showed that young adults who used to share meals with others were more likely to report increased intake of fruits and vegetables, whereas the "eating on the run" attitude was positively correlated with increased consumption of low-quality foods (Table 8.1a and b).

Although nowadays mealtimes are adapted to modern lifestyle, people living in the Mediterranean region are still attached to "eating well" and "drinking well." In a Mediterranean household, a person (usually the mother or grandmother) is responsible for preparing the family's daily dinner. Eating together may not happen several times of the day or even every day, but it is considered an essential part of family eating most days of the week and especially during weekends and holidays.

Cooking Practices

In the Mediterranean region, food was, and in some areas still is, predominately cooked at home by family and friends, rather than by commercial and industrial operators. Despite the fact that the effect of culinary practices on human health has not been thoroughly studied, these practices are thought to play an important role in individuals' nutritional status and health. Cooking can be a joyful practice, affecting people's dietary choices while bringing them together. Contrary to the popular belief that cooking is just clean, chop, and put the raw ingredients into a casserole, data suggest that there is much more to these procedures. Culinary practices are a matter of organization, concept, perception, and technique, and they seem to determine individuals' food-related behavior and dietary habits. Take children as an example. It is well documented that

children are much more open to try new foods if they were involved in the cooking. Finally, cooking is not the same for all; it is influenced by the person's socioeconomic level, the interaction with other people, and the degree of self-assertiveness regarding cooking skills.

Many studies have suggested that home cooking is positively associated with higher diet quality. The frequency of home-cooked meals has been associated with increased consumption of fruits, vegetables, and whole grains. Improving cooking skills has been related to reduced fast-food consumption, higher frequency of shared meals, and cooking using low-cost basic ingredients. Homemade meals are considered less energy-dense and contain lower concentrations of total fat and SFAs, dietary cholesterol, and sodium but have higher fiber, calcium, and iron content. Unfortunately, in modern societies when both parents work and most people have the feeling of "lack of time and need to rush," the frequency of home cooking has significantly decreased. Cooking at home has turned into a luxury procedure.

Agricultural products (fruits, vegetables, field crops) grow normally during certain times of the year (seasons). Figure 8.2 shows the seasonality of certain fruits and vegetables that are grown in the Mediterranean region. Fish consumption should also follow seasonality to ensure that the fish reproduction cycle is not disrupted.

> **Key Point**
> Home cooking is positively associated with higher diet quality.

Preference to seasonal products boosts local economies and amplifies the consumption of traditional goods. Fresh and locally grown species are considerably less expensive, compared to the imported ones, as no travel and storage expenses are added to the production cost. Nonseasonal products, especially if they come from other regions of the country or the world, require long-term storage in order to distribute them in markets year-round. As a consequence of the extended transportation and storage time, the concentration of vitamins, minerals, and other bioactive compounds may decrease. Moreover, based on the fact that plant-derived products, such as fruits and vegetables, are very vulnerable to rotting once ripened, long storage presupposes that those products may be subjected to various chemical processes to preserve them for longer periods of time. Domestic produce is usually delivered in markets and sold within 24–48 hours after its harvest, maintaining its optimum freshness, flavor, and ripeness.

> **Key Point**
> Preference to seasonal products boosts local economies and amplifies the consumption of traditional goods.

Seasonality in the diet and emphasis on plant-based nutrition ensures eco-friendliness. Plant-based diets have smaller carbon footprints compared to animal-based diets, resulting in less pollution. Conforming to seasonality and locality translates to minimum transport of products, fridge storage, and fewer greenhouses, as well as less need for irradiating fresh products for preservation purposes. All these lead to the yield of products

TABLE 8.1(a) Adjusted[a] daily mean dietary intakes by report of social eating among female and male young adult participants in Project EAT (Eating Among Teens)-II.

	Females			Males		
	Usually eat dinner with others			Usually eat dinner with others		
Intake	Disagree	Agree	P value[b]	Disagree	Agree	P value[b]
Foods (servings)						
Fruit	1.51	1.68	0.004	1.54	1.70	0.01
Vegetables	1.51	1.81	<0.001	1.26	1.51	<0.001
Dark-green and orange vegetables	0.38	0.46	0.01	0.28	0.33	0.008
Whole grains	0.69	0.76	0.12	0.91	0.91	0.43
Soft drinks	1.03	1.14	0.23	1.38	1.33	0.50
Fast-food intake (times/week)	1.95	1.65	0.10	2.20	2.21	0.75
Nutrients						
Energy (kcal)	1662	1.731	0.09	1986	2119	0.03
Energy from fat (%)	30.0	28.8	0.009	31.3	31.1	0.71
Energy from saturated fat (%)	10.3	9.9	0.05	11.0	10.8	0.32
Calcium (mg)	810	858	0.05	941	1,043	0.009
Sodium (mg)	2012	2028	0.83	2296	2477	0.03
Fiber (g)	13.6	14.4	0.05	14.3	15.7	0.009

[a] The weighted model is adjusted for race/ethnicity, student status, employment status, and report of eating on the run.

[b] P values represent testing to examine differences in intakes of young adults according to agreement with the statement: "I usually eat dinner with other people."

(Continued)

TABLE 8.1(b) Adjusted[a] daily mean dietary intakes by report of eating on the run among female and male young adult participants in Project EAT (Eating Among Teens)-II.

	Females			Males		
	Tend to eat on the run			Tend to eat on the run		
Intake	Disagree	Agree	P value[b]	Disagree	Agree	P value[b]
Foods (servings)						
Fruit	1.78	1.50	0.004	1.66	1.65	0.99
Vegetables	1.98	1.52	<0.001	1.48	1.40	0.44
Dark-green and orange vegetables	0.52	0.38	<0.001	0.33	0.30	0.19
Whole grains	0.73	0.75	0.85	1.00	0.83	0.02
Soft drinks	0.97	1.23	<0.001	1.22	1.44	0.002
Fast-food intake (times/week)	1.46	1.96	<0.001	1.67	2.64	<0.001
Nutrients						
Energy (kcal)	1696	1725	0.65	2009	2140	0.03
Energy from fat (%)	28.3	29.8	<0.001	30.2	32.0	<0.001
Energy from saturated fat (%)	9.6	10.3	<0.001	10.5	11.2	<0.001
Calcium (mg)	851	839	0.80	1043	991	0.36
Sodium (mg)	2023	2023	0.83	2373	2,470	0.09
Fiber (g)	15.1	13.5	0.001	15.2	15.4	0.62

[a] The weighted model is adjusted for race/ethnicity, student status, employment status, and report of "eating dinner with others."

[b] P values represent testing to examine differences in intakes of young adults according to agreement with the statement "I tend to 'eat on the run.'"

that are consistent with the idea of eco-friendliness. Eco-friendly products, such as organic fruits and vegetables, have higher nutritional value and negligible pesticide residues. Moreover, locality in food consumption is strongly correlated with biodiversity because producers whose target is a local market prioritize palatability and diversity instead of durability and loading efficiency of their produce.

In 2015, several health and professional organizations cooperated in the development of the Med Diet 4.0 framework, highlighting the four sustainable benefits of the Mediterranean diet: (i) major health and nutrition benefits; (ii) low environmental impact and richness in biodiversity; (iii) high sociocultural food values; and (iv) positive local economic returns (Figure 8.3).

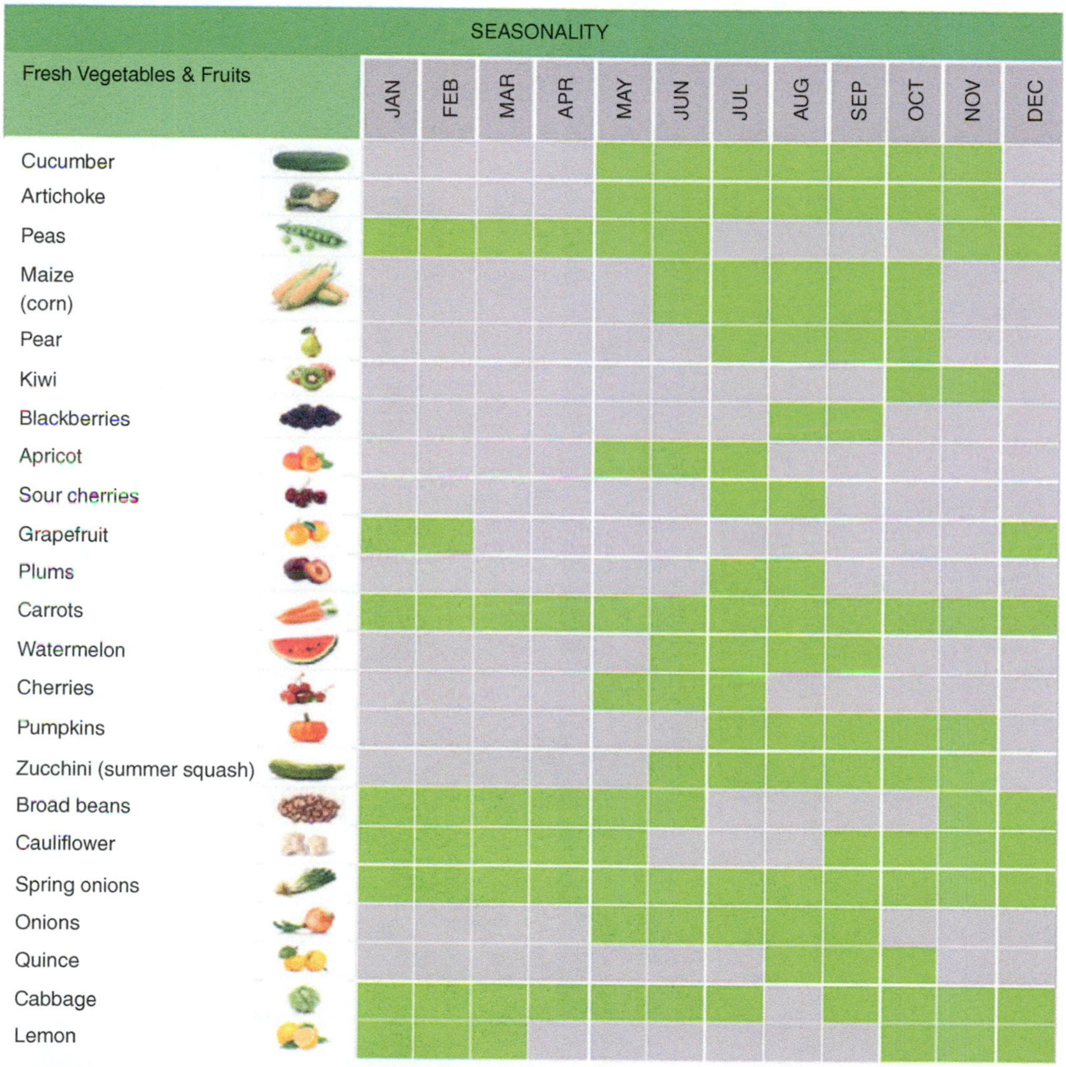

SEASONALITY												
Fresh Vegetables & Fruits	JAN	FEB	MAR	APR	MAY	JUN	JUL	AUG	SEP	OCT	NOV	DEC
Cucumber					■	■	■	■	■	■	■	
Artichoke					■	■	■	■	■			
Peas	■	■	■									■
Maize (corn)						■	■	■	■			
Pear								■	■	■		
Kiwi	■	■									■	■
Blackberries							■	■	■			
Apricot						■	■	■				
Sour cherries						■	■					
Grapefruit	■	■	■	■								■
Plums						■	■	■	■			
Carrots	■	■	■	■	■	■	■	■	■	■	■	■
Watermelon							■	■	■			
Cherries					■	■						
Pumpkins									■	■	■	
Zucchini (summer squash)					■	■	■	■	■			
Broad beans	■	■	■	■	■					■	■	■
Cauliflower	■	■	■							■	■	■
Spring onions	■	■	■	■	■				■	■	■	■
Onions	■	■	■	■	■	■	■	■	■	■	■	■
Quince									■	■	■	
Cabbage	■	■	■	■						■	■	■
Lemon	■	■	■	■							■	■

FIGURE 8.2 Seasonality of fruits and vegetables in the Mediterranean region (mainly Southern Europe). **Source:** Adapted from the Greek National Nutritional Guide for Adults (2014).

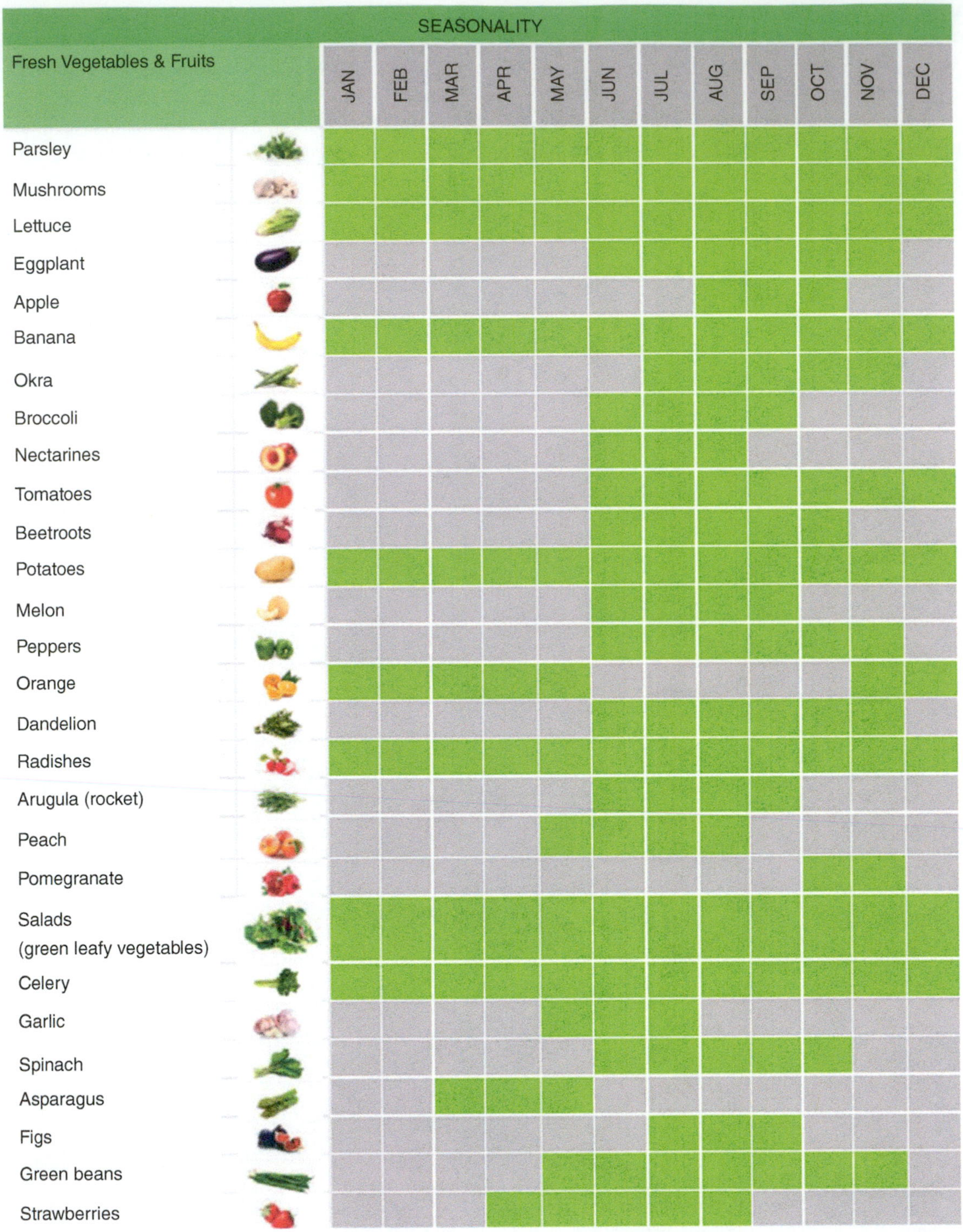

SEASONALITY

Fresh Vegetables & Fruits	JAN	FEB	MAR	APR	MAY	JUN	JUL	AUG	SEP	OCT	NOV	DEC
Parsley	●	●	●	●	●	●	●	●	●	●	●	●
Mushrooms	●	●	●	●	●	●	●	●	●	●	●	●
Lettuce	●	●	●	●	●	●	●	●	●	●	●	●
Eggplant						●	●	●	●	●	●	
Apple								●	●	●	●	●
Banana	●	●	●	●	●							
Okra								●	●	●		
Broccoli							●	●	●	●		
Nectarines							●	●	●			
Tomatoes						●	●	●	●	●	●	
Beetroots						●	●	●	●	●	●	
Potatoes	●	●	●	●			●	●	●	●	●	●
Melon						●	●	●	●			
Peppers						●	●	●	●	●	●	
Orange	●	●	●	●							●	●
Dandelion						●	●	●	●	●		
Radishes	●	●	●	●	●			●	●	●	●	●
Arugula (rocket)						●	●	●	●			
Peach					●	●	●	●	●			
Pomegranate										●	●	
Salads (green leafy vegetables)	●	●	●	●	●	●	●	●	●	●	●	●
Celery	●	●	●	●						●	●	●
Garlic	●	●	●	●	●							
Spinach	●	●	●	●					●	●	●	●
Asparagus			●	●	●							
Figs							●	●	●	●		
Green beans					●	●	●	●	●	●		
Strawberries			●	●	●	●	●	●				

FIGURE 8.2 *(continued)*

Med Diet 4.0

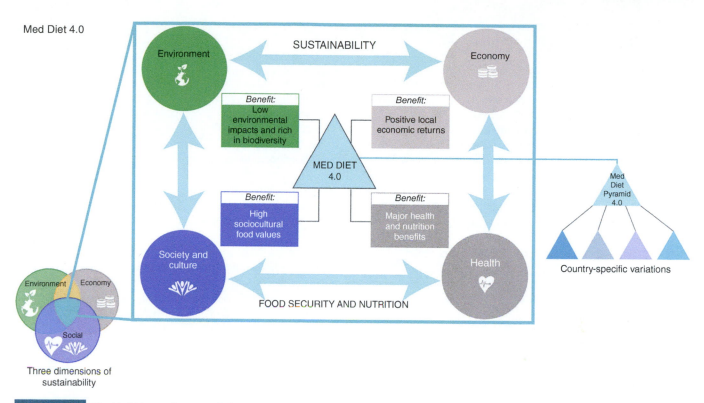

FIGURE 8.3 The Med Diet 4.0 framework that applies the principles of sustainability to the four dimensions of the Mediterranean diet.
Source: Reprinted from Dernini et al. (2017).

Take-Home Messages

- The MedD has been inextricably intertwined with other aspects of life – the daily engagement in physical activity, the conviviality of meals, deeply rooted religious consciousness, local cooking practices, the pattern of siesta, and the rich cultural heritage transmitted from one generation to another. The combination of all these idiosyncratic features synthesizes a complex and multifaceted concept – the Mediterranean lifestyle (MedL).
- MedL is the lifestyle paradigm encompassing the various components of the daily life of the people living in the Mediterranean basin.

- A significant aspect of the MedL is the conviviality of meals – the way people eat together.
- Food should be consumed with moderation and frugality, both key elements of the MedL.
- Culinary practices are a matter of organization, concept, perception, and technique and may determine individuals' food-related behavior and diet quality.
- The time that families dedicate to food preparation is now reduced, while pre-prepared foods or ready-made meals are widely available.

Self-Assessment Questions

1. Provide the definition of the Mediterranean lifestyle.
2. Fill in the blanks:
   a. The practice of eating your meals together with others in a pleasant environment is called _____, which is a very significant aspect of the MedL pattern.
   b. Homemade meals are considered _____ energy-dense.
   c. As a consequence of the extended transportation and storage time of nonseasonal products, the concentration of vitamins, minerals, and other bioactive compounds may _____.

   d. What makes the MedD so special is the fact that it was not constructed to improve health but was based on the _____ and was inextricably intertwined with _____.
3. List the four sustainable benefits of the MedD according to the Med Diet 4.0 framework.
4. How is cooking related to dietary habits and quality?
5. What are the benefits of consuming foods according to seasonality and locality?

Bibliography

Berge, J.M., MacLehose, R.F., Larson, N. et al. (2016). Family food preparation and its effects on adolescent dietary quality and eating patterns. *J. Adolesc. Health* 59 (5): 530–536.

Dernini, S. and Berry, E.M. (2015). Mediterranean diet: from a healthy diet to a sustainable dietary pattern. *Front. Nutr.* 2: 15.

Dernini, S., Berry, E.M., Serra-Majem, L. et al. (2017). Med Diet 4.0: the Mediterranean diet with four sustainable benefits. *Public Health Nutr.* 20 (7): 1322–1330.

Diolintzi, A., Panagiotakos, D.B., and Sidossis, L.S. (2019). From Mediterranean diet to Mediterranean lifestyle: a narrative review. *Public Health Nutr.* 22 (14): 2703–2713.

Engler-Stringer, R. (2010). Food, cooking skills, and health: a literature review. *Can. J. Diet. Pract. Res.* 71 (3): 141–145.

Gerber, M. and Hoffman, R. (2015). The Mediterranean diet: health, science and society. *Br. J. Nutr.* 113 (Suppl 2): S4–S10.

Greek National Nutritional Guide for Adults. (1999). *Archives of Hellenic Medicine* 16 (5): 516–524.

Hachem, F., Capone, R., Yannakoulia, M., Dernini, S., Hwalla, N., Kalaitzidis, C. (2016). The Mediterranean diet: a sustainable consumption pattern. Mediterra 2016. Zero Waste in the Mediterranean. Natural Resources, Food and Knowledge/International Centre for Advanced Mediterranean Agronomic Studies (CIHEAM) and Food and Agriculture Organization of the United Nations (FAO)–Paris: Presses de Sciences Po, 243.

Hershey, M.S., Sotos-Prieto, M., Ruiz-Canela, M. et al. (2021). The Mediterranean lifestyle (MEDLIFE) index and metabolic syndrome in a non-Mediterranean working population. *Clin. Nutr.* 40 (5): 2494–2503. doi: 10.1016/j.clnu.2021.03.026

Kavouras, S.A., Johnson, E.C., Bougatsas, D. et al. (2016). Validation of a urine color scale for assessment of urine osmolality in healthy children. *Eur. J. Nutr.* 55 (3): 907–915.

Larson, N.I., Nelson, M.C., Neumark-Sztainer, D. et al. (2009). Making time for meals: meal structure and associations with dietary intake in young adults. *J. Am. Diet. Assoc.* 109 (1): 72–79.

Maraki, M.I. and Sidossis, L.S. (2015). Physiology in medicine: update on lifestyle determinants of postprandial triacylglycerolemia with emphasis on the Mediterranean lifestyle. *Am. J. Physiol. Endocrinol. Metab.* 309 (5): E440–E449.

McGowan, L., Caraher, M., Raats, M. et al. (2017). Domestic cooking and food skills: a review. *Crit. Rev. Food Sci. Nutr.* 57 (11): 2412–2431.

Radd-Vagenas, S., Kouris-Blazos, A., Singh, M.F., and Flood, V.M. (2017). Evolution of Mediterranean diets and cuisine: concepts and definitions. *Asia Pac. J. Clin. Nutr.* 26 (5): 749–763.

Tiwari, A., Aggarwal, A., Tang, W., and Drewnowski, A. (2017). Cooking at home: a strategy to comply with U.S. dietary guidelines at no extra cost. *Am. J. Prev. Med.* 52 (5): 616–624.

Tosti, V., Bertozzi, B., and Fontana, L. (2018). Health benefits of the Mediterranean diet: metabolic and molecular mechanisms. *J. Gerontol. A Biol. Sci. Med. Sci.* 73 (3): 318–326.

U.S. Department of Health and Human Services and U.S. Department of Agriculture. (2015). *Dietary Guidelines for Americans, 2015*, 8e. Washington, DC: USDA.

Wolfson, J.A., Ramsing, R., Richardson, C.R., and Palmer, A. (2019). Barriers to healthy food access: associations with household income and cooking behavior. *Prev. Med. Rep.* 13: 298–305.

Wolfson, J.A., Leung, C.W., and Richardson, C.R. (2020). More frequent cooking at home is associated with higher healthy eating Index-2015 score. *Public Health Nutr.* 23 (13): 2384–2394.

CHAPTER 9

Physical Activity in the Mediterranean Region

All parts of the body, if used in moderation and exercised in labors to which each is accustomed, become thereby healthy and well developed and age slowly; but if they are unused and left idle, they become liable to disease, defective in growth, and age quickly.

Hippocrates (ancient Greek physician, often referred to as the "Father of Medicine")

Historical Perspective

Physical activity (PA) has been an integral part of human lifestyle since the beginning of time. The combined work of archeologists and medical anthropologists has established that our ancestors adopted a unique pattern of PA as part of their daily lives that was likely the norm for most of human existence and served many purposes besides survival. Investigations of preindustrial societies confirm that physical capacity was not just a necessity for success at gathering food and providing shelter and safety but was also considered as a component of religious, social, and cultural expression. Starting from the Paleolithic era, when humans grouped together in small societies and survived by gathering plants, fishing, hunting, or scavenging wild animals, hunters and gatherers performed a natural cycle of regularly intermittent PA; this typically involved one- or two-day periods of intense exertion for food foraging, followed by one- or two-day periods of rest and celebration, also including light PA.

The consequent Neolithic Agricultural Revolution allowed more people to live in larger group settings. The specialization of occupations reduced the intensity of work-related PA but still demanded a different PA pattern characterized by lower-intensity repetitive movements associated with cultivation and food production. Moving to historical times, PA remained a significant part of life in ancient human societies, including structured military training in the context of war preparation and training for participating in athletic competitions, such as the ancient Olympic Games.

Throughout much of recorded history, philosophers, scientists, physicians, and educators have promoted the idea that being physically active contributes to better health, improves physical functioning, and promotes longevity. Although some of these claims were based on personal opinions or clinical judgment, others were the result of systematic observation. However, scientific research in the field of PA is less than 100 years old, with the first investigations of the physiological effects of exercise beginning in the early twentieth century in Europe and the United States. More than 70 years of well-designed and executed epidemiologic and clinical studies have clearly documented a broad range of important health benefits associated with regular PA; over the last two decades, these observations have served as the basis for the development of evidence-based public health recommendations. At last, at the onset of the twenty-first century, PA has taken its rightful place in the mainstream of public health. PA is now considered an integral part of chronic disease prevention and health promotion efforts. Nevertheless, despite the accumulation of knowledge on the impact of PA on well-being, much remains to be done to ensure that attention and resource allocation within public health systems match the importance of PA and that the current global epidemic of sedentariness is properly addressed.

> **Key Point**
>
> Physical activity is now considered an integral part of chronic disease prevention and health promotion efforts.

Physical Activity: Definition, Terms, and Assessment

Physical activity is defined as any bodily movement produced by skeletal muscles that requires energy expenditure. PA can be classified into four domains: (i) occupational, i.e., work-related; (ii) domestic, i.e., housework; (iii) transportation, i.e., moving on foot from one place to another; and (iv) leisure time, i.e., occurs voluntarily and is not associated with obligatory activities of everyday life.

> **Key Point**
>
> Physical activity is defined as any bodily movement produced by skeletal muscles that requires energy expenditure.

PA can be further classified as either incidental or structured. Incidental PA is not planned and usually is the result of daily activities at work, at home, or during transportation. On the other hand, structured PA, also called exercise or exercise training, is a component of leisure-time PA and could be defined as planned, repetitive, and purposeful activity, in the sense that it is performed to improve or maintain one or more components of physical fitness (PF) (Table 9.1). It must be noted here that PA and PF, although highly related to each other, are two very different concepts. PF is defined as a set of attributes that people have or achieve, and being physically fit has been defined as "the ability to carry out daily tasks with vigor and alertness, without undue fatigue and with ample energy to enjoy leisure-time pursuits and to meet unforeseen emergencies." It comprises cardiorespiratory endurance, muscle endurance and muscle strength, flexibility, balance, agility, and coordination. Therefore, PF represents the ability of an individual to perform PA efficiently, while an important distinction between them is their pattern of change for each individual PA will undoubtedly vary on a daily or seasonal basis, whereas PF will remain relatively static, taking time and effort to change. In epidemiology, PA is usually what is subjectively reported regarding activity, while fitness is objectively measured.

The energy required for PA (EPA) represents one of the three fundamental parts of the total energy expenditure (TEE),

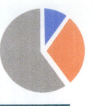

- Thermic Effect of Food (10%)
- Physical Activity Expenditure (15-30%)
- Resting Energy Expenditure (60-75%)

FIGURE 9.1 Components of total energy expenditure in most individuals.

i.e., the total amount of energy that a person expends on a daily basis to carry out all physiological functions; the other two are the resting energy expenditure (REE), i.e., the energy needed to maintain vital life functions (such as breathing and heart beating) during resting conditions, and the thermic effect of food (TEF), i.e., the obligatory energy expenditure that is associated with digestion and absorption of ingested foods (Figure 9.1). Therefore, EPA + REE + TEF = TEE. The REE and TEF are relatively stable, together determining 70–85% of TEE; on the other hand, EPA is a highly variable component, typically accounting for 15–30% of TEE. However, in extremely active individuals, EPA may constitute up to 60–70% of TEE. Therefore, the term PA basically incorporates any body movement that requires more energy than the resting state.

PA is commonly quantified by determining its energy expenditure, which is directly linked to its intensity, frequency, and duration, and can be expressed either in kilocalories (kcal) or in metabolic equivalents of task (MET). One kcal is equivalent to the energy needed to raise the temperature of 1 kg of water by 1°C (from 14.5° to 15.5° C). The human body requires oxygen to produce energy (even though small amounts of energy can be produced without oxygen – anaerobically). Approximately 5 kcal of energy are produced for each liter of oxygen consumed. Therefore, if a 70 kg individual walks for 30 minutes at an intensity requiring a rate of oxygen consumption of 1 l/min, the person would consume 30 l of oxygen. In this case, TEE (including REE) for those 30 minutes would be ~150 kcal (i.e., 30 l × 5 kcal/l). Accordingly, the total daily EPA would be the sum of all of the different physical activities performed on a given day.

> **Key Point**
>
> One kcal is equivalent to the energy needed to raise the temperature of 1 kg of water by 1°C (from 14.5° to 15.5° C).

MET is the objective measure of the ratio of the rate at which a person expends energy, relative to the energy expended when sitting quietly (set by convention at 3.5 ml of oxygen per kilogram per minute - i.e., 1 MET = 3.5 ml of oxygen per kilogram per minute). An activity with a MET value of 4 means you're exerting 4 times the energy that you would if you were sitting still. For example, a brisk walk at ~4 miles per hour has a value of 4 MET. Jumping rope, which is a

> **Key Point**
>
> Metabolic equivalents of task (MET) is the objective measure of the ratio of the rate at which a person expends energy, relative to the energy expended when sitting quietly (set by convention at 3.5 ml of oxygen per kilogram per minute).

TABLE 9.1   Physical activity domains.

Domain	Contextual definition or examples
Occupational	Work-related: involving manual labor tasks, walking, carrying or lifting objects
Domestic	Housework, yard work, child care, chores, self-care, shopping, incidental
Transportation	Purpose of going somewhere: walking, bicycling, climbing and descending stairs
Leisure time	Discretionary or recreational activities: sports, hobbies, exercise, volunteer work

Source: Adapted from Strath et al. (2013) and Warren et al. (2010).

TABLE 9.2   **Classification of physical activity intensity.**

Intensity	VO$_2$max (%) or HRR (%) *	Maximal HR (%)	RPE	Intensity	METs
	Relative intensity			Absolute intensity	
Very light	<25	<30	<9	Sedentary	1–1.5
Light	25–44	30–49	9–10	Light	1.6–2.9
Moderate	45–59	50–69	11–12	Moderate	3.0–5.9
Hard	60–84	70–89	13–16	Vigorous	≥6
Very hard	≥95	≥90	>16		
Maximal	100	100	20		

HR(R), heart rate (reserve); METs, metabolic equivalents of tasks; RPE, rating of perceived exertion; VO$_2$max, maximal aerobic capacity.
* HRR = [(maximal HR − resting HR) + resting HR].
Source: Adapted from Strath et al. (2013).

more vigorous activity, has a MET value of 12. In healthy adults, activities in the range of 1.0–1.5 MET are considered of very light intensity; 1.6–2.9 MET are considered as of low intensity; 3.0–5.9 MET as of moderate intensity, and ≥6.0 MET as of vigorous intensity (Table 9.2).

A collection of PA and its associated MET values has been published for adults and children, and it is frequently used to ascribe intensities in the analysis of self-report measures of PA. For example, the total daily volume associated with transportation for an individual who walked to and from work, each lasting 30 minutes and performed at an intensity of 3 METs, would be calculated as follows: 3 METs (intensity) × 30 minutes (duration) × 2 times per day (frequency) = 180 METmin per day. However, it should be mentioned that the published MET values should be used with caution in children, given that they have a higher oxygen consumption relative to body mass at rest. It may not be suitable for other groups either, such as obese people, in whom oxygen consumption expressed in relation to body weight is lower than in normal-weight individuals, and elderly people, in whom the basal metabolic rate is usually lower.

Another common measure of PA in epidemiological studies is the amount of time an individual spends in a specified PA intensity threshold range. For example, some PA assessment tools determine whether an individual is meeting specific PA guidelines, (e.g., 150 min per week of moderate-intensity PA or 75 min per week of vigorous-intensity PA). However, in order for the term *exercise intensity* to be meaningful, it must be further defined; PA intensity can be defined in both absolute and relative terms. Absolute intensity is determined by the work performed (e.g., running at an intensity of 6 miles per hour or cycling at an intensity of 50 W on a stationary bike). On the other hand, relative intensity is determined in relation to an individual's level of cardiorespiratory fitness, expressed as either maximal oxygen uptake (VO$_2$max – the maximum amount of oxygen the body is capable of using in 1 minute), or maximal heart rate (HRmax).

Standard definitions for both relative and absolute intensity are shown in Table 9.2. For example, walking is often described as a moderate-intensity PA; however, the actual intensity for an individual may vary. In absolute terms, walking at a speed of ~3 miles/h is equivalent to 3 METs, which meets the criteria for moderate-intensity PA. However, a difference can be noted when one compares individuals of different fitness levels (person A with a VO$_2$max of 17.5 mLO$_2$/kg/min [5 METs] vs. person B with a VO$_2$max of 42 mLO$_2$/kg/min [12 METs]) walking together at a speed of 3 mph. From an absolute standpoint, both person A and person B are performing at the same level of PA intensity (3 METs); however, from a relative standpoint, person A is performing at a high-intensity level (walking at 60% of VO$_2$max), whereas person B is performing at a low-intensity level (walking at 25% of VO$_2$max).

The precise estimation of PA is key to studies investigating PA trends and its association with health and disease. Several tools have been developed for PA evaluation, including both subjective and objective methods. Subjective methodologies rely on the individual's recollection of activities previously or usually performed, or a person's willingness to record activities as they occur in PA diaries and logs. Objective methodologies include wearable monitors that directly measure one or more biosignals indicative of an individual's PA level, such as acceleration (accelerometers), steps (pedometers), or heart rate (heart rate monitors), as well as techniques for the estimation of physical activity expenditure (PAE) (double-labeled water and indirect calorimetry) as PA occurs. Table 9.3 summarizes the basic characteristics, strengths, and weaknesses of the available methods for the assessment of PA. Feasibility and practicality, the availability of resources and administration considerations, and the desired outcome of the assessment guide the choice of the appropriate PA assessment tool, given that there is no single best instrument appropriate for every situation.

Key Point

Physical activity intensity can be defined in both absolute and relative terms.

TABLE 9.3   Overview of methods used to assess physical activity.

Characteristics	Strengths	Limitations
Doubly labeled water		
Known quantities of stable ^{18}O and ^{2}H isotopes are ingested as water. The difference in elimination rate between these isotopes represents the rate of CO_2 production, which is then used to calculate energy expenditure.	Gold standard measure for measuring TEE in free-living individuals, minimal burden to patients or participants, suitable for all populations.	Expensive; technical equipment and trained personnel required; measures of REE and thermic effect of food required to derive PAE; unable to discern dimensions or domains.
Indirect calorimetry		
The amounts of O_2 consumed and CO_2 produced are measured at an open-circuit system in which a person breathes either room air or a mixture of gases of known concentration.	Highly accurate and reliable measure of physical activity and energy expenditure; suitable for all populations.	Expensive; high degree of technical expertise required; short time assessment only permissible.
Direct observation		
A trained observer watches an individual to monitor and record physical activity mode, duration, and intensity. It is more commonly used with children than with adults.	No respondent burden; provides detailed quantitative and qualitative information on dimensions and domains; suitable for all populations.	High burden on the observer; training is essential to successfully administer this technique; can alter individual behavior of the one being assessed due to the observer presence.
Questionnaire		
Identification of physical activity dimensions and domains from either self-reported responses or interviews. Questionnaires vary from a few item tools that give a global overview of activity to a long, detailed quantitative history of activity over the past year or even a lifetime.	Low cost, low burden; applicable to large numbers of individuals; valid to assess exercise; can successfully rank into high/low categories, and can assess different dimensions and domains.	Recall and social desirability bias can occur; needs to be population and culture specific; low validity for assessing incidental or lifestyle physical activity.
Diary/log		
Detailed hour-by-hour or activity-by-activity record of one's physical activity and sedentary behaviors. Usually completed by the user.	Low-cost, detailed information on dimension and domains; not subjected to memory or recall; provides a good subjective measure of PAE and TEE.	Very high burden on patients and participants; complex and time-consuming data reduction and analysis; similar to questionnaires, they should be population and culture specific.
Heart rate monitoring		
A device (small wrist-worn receiver) accepts signals wirelessly from electrodes secured to a chest strap. Alterations in heart rate are indicative of cardiorespiratory stress during physical activity.	Low burden for short periods; relatively inexpensive; correlates strongly with moderate-to-vigorous-intensity exercise; suitable for all populations.	Affected by nonactivity stimuli (emotion, medication, caffeine); weak relationship at the low end of intensity realm; subject to interference with signal.
Accelerometer		
A device attached to the body (either at the hip, ankle, wrist, or lower back) that provides a measure of accelerations of the body during movement. Acceleration can be measured in 1–3 planes (vertical, mediolateral, and anterior–posterior).	Concurrent measure of movement; provides detailed intensity, frequency, and duration data; can store data for weeks at a time; low burden, relatively inexpensive, suitable for all populations.	Cannot account for all activities, such as cycling, stair use, or activities that require lifting a load; upper-body activities neglected with hip or lower-back wear; data processing takes time.

(continued)

TABLE 9.3   *(continued)*

Characteristics	Strengths	Limitations
Pedometer		
Simple and inexpensive typically belt- or waistband-worn motion sensor that records movement during regular gait cycles and is used to assess walking behavior. Early models used a mechanical gear, whereas newer versions are electronic.	Low cost, low burden, easy data processing, applicable to large numbers of individuals, can also be used to motivate people to increase physical activity, suitable for all populations.	Simple pedometers cannot measure intensity/duration, cannot measure mode/type; not accurate for energy expenditure; degree of accuracy differs between devices; false steps can be recorded; some brands require user to write steps down.
Multisensing unit		
A device designed to assess multiple parameters, usually combining accelerometry and heart rate monitoring. The pros of each method are combined, thereby negating some of their individual limitations.	Improved accuracy compared with single sensing assessments; suitable for all populations.	Higher cost; increased burden of wear for some devices, depending on device technical expertise; complex data analysis.

CO_2, carbon dioxide; ^{18}O, oxygen-18; O_2, oxygen; PAE, physical activity expenditure; REE, resting energy expenditure; TEE, total energy expenditure; ^{2}H, deuterium.
Source: Adapted and modified from Strath et al. (2013) and Warren et al. (2010).

Global Health Implications and Trends of Physical Activity

The fundamental role of PA in well-being was recognized as early as the fifth century BCE by the Greek physician and "Father of Medicine" Hippocrates. With the decline of the Hellenic civilization, this concept faded, and for centuries PA and PF were considered relevant primarily for military purposes. After the 1950s, exercise science gradually started to blossom. Seven decades of intense investigation of the effects of PA on health and disease has produced significant evidence that an active lifestyle has several important health benefits. In contrast, a sedentary lifestyle is associated with an increased risk of NCDs and decreased longevity, as highlighted in all current public health guidelines regarding health promotion.

> **Key Point**
>
> The fundamental role of PA in well-being was recognized as early as the fifth century BCE by the Greek physician and "Father of Medicine" Hippocrates.

In the 1950s, Jeremy Morris et al. showed that the incidence of coronary heart disease in physically active bus conductors (i.e., those who climbed up and down stairs of double-deck buses collecting tickets) and postal carriers (i.e., those who delivered the mail on foot) was significantly lower compared to the relatively inactive bus drivers or postal office workers who worked in the office. The same findings were apparent when the effect of leisure-time PA was explored. Over a period of nine years, men who engaged in vigorous PA (i.e., those who participated in vigorous sports or did considerable amounts of cycling or rated the pace of their regular walking as fast) had 50% less incidence of nonfatal and fatal coronary heart disease episodes, compared to their colleagues who reported no engagement in vigorous exercise.

The Harvard College alumni studies by Paffenbarger et al. (1993) confirmed the strong beneficial effect of PA on all-cause mortality and cardiovascular health. Walking, stair climbing, and playing sports related inversely to total mortality, primarily to death due to cardiovascular or respiratory causes; death rates decline steadily as PAE increases from <500 to >3500 kcal per week. The study also highlighted that the long-term maintenance of a physically active lifestyle is essential for good health. Ex-varsity athletes who became sedentary alumni had high total and cardiovascular disease–related risk compared to those who were regularly physically active or those who were sedentary as students and then became physically active adults.

> **Key Point**
>
> Death rates decline steadily as PAE increases from <500 to >3500 kcal per week.

There are thousands of published reports in peer-reviewed journals documenting the benefits of being physically active. The available evidence suggests a dose–response relationship between PA and beneficial health outcomes, in a way that being active – even to a modest level – is preferable to being inactive; the greatest health benefits are commonly acquired from previously sedentary individuals assuming a more active lifestyle. Specifically, based on data from systematic reviews and meta-analyses of numerous epidemiological and interventional studies conducted over the last decades, adequate levels of PA among adults have been associated with reduced total mortality and disease-specific mortality (mostly malignancy- and cardiovascular-related); a beneficial cardiometabolic profile (i.e., improved blood lipid profile, blood pressure levels, glucose homeostasis, and inflammatory markers); and lower risk for metabolic syndrome, cardiovascular disease (coronary heart disease, heart failure, and cerebrovascular disease), insulin resistance, T2DM, and gestational diabetes mellitus, cancer (esophageal, gastric, colorectal, pancreatic, renal, lung, bladder, endometrial, ovarian, prostate, breast, and thyroid), and liver disease.

Adequate levels of PA are also considered as a key determinant of energy expenditure, and thus are fundamental to energy balance and body weight regulation. The same applies to older adults and the elderly, in whom adequate PA has been associated with the following:

- Reduced total and disease-specific mortality
- Improved physical functioning and performance capabilities (coordination, flexibility, strength, speed, and endurance)
- Psychological health and quality of life (autonomy and vitality)
- Reduced disability and fall-related injuries
- Improved cognitive function in terms of both reduced age-related cognitive decline and reduced risk for neurological disorders, such as Alzheimer's disease.

Although available scientific data for children and adolescents are more limited, the beneficial effects of PA on their physical, psychological, and mental health are also evident, in terms of body weight regulation, cardiometabolic health, bone density and strength, as well as achievement and cognitive outcomes, self-esteem, self-concept, and depression.

Evolution and Current Trends in Physical Activity Recommendations

Although the evidence that a physically active way of life has many pronounced health benefits has been very convincing since the 1970s, the specific dose of PA necessary for good health and well-being in the various age groups remains to be determined. Continued debate as to how much, what type, how often, what intensity, and how long the PA should be has led to the development of numerous public health and clinical recommendations. Some of the inconsistency among PA recommendations is due to the inherent uncertainties of biomedical science, augmented by methodological differences in collecting and interpreting the data, whereas some is due to a focus on different health outcomes by different groups.

The earliest unofficial recommendations for PA to achieve fitness were based on systematic comparisons of effects from different profiles of exercise training in the 1950s and 1960s. Karvonen and colleagues are credited with having carried out the first controlled exercise training experiment by evaluating the effects of two different exercise intensities on adaptations in exercise capacity. They reported that a training intensity corresponding to 70% of HRmax resulted in greater improvement in physical work capacity than did a training intensity at 60% HRmax, thus providing the first recommendation on PA intensity to gain functional benefits. Many other researchers conducted similar small-scale investigations over the next few years, determining the dose of exercise that is required to improve physical work capacity. A common finding among these studies was that higher-intensity exercise produced greater gains in fitness than lower-intensity exercise of the same duration.

Based on available scientific data, the American College of Sports Medicine (ACSM) has been publishing guidelines for PA since 1975. An overview of the ACSM recommendations for the frequency, intensity, and duration of exercise is shown in Table 9.4. In total, the exercise recommendations of the ACSM were quite specific and strict and led to somewhat regimented thinking about how much exercise should be recommended, possibly leading to the conclusion that a PA level not meeting these specific criteria (i.e., high-intensity PA) would be of limited or no value.

While controlled exercise studies have been critical to defining the cardiovascular responses to PA prescriptions, they lack long-term data and do not provide any guidance on the amount and intensity of beneficial lifestyle activity, which is typically explored in the context of long-term epidemiological studies. Interestingly, the 1990 ACSM position represented the beginning of a shift of guidelines away from an exclusively "performance-related fitness" paradigm to one that includes PA recommendations for both performance and health-related outcomes as evident for the first time in 2000: "ACSM recognizes the potential health benefits of regular exercise performed more frequently and for longer duration, but at lower intensities than prescribed in this position statement."

TABLE 9.4   Evolution of physical activity recommendations by the American College of Sports Medicine.

Year	Physical activity recommendation			Objective
	Frequency (days/week)	Duration (min/day)	Intensity (% of maximal HR)	
1975[a]	3–5	20–45	70–90	Cardiorespiratory fitness
1978[b]	3–5	15–60	50–80	Cardiorespiratory fitness
1980[c]	3–5	15–60	50–80	Cardiorespiratory fitness
1986[d]	3–5	15–60	50–80	Cardiorespiratory fitness
1990[e]	3–5	20–60	50–80	Cardiorespiratory fitness
1991[f]	3–5	15–60	40–80	Cardiorespiratory fitness
1995[g]	3–5	20–60	40–90	Cardiorespiratory fitness
1998	5 (aerobic exercise) 3 (aerobic exercise) 2–3 (muscle strengthening)	30 20	40 80	Health promotion
2000[h]	7 2–3 (muscle strengthening)	≥20	40–80	Health promotion
2011	5 (aerobic exercise) 3 (aerobic exercise) >2 (muscle strengthening)	30 20	40 80	Health promotion

ACSM, American College of Sports Medicine; HR, heart rate.
[a] American College of Sports Medicine (1975). [b] American College of Sports Medicine (1978). [c] American College of Sports Medicine (1980). [d] American College of Sports Medicine (1986). [e] American College of Sports Medicine (1990). [f] American College of Sports Medicine (1991). [g] American College of Sports Medicine (1995). [h] American College of Sports Medicine (2000). **Source:** Adapted from Blair et al. (2004).

This change in the perception of PA recommendations that further evolved in following years was in line with the findings of interventional studies, suggesting that even moderate-intensity PA produces significant improvements in work capacity, and that exercising at higher intensities or volumes has only modest additional effects. These findings are very important; now it is clear that even people who cannot perform high-intensity or prolonged exercise can benefit from doing any kind of PA.

As a result, the focus of public health PA guidelines gradually shifted to a lower-intensity, longer-duration lifestyle PA model, with the goal of protecting against NCDs. Accumulated evidence regarding the cardioprotective effects of regular exercise identified physical inactivity as the fourth major modifiable coronary heart disease risk factor, joining smoking, hypertension, and dyslipidemia. An important feature of

this report was the recognition of the health value of moderate amounts and intensities of exercise. Evidence cited in the report supported the conclusion that there is an inverse and graded dose–response association between exercise and the risk of coronary heart disease, and that high levels of exercise training were not required for a person to gain the health-related benefits of exercise.

The next major development in public health recommendations for PA was the 1995 report by the CDC and ACSM, emphasizing the need for accumulation of ≥30 min of moderate-intensity PA each day. Similar recommendations by others, such as the WHO in 1995, the US Surgeon General in 1996, and the National Institutes of Health (NIH) in 1996, soon followed. The rationale behind the concept of ≥30 min of daily moderate-intensity PA was based on both practical and health-related issues. From the practical point of view, even small amounts of moderate-intensity PA are considered fundamental for sedentary individuals, given that they are unlikely to have the physical capacity to engage in greater quantities of high-intensity PA. From the health-related point of view, even

Key Point

There is an inverse and graded dose–response association between exercise and the risk of coronary heart disease.

Key Point

Moderately fit women and men have approximately half the mortality rate of their unfit peers.

Key Point

Individuals already meeting the basic recommendation could gain additional health benefits by doing more exercise.

Key Point

Health screening, appropriate to the health and PA status of the individual, is mandatory before the initiation of any exercise program

relatively small increases in PA or PF levels in sedentary individuals might produce large reductions in disease risk. Indeed, according to data published around that time, moderately fit women and men have approximately half the mortality rate of their unfit peers, while this moderate level of PF could actually be attained by meeting the consensus recommendation for 30 minutes of moderate-intensity PA on ≥5 days/week. In other words, the 1995 CDC/ACSM report recommended a dose of PA that would likely be achievable by the primary target population (i.e., sedentary individuals at risk for NCDs) and that was supported by a large evidence base as being efficacious for disease risk reduction among a significant proportion of the general population. The report also highlighted the dose–response character of the relationship between PA and health and suggested that individuals already meeting the basic recommendation could gain additional health benefits by doing more exercise.

In 2018, the ACSM and the US CDC published new guidelines regarding the optimal dose of PA for the various age groups (Table 9.5). It is important to emphasize that before starting an exercise program, all adults, especially those with health concerns, should have a health screening by a qualified professional (Figure 9.2).

Physical Activity in the Mediterranean Lifestyle: History and Characteristics

As previously described, the Mediterranean lifestyle is a holistic way of living, incorporating social, cultural, religious, and other aspects of life, all pointing synergistically toward a mode of living that promotes wellness. Among the various components of lifestyle, regular PA is an essential part of the Mediterranean lifestyle and a key element to its well-established health benefits.

The Mediterranean diet has been a subject of intense interest since antiquity, with numerous investigations dating back to the 1940s and 1950s demonstrating its superiority over dietary habits of other populations. In contrast, traditional PA patterns of the populations of the Mediterranean region have not been systematically recorded and evaluated. Such an evaluation was difficult even 20 years ago due to the absence of standardized instruments for the assessment of PA. Nevertheless, it is believed that the Mediterranean lifestyle historically included regular PA, mostly through daily tasks rather than structured exercise.

Walter Willet, professor of epidemiology and nutrition at Harvard T.H. Chan School of Public Health, described the PA patterns of the Mediterranean populations from observations made during his visits in the region: "In the 1960s and 1970s during my visits there, much of the work was done by hand, including the harvesting and threshing of grain. Travel was often by foot or donkey." As Willet has suggested, part of the health benefits of the Mediterranean diet documented in numerous investigations over the last decades may have

TABLE 9.5   Recommendations for physical activity per age group.

	Duration/intensity	Intensity	Muscle strength activities
Preschool aged children (3–5 years)	Physical activity in the form of play every day, throughout the day	Active play through a variety of enjoyable physical activities	Not recommended
Children and adolescents (6–17 years)	60 minutes or more of moderate-to-vigorous intensity enjoyable physical activities	As part of the 60 minutes, on at least 3 days a week, vigorous activity such as running or soccer	Activities that strengthen muscles such as climbing or push-ups; activities that strengthens bones such as gymnastics or jumping rope
Adults (18–64 years)	At least 150 minutes per week	Moderate-intensity activity such as brisk walking	At least 2 days per week of activities that strengthen muscles
Older adults (65 years and older)	At least 150 minutes per week	Moderate-intensity activity such as brisk walking	At least 2 days per week of activities that strengthen muscles and activities to improve balance such as standing on one foot

Source: Adapted from American College of Sports Medicine (2018). *ACSM's Guidelines for Exercise Testing and Prescription*. Philadelphia, PA: Lippincott Williams & Wilkins.

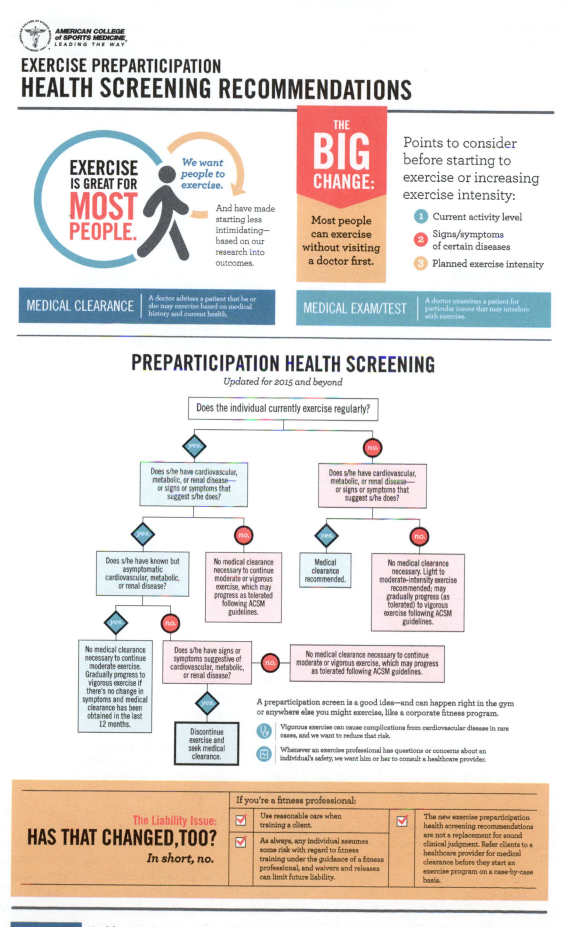

TABLE 9.6	The Keys' dietary advice for prevention of coronary heart disease (1959) compared with the US dietary guidelines (1980).
Keys' advice	Do not get fat; if you are fat, reduce.
	Restrict saturated fats; the fats in beef, pork, lamb, sausages, margarine, and solid shortenings; and the fats in dairy products.
	Prefer vegetable oils to solid fats, but keep total fats under 30% of your diet calories.
	Favor fresh vegetables, fruits, and nonfat milk products.
	Avoid heavy use of salt and refined sugar.
	Good diets do not depend on drugs and fancy preparations.
	Get plenty of exercise and outdoor recreation.
	Be sensible about cigarettes, alcohol, excitement, and business strain.
	See your doctor regularly and do not worry.
US dietary guidelines	Eat a variety of foods.
	Maintain ideal weight.
	Avoid too much fat, saturated fat, and cholesterol.
	Eat foods with adequate starch and fiber.
	Avoid too much sugar.
	Avoid too much sodium.
	If you drink alcohol, do so in moderation.

Source: Adapted and modified from Nestle (1995).

weight, and attain the numerous health benefits of PA. What distinguishes the Mediterranean lifestyle PA recommendations from other formal guidelines is the promotion of the social character of PA, achieved through practicing leisure activities outdoors, preferably with company, thus making them more enjoyable and strengthening the sense of community. This is in accordance with the overall concept of conviviality and socialization of the Mediterranean lifestyle, which promotes the social and cultural value of lifestyle habits, characteristics that are considered crucial for the long-term maintenance of healthy behaviors and, consequently, the promotion of well-being.

> **Key Point**
> What distinguishes the Mediterranean lifestyle PA recommendations is the promotion of the social character of PA.

The concept of *lifestyle PA* gradually emerged as a result of the evolution of PA guidelines during the 1990s, in order to highlight the role of simple activities embedded into daily life. A widely accepted definition of the term was provided in 1998 by Dunn et al.: "Lifestyle PA is the daily accumulation of ≥ 30 min of self-selected activities, including all leisure, occupational, or household activities that are at least of moderate to vigorous intensity and that are part of everyday life." A critical point in this definition is that these are activities that the individual selects instead of being prescribed, and they can be either planned by a person or unplanned by manipulation of the environment (e.g., signs by the elevators suggesting that individuals should climb stairs instead of using the elevator).

> **Key Point**
> Lifestyle PA is the daily accumulation of ≥ 30 min of self-selected activities.

As shown in Figure 9.5, lifestyle activities are accumulated in several short bouts during the day rather than performed in one long bout of continuous activity. In practice, lifestyle PA usually involves active transportation (such as walking), gardening, mopping the floors, etc. In contrast to traditional exercise, lifestyle PA does not require the use of specific accommodations or equipment. This type of activity may appeal to individuals who would not consider undertaking traditional exercise and serves as an important element of public health efforts to make more people active.

The determinants of PA are numerous, and the overall PA level of an individual is the result of the complex interaction between opportunities/facilitators and difficulties/barriers associated with both intrapersonal and environmental factors. A multilevel model, depicted in Figure 9.6, was developed by Sallis et al. to capture the complexity of influences on active living around all four domains of PA, i.e., the occupational, the domestic, the transportation, and the leisure-time domain, with multiple levels of influences specific to each domain. Interestingly, several of these positive and negative influences (highlighted in black frames) can be enhanced or moderated, respectively, by the PA pattern proposed by the Mediterranean

been not an effect of diet alone but also due to other aspects of the Mediterranean lifestyle, including PA. Interestingly, in the cookbook published in 1959, Ancel Keys and his wife, Margaret, did not focus only on the diet aspect of Mediterranean healthy living. Based on their observations in the region, they provided a more holistic approach to a healthy lifestyle, including the suggestion for "plenty of exercise and outdoor recreation" (Table 9.6). Therefore, it is not surprising that the concept of PA, as an integral part of the Mediterranean lifestyle, was always part of the Mediterranean diet pyramid (Figure 9.3).

The latest version of the Mediterranean diet pyramid, described in detail in Chapter 7, also recommended PA as a practice for a healthy way of living (Figure 9.4). Specifically, regular practice of moderate PA, i.e., ≥30 min throughout the day, is recommended as a fundamental complement to healthy dietary habits (in accordance with the Mediterranean diet) as a means to balance energy intake, maintain a healthy body

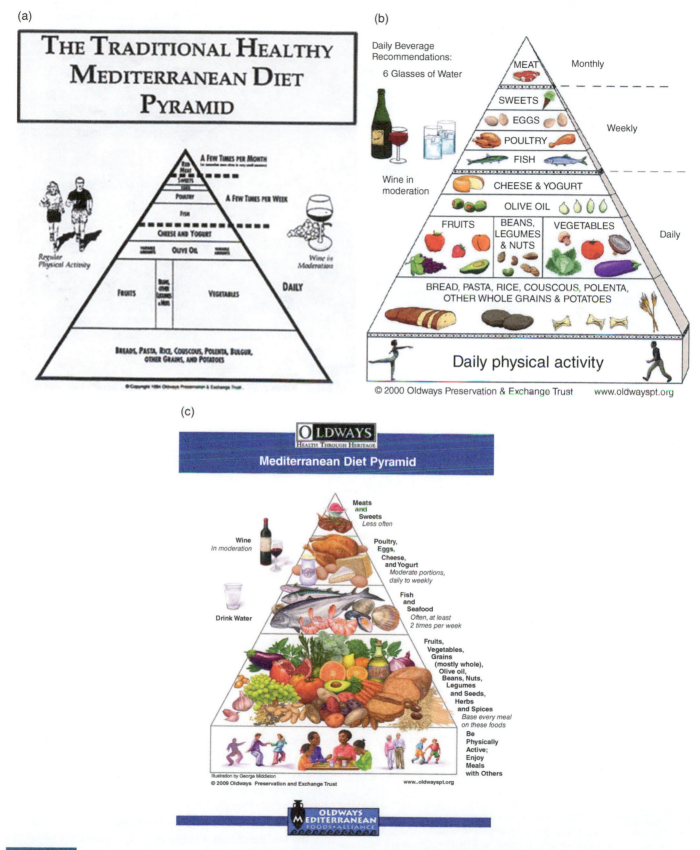

FIGURE 9.3 The evolution of the Mediterranean diet pyramid. In 1993, OLDWAYS, the Harvard School of Public Health, and the European Office of the World Health Organization introduced the classic Mediterranean diet pyramid (a). Many updates were published since 1993, including those in 2000 (b) and 2009 (c). The recommendation for physical activity was always part of the Mediterranean diet pyramid, as an integral part of the Mediterranean lifestyle.

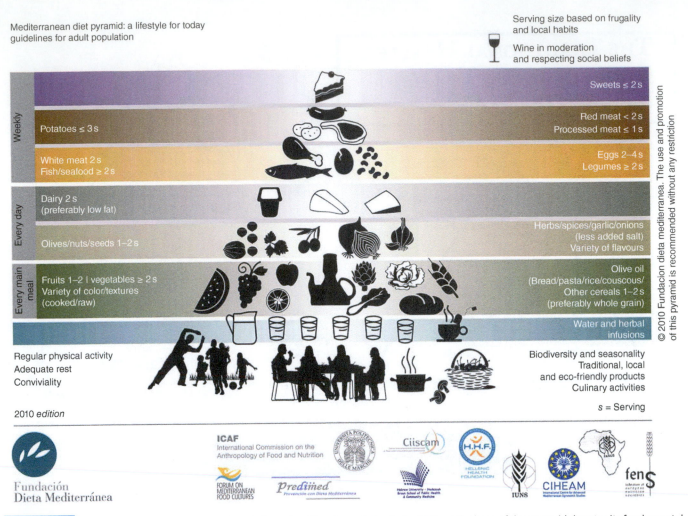

FIGURE 9.4   Mediterranean diet pyramid: a lifestyle for today. The place of physical activity at the base of the pyramid denotes its fundamental role in the Mediterranean lifestyle. **Source:** Reprinted from Bach-Faig et al. (2011).

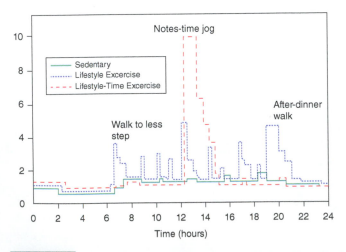

FIGURE 9.5   Conceptual figure of daily energy expenditure for a sedentary person (solid line), a person engaging in planned vigorous exercise during leisure time (dashed line), and lifestyle physical activity accumulated in moderate-intensity bouts over the course of the day (dotted line). **Source:** Reprinted from Dunn et al. (1998). Copyright © 1998 American Journal of Preventive Medicine. Published by Elsevier Inc.

lifestyle. Specifically, among the determinants of PA, convenience, comfort, attractiveness, and accessibility are considered important. This notion is supported by data suggesting that barriers for PA include limited time to exercise, limited access to sports or recreation facilities, and displeasure against vigorous exercise and the imposed conformity or adherence to gymnasium-based exercise. On the other hand, enjoyment of the activity performed, perceived competence, and social environment characteristics, such as the parallel participation of and the support from friends and family, have been identified as significant positive correlates of PA. It is obvious that the Mediterranean lifestyle actively promotes a physically active way of life over prescribed and structured exercise programs, through proposing a simple and sustainable lifestyle PA pattern that is not forced but rather enjoyable in the context of everyday social life.

> **Key Point**
>
> The Mediterranean lifestyle actively promotes a physically active way of life over prescribed and structured exercise programs.

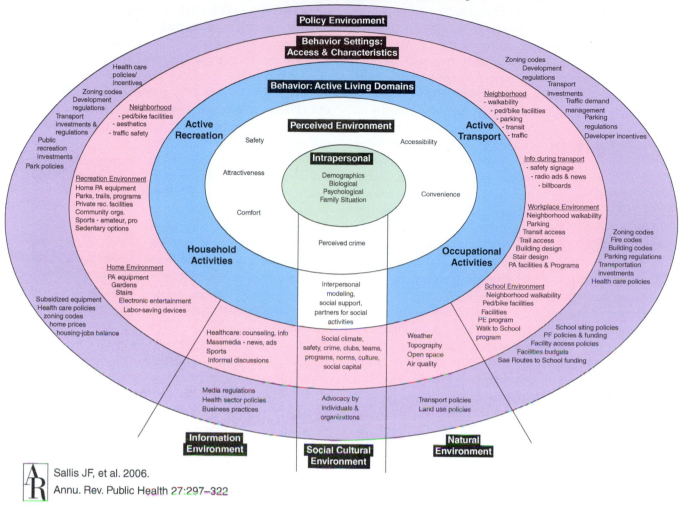

Ecological Model of Four Domains of Active Living

Sallis JF, et al. 2006.
Annu. Rev. Public Health 27:297–322

FIGURE 9.6 Ecological model of four domains of active living. Broad categories of intrapersonal variables are shown at the center to represent the individual, while individuals' perceptions of environments are distinguished from more objective aspects of environments; both are likely to be important influences. Behavior represents the interaction of the person and the environment, with the domains of active living shown at this boundary. The four active living domains of recreation, transport, occupation, and household are consistent with contemporary concepts and are useful for identifying the variety of environments and policies that may influence active living. Black frames indicate influences of physical activity that could be positively modified in the context of the Mediterranean lifestyle toward a physically active way of living.
Source: Reprinted from Sallis et al. (2015). Copyright © 2006 ANNUAL REVIEWS, INC.

Physical Activity in the Mediterranean Lifestyle: Clinical Significance

Despite the lack of data on the effects of PA as a component of the Mediterranean lifestyle, i.e., everyday simple activities performed indoors and outdoors, valuable information can be drawn from indirect data regarding the effects of nonstructured vs. structured PA programs on human health. For example, it has been shown that the prevalence of the metabolic syndrome decreases as steps/day increase in adults. Moreover, Hamer et al. (2008) demonstrated a robust protective effect of active

commuting (walking and cycling) on cardiovascular mortality, incidence of coronary heart disease, stroke, hypertension, and T2DM. Samitz et al. in 2011 analyzed the combined results from 80 scientific studies with 1,338,143 adult participants; they found that people with the highest levels of PA had 20–40% lower relative risk for all-cause mortality compared to people with low levels of PA. The aforementioned studies indicate that lifestyle PA is associated with substantial health benefits; however, given their epidemiological design, the possibility of residual confounding factors warrants the implementation of well-designed prospective clinical studies to determine the effect of lifestyle PA on human health.

In the context of lifestyle PA and its effect on health, it is important to consider the notion of nonexercise activity thermogenesis (NEAT). NEAT is defined as the energy expended for walking to work, standing, performing yard work, undertaking agricultural tasks, fidgeting, and other daily PA; i.e., everything that is not sleeping, eating, or sports-like exercise. Factors that impact a person's NEAT include environmental factors, such as occupation or dwelling, and biological factors, such as body weight, body composition, and gender. The combined impact of these factors explains the substantial variance in human NEAT that can reach 2000 kcal per day, depending mostly on occupation and leisure-time PA. This large variability in NEAT might be viewed as random; however, human and animal data contradict this notion. There is now evidence to at least suggest that hypothalamic factors may regulate NEAT; in this case, spontaneous PA may not be spontaneous at all but carefully programmed into our genes. It has been hypothesized that changes in NEAT subtly accompany experimentally induced changes in energy balance and are important in the physiology of weight regulation, as shown in Figure 9.7. Indeed, the strong negative correlation between increases in NEAT and fat gain supports this contention, as do the consistent findings from studies demonstrating that PA and NEAT decrease during periods of negative energy balance, such as during weight loss. Under this scope, accumulated data support the central hypothesis that NEAT is pivotal in the regulation of human energy expenditure and body weight regulation and that NEAT is important for designing effective treatments for overweight and obesity.

In line with the development of the lifestyle concept of PA, lifestyle PA interventions have slowly started to be included in public health policy over the past two decades. They focus mainly on promoting a physically active lifestyle, taking into account the cultural and environmental characteristics of each population. This approach provides opportunities and options for tailoring PA to the individual's preferences, regardless of their current lifestyle, and is of great importance for those who are considered sedentary or not adequately active. It is well established that even small increases in everyday PA result in substantial health benefits. Indeed, lifestyle PA interventions have been shown to be effective at increasing and maintaining levels of PA that meet or even exceed public health guidelines for PA.

As previously mentioned, more recent well-designed interventional studies have questioned the early, strict exercise recommendations. Subjects assigned to either lifestyle PA or structured exercise exhibited similar increase in PF and participation in PA, similar decrease in blood pressure and blood lipids, and lost similar amounts of body weight and fat compared to baseline. These clinical trials support the effectiveness of an unstructured lifestyle approach for increasing PA and improving

> **Key Point**
>
> Spontaneous physical activity may not be spontaneous at all but carefully programmed into our genes.

> **Key Point**
>
> Clinical trials support the effectiveness of an unstructured lifestyle approach for increasing PA.

health indices; this is indirect evidence for the beneficial effect of the Mediterranean lifestyle PA pattern on health.

A few studies have attempted to determine the minimum exercise volume to confer health benefits. For example, Ebisu in 1985 was the first to show that splitting the same total amount of exercise into three shorter sessions results in similar improvements in PF and significantly greater improvements in blood HDL cholesterol levels, as compared with one or two session(s). Since then, many others have studied the effectiveness of splitting exercise into several shorter sessions throughout the day in various populations. For example, Jakicic et al. assigned obese women to either one long 30- to 40-minute bout of continuous exercise or intermittent exercise, i.e., 3–4 short 10-minute bouts of moderate PA. They found greater improvements in exercise adherence, a slightly greater weight loss, and similar improvements in PF indices (VO$_2$max and resting heart rate) and blood pressure levels in the intermittent exercise group, compared to the continuous exercise group. Subsequent studies have confirmed the beneficial effects of intermittent exercise on exercise adherence, cardiorespiratory fitness, body composition, and cardiometabolic indices. In total, available data suggest that PA performed in small bouts, similar to spontaneous everyday life activities as part of the Mediterranean lifestyle, may be superior to structured exercise programs, possibly due to better long-term adherence to PA.

Another issue that needs to be addressed in the context of evaluating the clinical significance of the Mediterranean PA pattern is the recommendation for outdoor activities. Available studies are characterized by significant heterogeneity with regard to outcome measures employed and have followed relatively poor methodology. Nevertheless, most studies have demonstrated that exercising outdoors improves self-reported mental well-being and is associated with better feelings of revitalization and positive engagement. Furthermore, outdoors PA decreases tension, confusion, anger, and depression and increases energy, compared to exercising indoors. Finally, although differences in adherence rates between indoor and outdoor PA have not been systematically assessed, the latter has been found to result in greater enjoyment and satisfaction, as well as a greater intent to repeat the activity at a later date. These factors can predict a better adherence to a PA pattern characterized by outdoor activities.

The exact reasons why outdoor PA results in improved mental well-being are not fully understood; however, exposure to natural environment might be associated with an increased level of vitality, defined as a positive state of physical and mental

> **Key Point**
>
> Studies have confirmed the beneficial effects of intermittent exercise on exercise adherence, cardiorespiratory fitness, body composition, and cardiometabolic indices.

> **Key Point**
>
> Exposure to natural environment might be associated with an increased level of vitality.

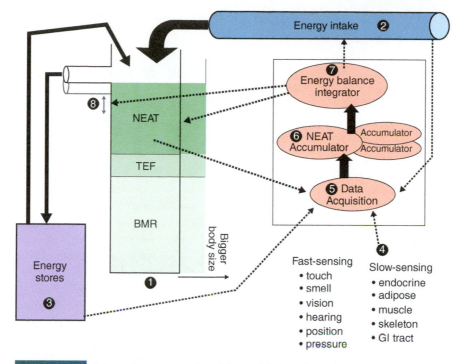

FIGURE 9.7 *Schematic representation of the modulation of NEAT in the context of human energy balance. Continuous arrows represent energy flow through the system; broken lines represent putative signaling pathways (neuronal or blood-borne). The components of energy expenditure are shown in (1). The balance among energy intake (2), energy stores (3), and energy expenditure is in constant flux, and data from each component are sensed. This is self-evident; otherwise, we would never stop eating, or know that after a day of hanging plasterboard, we are exhausted. It seems likely that NEAT signals are derived from known pathways (4), and it is likely that there are numerous NEAT-sensing pathways, since NEAT has many environmental cues and includes many behaviors. The signals can be divided into fast-response elements, such as the startle response, and slow-response elements, such as thyroid hormone. These signals converge at a data acquisition center (5) that is likely to lie within a primal part of the brain, such as the hypothalamus, because all animals regulate energy balance. Once the data on the various NEAT signals are rectified into a common signal, the data acquisition center signals the NEAT accumulator (6), which is an invented concept to allow the ready explanation of energy balances. The NEAT accumulator is constantly summing the net amount of NEAT per unit time. NEAT: non-exercise activity thermogenesis, TEF: thermic effect of food, BMR: basal metabolic rate, GI: gastrointestinal.* **Source:** Reprinted from Levine (2004). Copyright © 2004 by American Physiological Society.

energy, characterized by a sense of enthusiasm, aliveness, and vigor. In his poem, John Muir (1901) highlights the stimulating effects of immersing oneself in nature, stating that natural elements bestow a sense of wellness and energy: "Climb the mountains and get their good tidings. Nature's peace will flow into you as sunshine flows into trees. The winds will blow their own freshness into you, and the storms their energy."

It is noteworthy that a number of studies have explored the question of whether exposure to outdoors or natural environments influences the sense of vitality. These studies suggest that engagement in outdoor experiences and activities is essential to avoiding exhaustion and devitalization, contributes to feeling more alive and engaged with the world, and promotes the experience of aliveness and energy. The aforementioned positive influences have been demonstrated

above and beyond the effects of PA or social interactions that can take place in natural settings, suggesting that there may be potential additive benefits of undertaking PA in nature.

Despite the scarce scientific data on the effects of the Mediterranean PA pattern on health, evidence from lifestyle PA interventions shed light into its clinical significance and its potential applications in public health strategies for promoting PA, health, and well-being. Most importantly, the combination of such a sustainable and health-promoting PA pattern with all other lifestyle characteristics of the Mediterranean lifestyle can undoubtedly serve as a unique tool for healthcare providers in the context of promoting individuals' health in everyday clinical practice. It can also help health policy makers in designing and implementing efficient strategies for the management of the global sedentariness and NCD epidemic.

Take-Home Messages

- TEE is the arithmetic sum of REE, i.e., the energy required for a 24-hour period by the body during resting conditions EPA, i.e., the energy required for any body movement, and TEF, i.e., the obligatory energy expenditure that is associated with digestion and absorption of ingested foods.
- PA can be classified as either incidental (the result of daily activities at work, at home, or during transport) or structured (also called exercise or exercise training – usually planned, structured, repetitive, and purposeful).
- PA expenditure is directly linked to its intensity, frequency, and duration and can be expressed either in kcal expended or in MET.
- A collection of PA and its associated MET values for adults and children has been published, and it is being used to ascribe intensities in the analysis of self-reported measures of PA.
- A commonly used measure of PA is simply the amount of time an individual spends in a specified PA intensity. PA intensity can be defined in both absolute and relative terms; absolute intensity is determined by the work performed (e.g., running at an intensity of 6 miles per hour or cycling at an intensity of 50 W on a stationary bike), whereas relative intensity is relative to an individual's level of cardiorespiratory fitness,

expressed as percent of maximal oxygen uptake (VO_2max) or percent of maximum heart rate (HRmax) (e.g., running at an intensity corresponding to 70% VO_2max or cycling at an intensity corresponding to 85% of HRmax).
- Available evidence suggests that there is a dose–response relationship between PA and beneficial health outcomes; however, being even minimally active is preferable to being completely inactive.
- Public health PA guidelines have gradually shifted to a lower-intensity, longer-duration lifestyle PA model, with the goal of protecting against NCDs.
- According to the 2011 Mediterranean diet pyramid, regular practice of moderate lifestyle PA, i.e., ≥30 min throughout the day, is suggested as a fundamental complement to healthy dietary habits in order to balance energy intake, maintain a healthy body weight, and experience the numerous health benefits of PA.
- The combination of the Mediterranean PA pattern with all the other lifestyle characteristics of the Mediterranean lifestyle – i.e., the Mediterranean diet, healthy sleeping patterns, conviviality, and stress relief – can undoubtedly serve as a unique tool for health-care providers in the context of promoting individuals' health in everyday clinical practice.

Self-Assessment Questions

1. How is the total energy expenditure (TEE) of a person calculated?
2. Which of the following is a structured physical activity?
   a. daily activities at work
   b. activities at home
   c. activities during transportation
   d. jogging for 1 hour
3. Fill in the blanks:
   a. An activity with a MET value of 4 means that you're exerting _____ that you would if you were sitting still.
   b. Intensity, frequency, and _____ are directly linked with physical activity expenditure.
   c. Simple pedometers cannot measure _____.
   d. Relative intensity describes the intensity of exercise relative to an individual's _____.
4. Give the definition of nonexercise activity thermogenesis.
5. Briefly discuss the available methods for the assessment of physical activity.
6. What is the physical activity recommendation for older adults (65 years and older)?
7. How can outdoor physical activity improve mental well-being?
8. Choose the correct statement:
   a. There is a dose–response relationship between physical activity and beneficial health outcomes.
   b. The overall physical activity level of an individual is not affected by environmental factors.
   c. Indirect calorimetry does not require technical expertise.
   d. When maximal heart rate is 50–69%, the exercise is vigorous.
9. Discuss the physical activity recommendations according to the 2011 Mediterranean diet pyramid.
10. How can the MedL paradigm promote physical activity?
11. How have PA recommendations evolved over time?
12. Briefly discuss the health benefits of PA across lifespan.

Bibliography

American College of Sports Medicine. (1975). *Guidelines for Graded Exercise Testing and Exercise Prescription*. Philadelphia: Lea & Febiger.

American College of Sports Medicine. (1978). American College of Sports Medicine position statement on the recommended quantity and quality of exercise for developing and maintaining fitness in healthy adults. *Med. Sci. Sports* 10 (3): vii–x.

American College of Sports Medicine. (1980). *Guidelines for Graded Exercise Testing and Exercise Prescription*. Philadelphia: Lea & Febiger.

American College of Sports Medicine. (1986). *Guidelines for Exercise Testing and Prescription*. Philadelphia: Lea & Febiger.

American College of Sports Medicine. (1990). Position stand: the recommended quantity and quality of exercise for developing and maintaining cardiorespiratory and muscular fitness in healthy adults. *Med. Sci. Sports Exerc.* 22 (2): 265–274.

American College of Sports Medicine. (1991). *Guidelines for Exercise Testing and Prescription*. Philadelphia: Lea & Febiger.

American College of Sports Medicine. (1995). *ACSM's Guidelines for Exercise Testing and Prescription*. Media, PA: Williams & Wilkins.

American College of Sports Medicine. (2000). *ACSM's Guidelines for Exercise Testing and Prescription*. Philadelphia, PA: Lippincott Williams & Wilkins.

American College of Sports Medicine. (2018). *ACSM's Guidelines for Exercise Testing and Prescription*. Philadelphia, PA: Lippincott Williams & Wilkins.

Aune, D., Norat, T., Leitzmann, M. et al. (2015). Physical activity and the risk of type 2 diabetes: a systematic review and dose-response meta-analysis. *Eur. J. Epidemiol.* 30 (7): 529–542.

Bach-Faig, A., Berry, E.M., Lairon, D., et al. (2011). Mediterranean diet pyramid today. Science and cultural updates. *Public Health Nutr.* 14 (12A): 2274–2284.

Bathrellou, E., Lazarou, C., Panagiotakos, D.B., and Sidossis, L.S. (2007). Physical activity patterns and sedentary behaviors of children from urban and rural areas of Cyprus. *Cent. Eur. J. Public Health* 15 (2): 66–70.

Bauman, A., Finegood, D.T., and Matsudo, V. (2009). International perspectives on the physical inactivity crisis – structural solutions over evidence generation? *Prev. Med.* 49 (4): 309–312. doi: 10.1016/j.ypmed.2009.07.017

Bauman, A.E., Nelson, D.E., Pratt, M. et al. (2006). Dissemination of physical activity evidence, programs, policies, and surveillance in the international public health arena. *Am. J. Prev. Med.* 31 (4 Suppl): S57–65. doi: 10.1016/j.amepre.2006.06.026

Bauman, A.E., Reis, R.S., Sallis, J.F. et al. (2012). Correlates of physical activity: why are some people physically active and others not? *Lancet* 380 (9838): 258–271.

Bellou, E., Magkos, F., Kouka, T. et al. (2013). Effect of high-intensity interval exercise on basal triglyceride metabolism in non-obese men. *Appl. Physiol. Nutr. Metab.* 38 (8): 823–829.

Bellou, E., Siopi, A., Galani, M. et al. (2013). Acute effects of exercise and calorie restriction on triglyceride metabolism in women. *Med. Sci. Sports Exerc.* 45 (3): 455–461.

Blair, S.N., LaMonte, M.J., and Nichaman, M.Z. (2004). The evolution of physical activity recommendations: how much is enough? *Am. J. Clin. Nutr.* 79 (5): 913S–920S.

Borjesson, M., Onerup, A., Lundqvist, S., and Dahlof, B. (2016). Physical activity and exercise lower blood pressure in individuals with hypertension: narrative review of 27 RCTs. *Br. J. Sports Med.* 50 (6): 356–361.

Caspersen, C.J., Powell, K.E., and Christenson, G.M. (1985). Physical activity, exercise, and physical fitness: definitions and distinctions for health-related research. *Public Health Rep.* 100 (2): 126–131.

CDC. 2020. Physical activity recommendations for different age groups. https://www.cdc.gov/physicalactivity/basics/age-chart.html.

Cliff, D.P., Jones, R.A., Burrows, T.L. et al. (2014). Volumes and bouts of sedentary behavior and physical activity: associations with cardiometabolic health in obese children. *Obesity (Silver Spring)* 22 (5): E112–118. doi: 10.1002/oby.20698

Cliff, D.P., Okely, A.D., Burrows, T.L. et al. (2013). Objectively measured sedentary behavior, physical activity, and plasma lipids in overweight and obese children. *Obesity (Silver Spring)* 21 (2): 382–385. doi: 10.1002/oby.20005

de Rezende, L.F., Rodrigues Lopes, M., Rey-Lopez, J.P. et al. (2014). Sedentary behavior and health outcomes: an overview of systematic reviews. *PLoS One* 9 (8); e105620. doi: 10.1371/journal.pone.0105620.

Dunn, A.L., Andersen, R.E., and Jakicic, J.M. (1998). Lifestyle physical activity interventions: history, short-and long-term effects, and recommendations. *Am. J. Prev. Med.* 15 (4): 398–412.

Ebisu, T. (1985). Splitting the difference of endurance running: on cardiovascular endurance and blood lipids. *Jap. J. Phys. Educ.* 30: 37–43.

Echouffo-Tcheugui, J.B., Butler, J., Yancy, C.W., and Fonarow, G.C. (2015). Association of physical activity or fitness with incident heart failure: a systematic review and meta-analysis. *Circ. Heart Fail.* 8 (5): 853–861.

Garland, T. Jr., Schutz, H., Chappell, M.A. et al. (2011). The biological control of voluntary exercise, spontaneous physical activity and daily energy expenditure in relation to obesity: human and rodent perspectives. *J. Exp. Biol.* 214 (Pt 2): 206–229.

Gill, J.M. (2007). Physical activity, cardiorespiratory fitness and insulin resistance: a short update. *Curr. Opin. Lipidol.* 18 (1): 47–52.

Hall, K.D., Heymsfield, S.B., Kemnitz, J.W. et al. (2012). Energy balance and its components: implications for body weight regulation. *Am. J. Clin. Nutr.* 95 (4): 989–994.

Hamer, M. and Chida, Y. (2008). Active commuting and cardiovascular risk: a meta-analytic review. *Prev. Med.* 46 (1): 9–13.

Harrell, J.S., McMurray, R.G., Baggett, C.D. et al. (2005). Energy costs of physical activities in children and adolescents. *Med. Sci. Sports Exerc.* 37 (2): 329–336.

He, D., Xi, B., Xue, J. et al. (2014). Association between leisure time physical activity and metabolic syndrome: a meta-analysis of prospective cohort studies. *Endocrine* 46 (2): 231–240.

Hills, A.P., Street, S.J., and Byrne, N.M. (2015). Physical activity and health: "what is old is new again." *Adv. Food Nutr. Res.* 75: 77–95.

Jakicic, J.M., Wing, R.R., Butler, B.A., and Robertson, R.J. (1995). Prescribing exercise in multiple short bouts versus one continuous bout: effects on adherence, cardiorespiratory fitness, and weight loss in overweight women. *Int. J. Obesity Related Metabolic Disorders* 19 (12): 893–901.

Karvonen, M.J., Kentala, E., and Mustala, O. (1957). The effects of training on heart rate; a longitudinal study. *Ann. Med. Exp. Biol. Fenn.* 35 (3): 307–315.

Kavouras, S.A., Sarras, S.E., Tsekouras, Y.E., and Sidossis, L.S. (2008). Assessment of energy expenditure in children using the RT3 accelerometer. *J. Sports Sci.* 26 (9): 959–966.

Keys, A. and Keys, M. (1959). *Eat Well and Stay Well*. New York: Doubleday & Company.

Kokkinos, P., Faselis, C., Franklin, B. et al. (2019). Cardiorespiratory fitness, body mass index and heart failure incidence. *Eur. J. Heart Fail.* 21 (4): 436–444.

Kokkinos, P.F., Giannelou, A., Manolis, A., and Pittaras, A. (2009). Physical activity in the prevention and management of high blood pressure. *Hell. J. Cardiol.* 50 (1): 52–59.

Kokkinos, P. and Myers, J. (2010). Exercise and physical activity: clinical outcomes and applications. *Circulation* 122 (16): 1637–1648.

Konidari, S., Sidossis, L.S., and Geladas, N. (2008). Relation between levels of physical activity and body fat in 9 to 12 years old Greek boys. *Gazz. Med. Ital.* 167 (6): 283–291.

Lee, I.M., Shiroma, E.J., Lobelo, F. et al. (2012). Effect of physical inactivity on major non-communicable diseases worldwide: an analysis of burden of disease and life expectancy. *Lancet* 380 (9838): 219–229.

Levine, J.A. (2004). Nonexercise activity thermogesis (NEAT): environment and biology. *Am. J. Physiol-Endoc. M.* 286 (5): E675–E685. http://activeworking.com/pdfs/research/64.pdf.

Magkos, F. and Sidossis, L.S. (2008). Exercise and insulin sensitivity – where do we stand? You'd better run! *Eur. Endocrinol.* 4 (1): 22–25.

Magkos, F., Tsekouras, Y., Kavouras, S.A. et al. (2008). Improved insulin sensitivity after a single bout of exercise is curvilinearly related to exercise energy expenditure. *Clin. Sci. (Lond.)* 114 (1): 59–64.

Magkos, F., Tsekouras, Y.E., Prentzas, K.I. et al. (2008). Acute exercise-induced changes in basal VLDL-triglyceride kinetics leading to hypotriglyceridemia manifest more readily after resistance than endurance exercise. *J. Appl. Physiol.* 105 (4): 1228–1236.

Magkos, F., Yannakoulia, M., Kavouras, S.A., and Sidossis, L.S. (2007). The type and intensity of exercise have independent and additive effects on bone mineral density. *Int. J. Sports Med.* 28 (9): 773–779.

Maraki, M., Christodoulou, N., Aggelopoulou, N. et al. (2009). Exercise of low energy expenditure along with mild energy intake restriction acutely reduces fasting and postprandial triacylglycerolaemia in young women. *Br. J. Nutr.* 101 (3): 408–416.

Micheli, L., Mountjoy, M., Engebretsen, L. et al. (2011). Fitness and health of children through sport: the context for action. *Br. J. Sports Med.* 45 (11): 931–936. doi: 10.1136/bjsports-2011-090237

Morris, J.N. (2005). Exercise versus heart attack: history of a hypothesis. In: *Coronary Heart Disease Epidemiology: From Etiology to Public Health,* 2e, 275–90. Oxford: Oxford University Press.

Mountjoy, M., Andersen, L.B., Armstrong, N. et al. (2011). International Olympic Committee consensus statement on the health and fitness of young people through physical activity and sport. *Br. J. Sports Med.* 45 (11): 839–848. doi: 10.1136/bjsports-2011-090228

Muir, J. (1901). *Our National Parks*, 56. Boston, MA: Houghton Mifflin.

Nassis, G.P., Papantakou, K., Skenderi, K. et al. (2005). Aerobic exercise training improves insulin sensitivity without changes in body weight, body fat, adiponectin, and inflammatory markers in overweight and obese girls. *Metabolism* 54 (11): 1472–1479.

Nestle, M. (1995). Mediterranean diets: historical and research overview. *Am. J. Clin. Nutr.* 61 (6 Suppl): 1313S–1320S.

OLDWAYS Preservation and Exchange Trust. (1997; 2000; 2009). The traditional healthy Mediterranean Diet pyramid; first version presented in 1993. http://www.oldwayspt.org/traditional-diets/mediterranean-diet.

Ozemek, C., Lavie, C.J., and Rognmo, O. (2019). Global physical activity levels – need for intervention. *Prog. Cardiovasc. Dis.* 62 (2): 102–107.

Paffenbarger, R.S. Jr., Hyde, R.T., Wing, A.L. et al. (1993). The association of changes in physical-activity level and other lifestyle characteristics with mortality among men. *N. Engl. J. Med.* 328 (8): 538–545.

Paffenbarger, R.S. Jr., Hyde, R.T., Wing, A.L., and Hsieh, C.C. (1986). Physical activity, all-cause mortality, and longevity of college alumni. *N. Engl. J. Med.* 314 (10): 605–613.

Pitsavos, C., Panagiotakos, D.B., Tambalis, K.D. et al. (2009). Resistance exercise plus to aerobic activities is associated with better lipids' profile among healthy individuals: the ATTICA study. *QJM* 102 (9): 609–616.

Pratt, M., Epping, J.N., and Dietz, W.H. (2009). Putting physical activity into public health: a historical perspective from the CDC. *Prev. Med.* 49 (4): 301–302.

Riebe, D., Franklin, B.A., Thompson, P.D. et al. (2015). Updating ACSM's recommendations for exercise preparticipation health screening. *Med. Sci. Sports Exerc.* 47 (11): 2473–2479.

Rossi, A., Dikareva, A., Bacon, S.L., and Daskalopoulou, S.S. (2012). The impact of physical activity on mortality in patients with high blood pressure: a systematic review. *J. Hypertens.* 30 (7): 1277–1288.

Russo, L.M., Nobles, C., Ertel, K.A. et al. (2015). Physical activity interventions in pregnancy and risk of gestational diabetes mellitus: a systematic review and meta-analysis. *Obstet. Gynecol.* 125 (3): 576–582.

Sallis, J.F., Owen, N., and Fisher, E. (2015). Ecological models of health behavior. In: *Health Behavior: Theory, Research, and Practice*, 5e, 43–64. San Francisco, CA: Jossey-Bass.

Samitz, G., Egger, M., and Zwahlen, M. (2011). Domains of physical activity and all-cause mortality: systematic review and dose–response meta-analysis of cohort studies. *Int. J. Epidemiology* 40 (5): 1382–1400.

Sanabria-Martinez, G., Garcia-Hermoso, A., Poyatos-Leon, R. et al. (2015). Effectiveness of physical activity interventions on preventing gestational diabetes mellitus and excessive maternal weight gain: a meta-analysis. *BJOG* 122 (9): 1167–1174.

Sattelmair, J., Pertman, J., Ding, E.L. et al. (2011). Dose response between physical activity and risk of coronary heart disease: a meta-analysis. *Circulation* 124 (7): 789–795.

Strath, S.J., Kaminsky, L.A., Ainsworth, B.E. et al. (2013). Guide to the assessment of physical activity: clinical and research applications: a scientific statement from the American Heart Association. *Circulation* 128 (20): 2259–2279.

Tambalis, K., Panagiotakos, D.B., Kavouras, S.A., and Sidossis, L.S. (2009). Responses of blood lipids to aerobic, resistance, and combined aerobic with resistance exercise training: a systematic review of current evidence. *Angiology* 60 (5): 614–632.

Tobias, D.K., Zhang, C., van Dam, R.M. et al. (2011). Physical activity before and during pregnancy and risk of gestational diabetes mellitus: a meta-analysis. *Diabetes Care* 34 (1): 223–229.

Tsekouras, Y.E., Magkos, F., Kellas, Y. et al. (2008). High-intensity interval aerobic training reduces hepatic very low-density lipoprotein-triglyceride secretion rate in men. *Am. J. Physiol. Endocrinol. Metab.* 295 (4): E851–E858.

Tsekouras, Y.E., Magkos, F., Prentzas, K.I. et al. (2009). A single bout of whole-body resistance exercise augments basal

VLDL-triacylglycerol removal from plasma in healthy untrained men. *Clin. Sci. (Lond.)* 116 (2): 147–156.

Tsekouras, Y.E., Yanni, A.E., Bougatsas, D. et al. (2007). A single bout of brisk walking increases basal very low-density lipoprotein triacylglycerol clearance in young men. *Metabolism* 56 (8): 1037–1043.

Villablanca, P.A., Alegria, J.R., Mookadam, F. et al. (2015). Nonexercise activity thermogenesis in obesity management. *Mayo Clin. Proc.* 90 (4): 509–519.

Warren, J.M., Ekelund, U., Besson, H. et al. (2010). Assessment of physical activity – a review of methodologies with reference to epidemiological research: a report of the exercise physiology section of the European Association of Cardiovascular Prevention and Rehabilitation. *Eur. J. Cardiovasc. Prev. Rehabil.* 17 (2): 127–139.

Willett, W.C. (2006). The Mediterranean diet: science and practice. *Public Health Nutr.* 9 (1A): 105–110.

Yin, Y.N., Li, X.L., Tao, T.J. et al. (2014). Physical activity during pregnancy and the risk of gestational diabetes mellitus: a systematic review and meta-analysis of randomised controlled trials. *Br. J. Sports Med.* 48 (4): 290–295.

Zhong, S., Jiang, T., Ma, T. et al. (2014). Association between physical activity and mortality in breast cancer: a meta-analysis of cohort studies. *Eur. J. Epidemiol.* 29 (6): 391–404.

Zotou, E., Magkos, F., Koutsari, C. et al. (2010). Acute resistance exercise attenuates fasting and postprandial triglyceridemia in women by reducing triglyceride concentrations in triglyceride-rich lipoproteins. *Eur. J. Appl. Physiol.* 110 (4): 869–874.

CHAPTER 10

The Need for Sleep and Its Effect on Health

There is a time for many words, and there is also a time for sleep.

Homer, *The Odyssey (800–600 BCE)*

The Chronicle of Sleep Research

Sleep is a basic element of life, as people spend one third of their lives sleeping. The study of sleep has attracted the interest of philosophers, physicians, and scientists since ancient and prehistoric times. Furthermore, the functions of sleep, the mechanisms that regulate sleep physiology, and its role in physical and mental health have been the subjects of debate since the fourth century BCE. Homer in his epic poem *The Odyssey* wrote: "In your first sleep, call up your hardiest cheer," referring to the segmented sleeping patterns during the night. The ancient Greek philosopher and physician *Alcmaeon* (500–450 BCE) opposed the popular belief that sleep was a stage of unconsciousness occurring when the vessels near the surface of the human body run out of blood. *Hippocrates, the father of medicine,* described the first sleep disorder while examining the mechanism of infant death during sleep.

The first reference to "the circadian rhythm" has been found in the scripts of *Androsthenes of Thasos*, a ship captain serving under Alexander the Great. Androsthenes described in detail diurnal leaf movements of the tamarind tree. An observation of a circadian rhythm in humans is mentioned in Chinese medical texts dated back to the thirteenth century, including the Noon and Midnight Manual and the Mnemonic Rhyme to Aid in the Selection of Acu-points. In the eighteenth century, *Jean-Jacques d' Ortous de Mairan*, a French geophysicist, astronomer, and chronobiologist, observed that the leaves of the heliotrope were open during the day and closed during the night, even when the plant remained in the dark. This was a big step forward in defining circadian rhythm. In the middle of the nineteenth century, *William Ogle* observed a cyclical variation of body temperature that could not be attributed to environmental factors. Furthermore, *Wilhelm Griesinger*, a German psychiatrist, proposed that sleep is an active rather than an inert process, after recording eye movements both at the beginning of sleep and during dreams. Even though *Griesinger* was the first who observed this phenomenon, the term *rapid eye movement* (REM) was not coined until 1953. *Richard Caton* made his own contribution by detecting cerebral electrical waves, making an important step in the development of the electroencephalograph (EEG).

The invention of Thomas Edison's incandescent light bulb, introduced approximately the same period, changed sleeping habits forever, allowing light to be extended into the night. It has been estimated that since the advent of the incandescent light bulb, the average American gets approximately 2 hours less sleep.

> **Key Point**
>
> Since the advent of the incandescent light bulb, the average American gets approximately 2 hours less sleep.

Research during the first half of the twentieth century focused on sleep, brain activity during sleep, dreams, and circadian rhythms. In 1913, *Henri Pieron* published a seminal paper titled *Le Probleme Physiologique du Sommeil*, dedicated to the physiological features of sleep. Twelve years later, in 1925, Dr. *Nathaniel Kleitman*, the "father of modern sleep research," developed the first sleep laboratory. His research revolved around the circadian rhythms, the dipole sleep–wakefulness, and sleep deficiency. Dr. *Kleitman* discovered REM sleep and authored the pioneering work "Sleep and Wakefulness." In 1937, the use of the EEG enabled the description of sleep structure. In the years that followed, mounting scientific evidence documented several aspects of sleep, such as the cyclical pattern of sleep and the repetition of its stages during nighttime, the discovery of the hormone melatonin as a regulator of sleep and wakefulness, and the establishment of the term *circadian* by *Franz Helberg*, the "father of chronobiology." Moreover, Dr. Anthony Kales described patterns of sleep and waking in humans and laid the basis for pharmacologic studies in sleep. Dr. Kales, together with Dr. Rechtschaffen from the University of Chicago, chaired a group that established the first atlas for scoring human sleep in 1967.

Sleep research spiked over the last five decades; the first "clock" gene related to the circadian clock, the "per," was isolated from the fruit fly Drosophila and investigation begun on the genetic determinants of sleep and wakefulness. It was discovered that circadian rhythms are present in cells throughout the body; in the brain, a small group of hypothalamic nerve cells, called "the suprachiasmatic nucleus (SCN)," functions as a master circadian pacemaker. This group of cells controls the sleep–wake cycle and works together, along with the circadian rhythms in other brain areas and other tissues, to enhance behavioral adaptation.

In 1963, the 7-Eleven store near the University of Texas at Austin football stadium stayed open past its closing time of 11 p.m. in order to serve the game fans. After considering how well their sales did that night, the manager decided to keep the store open 24 hours per day, 7 days per week (24/7), permanently. Soon, numerous other stores across the nation followed this trend. The fact that society wanted stores to operate 24 hours per day suggests that sleeping habits had already changed by that time. Later, it was revealed that when humans are exposed to artificial light, the secretion of melatonin is suppressed, and so is the need for sleep. Average sleep time has decreased over the last century by 1.5 – 2 hours. At least 30% of Americans aged 30–64 report sleeping less than 6 hours per night.

The Need for Sleep

Sleep is not just a simple absence of wakefulness. It is considered a physiologically active state in which specific processes and metabolic pathways are activated that are essential for the regulation of daytime functioning and overall well-being. The quantity and quality of sleep determine people's performance and

> **Key Point**
>
> Sleep is not just a simple absence of wakefulness.

quality of life during the day and vice versa, suggesting that adequate sleep is essential for a well-functioning body. Sleep happens in regular intervals and is homeostatically regulated. Sleep deprivation (e.g., below 6 hours for adults) and sleep disruptions cause severe cognitive and emotional problems. Furthermore, they are detrimental to glucose metabolism and secretion of several hormones, linking sleep deprivation

with increased risk of obesity and T2DM as well as CVD and mortality.

Sleep remains one of the great challenges of mammalian biology, as many mechanisms regulating sleep physiology are still unknown. Several theories about the necessity of sleep have been proposed. Following are the predominant theories explaining the need for sleep.

Inactivity Theory

Inactivity theory, also known as the adaptive or revolutionary theory, suggests that inactivity at nighttime may protect mammals from dangerous situations arising during darkness. It has been proposed that animals that can remain motionless during these hours of increased danger have fewer accidents and casualties from predators. It is believed that sleep, as we know it today, is the evolution of this behavior. Opponents of this theory claim that if safety is the primary concern, it is probably safer being awake and alert than sleeping at night.

Energy Conservation Theory

The energy conservation theory proposes that the antagonism for energy resources and their beneficial exploitation are of paramount importance. Therefore, this theory speculates that sleep is a way for the organism to conserve energy, mainly during the hours that it is not possible to search or hunt for food. This theory is supported by the fact that energy metabolism and body temperature decrease during sleep in humans and many other species.

Restorative Theory

Another theory concerning the necessity for sleep is that it contributes to energy restoration, i.e., it helps the organism to repair small injuries that occur when the organism is awake and active. Evidence from human and animal studies supports this theory; animals subjected to complete sleep deprivation die within a few weeks due to loss of immunity. The fact that the main body-repairing activities, including tissue repair, protein synthesis, and the release of growth hormone, take place mainly during sleep offers further support to this theory.

During wakefulness, adenosine is accumulated in the brain as a byproduct of neuronal activity and ATP breakdown. It has been suggested that adenosine accumulation causes fatigue and exhaustion, and accordingly, the incentive to sleep. Sleep can counteract this effect as adenosine concentration decreases during sleep; as a consequence, when we wake up we feel fresh and alert.

Brain Plasticity Theory

The contemporary theory on sleep comes from historical and enduring associations of sleep with processes that require brain plasticity, meaning structural and organizational processes as well as adjustments that take place in the brain during sleep.

Although not fully elucidated, the brain plasticity theory is supported by the findings that sleep makes a major contribution to learning, memory, and neurodevelopment, especially in infants and young children but also in adults. It has been estimated that infants spend half of their total daily sleeping hours (12–14 hours/day) in the phase of REM sleep (see next section for the definition of REM and non-REM sleep phases). This connection between sleeping hours and brain plasticity is being studied in adults in terms of learning ability and tasks performance.

> **Key Point**
>
> Infants spend half of their total daily sleeping hours (12–14 hours/day) in the phase of REM sleep.

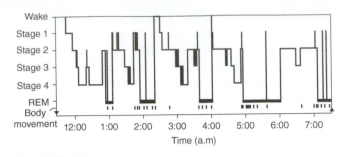

FIGURE 10.1 Progression of sleep states across a single night in a young adult. **Source:** Reprinted from Carskadon and Dement (2005). Copyright © 2005 by Elsevier Saunders.

The Phases of Sleep

Sleep can be separated into two phases: the rapid-eye-movement phase (REM; also known as desynchronized sleep or active sleep), associated mostly with dreaming, and non-REM (NREM; also known as synchronized sleep). The REM and NREM phases rotate following a cyclical pattern of 70–120 minutes. As the night progresses, fewer NREM stages occur while longer REM sleep episodes follow, lasting from less than 1 up to 30 minutes or more.

NREM sleep is the first phase of sleep experienced by adults. It is further divided into distinct stages that are characterized by the ability of the person to respond to exogenous disturbances; stages N1, N2, and N3 (some researchers have further divided stage 3 into two stages: stage 3 and stage 4; see Figure 10.1)

The transition between wakefulness and sleep is the N1 phase of NREM sleep and lasts approximately 1–7 minutes. Then, the N2 follows lasting 10–25 minutes; finally comes the N3 stage, or "deep" sleep, lasting 20–40 minutes. As the body passes from the first to the latter phases of NREM sleep, the cerebral ability to respond to environmental stimuli declines, and it becomes very difficult to arouse someone from sleep. Figure 10.1 summarizes the physiologic alterations occurring during the various phases of sleep, with stages 1–4 comprising NREM sleep, whereas stage 5 represents the REM sleep stage.

The NREM sleep stages are quiet and stable, compared to REM sleep. REM sleep is associated with dreaming, and although the EEG is similar to the waking state, is not accompanied by active muscle tone. In REM sleep, the muscles located in the limbs of the body are transiently atonic, which explains the inability to react to our dreams. NREM has been associated with a condition of sensory deprivation, whereas REM is the condition during which cortical excitation is restored to some extent via homeostatic mechanisms. This is why REM is considered to be a status of sensorial stimulation. REM sleep is believed to provide the adequate sensory stimulation for learning processes, such as memory, brain genetic printing, and brain reprogramming.

> **Key Point**
>
> In REM sleep, the muscles located in the limbs of the body are transiently atonic, which explains the inability to react to our dreams.

Many physiological changes occur during sleep; body temperature declines slightly before sleep, while during sleep it decreases further by 1–2 °F; the most significant decrease in body temperature occurs during REM sleep. Breathing rate also changes during sleep; during wakefulness respiration varies based on several conditions such as speech, emotions, and physical activity. However, in the NREM phase breathing rate tends to decrease, while in the REM phase, breathing becomes more intense and its frequency varies.

Similar to breathing, cardiovascular activity declines during NREM sleep, as a result of decreases in cardiac frequency and blood pressure. In contrast, REM sleep is characterized by both augmented heart rate and blood pressure. The activity of kidneys diminishes during sleep, whereas the release of growth hormone (GH) by the anterior pituitary gland follows a pulsatile pattern; the highest GH peaks (i.e., nearly 50% of GH secretion) occurs during the third and fourth NREM sleep stages. A number of other biological functions linked to digestion, cell repair, and growth are also enhanced during sleep. This is why it is believed that cell repair and growth are among the most significant functions of sleep.

Mediterranean Lifestyle and Sleep Recommendations

Sleep is an important component of the Mediterranean lifestyle, as highlighted in the latest version of the Mediterranean diet pyramid. Sleeping doesn't occur only at night but also during the day in the form of short naps or siestas.

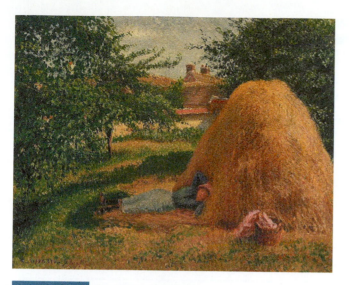

FIGURE 10.2 *The Siesta*, Camille Pissarro, 1899.

Siesta is a Spanish word, derived from the Latin *sexta (hora),* which means sixth (hour). That is midday, because counting from dawn, midday is approximately the sixth hour. The word *siesta* has been used to express the midday or afternoon rest or nap, which is taken usually after the midday meal, as depicted by various famous artists in the past, such as *The Siesta* from *Camille Pissarro* (Figure 10.2) and *La Siesta* from *Vincent van Gogh* (Figure 10.3).

Afternoon napping or siesta is common in many Mediterranean populations but also in China and other countries where the Spanish had colonies, like the Philippines. The practice of siesta was very prevalent in the agricultural regions of the Mediterranean and other areas of the world with warm climates, where the midday meal was usually the biggest meal of the day. Under the warm sun, agricultural labor had to stop for a while for the farmers to get some rest, get protection from the sun, and enjoy their lunch.

Siesta lasts approximately 20–40 minutes; longer sleep brings people to the stage of deeper stages of sleep from which it is more difficult to awake. Midday voluntary naps offer various benefits such as memory consolidation, subsequent learning, and executive functioning enhancement and emotional stability. Even if sleep during the previous night was adequate and of good quality, these benefits are maintained, while midday naps have been shown to "recover" the reduced cognitive abilities caused by sleep deprivation. However, frequent napping should be treated distinctly from planned, voluntary siesta, as it might be a marker of underlying disease. Indeed, frequent napping has also been associated with numerous negative outcomes such as hypertension and T2DM, particularly in older populations, as we will further discuss later in this chapter.

In 2015, the National Sleep Foundation (NSF) published recommendations for sleep (Figure 10.4). As age progresses, people require less nocturnal sleep. According to these recommendations, infants aged 0–3 months should sleep between 14 and 17 hours daily, infants (4–11 months) from 12 to 15 hours, toddlers (1–2 years old) between 11 and 14 hours, and preschoolers (3–5 years old) 10–13 hours per day. Children (6–13 years old) should sleep 9–11 hours, while adolescents are advised to sleep 8–10 hours daily. Adults (18–64 years old) are advised to sleep 7–9 hours per day, whereas for the elderly, 7–8 hours of sleep per day are associated with desired health benefits. The elderly have more difficulty sleeping at night but greater propensity for naps during the day, whereas hypersomnia (as explained below) in adults usually indicates an underlying disease.

The Effects of Sleep on Health

Learning and Memory Consolidation during Sleep

The amount and quality of sleep play a critical role in the process of learning and memory stabilization. It appears that sleep enhances these processes in two ways; first, individuals who are sleep deprived cannot focus on what they learn and, as a consequence, they are not able to acquire knowledge efficiently. Second, sleep contributes greatly to the integration of memory, which in turn is robustly associated with the learning process.

The mechanistic pathways through which learning and memory occur are not fully understood, but they probably transpire via encoding, consolidation, and retrieval. The first stage, encoding, refers to the insertion of new data into the brain. Consolidation refers to the process through which this newly acquired information is being stabilized. The third stage, retrieval, describes the capacity for accessing and recalling this information after it has been acquired and stored. Of note, the

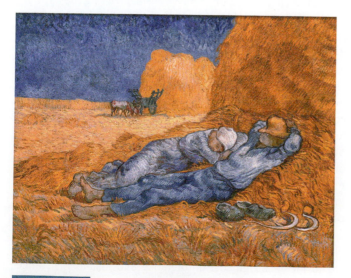

FIGURE 10.3 *La Siesta*, Vincent van Gogh, 1890.

Age	Recommended, h	May be appropriate, h	Not recommended, h
Newborns 0-3 mo	14 to 17	11 to 13 18 to 19	Less than 11 More than 19
Infants 4-11 mo	12 to 15	10 to 11 16 to 18	Less than 10 More than 18
Toddlers 1-2 y	11 to 14	9 to 10 15 to 16	Less than 9 More than 16
Preschoolers 3-5 y	10 to 13	8 to 9 14	Less than 8 More than 14
School-aged children 6-13 y	9 to 11	7 to 8 12	Less than 7 More than 12
Teenagers 14-17 y	8 to 10	7 11	Less than 7 More than 11
Young adults 18-25 y	7 to 9	6 10 to 11	Less than 6 More than 11
Adults 26-64 y	7 to 9	6 10	Less than 6 More than 10
Older adults ≥65 y	7 to 8	5 to 6 9	Less than 5 More than 9

FIGURE 10.4   Schematic representations of sleep recommendations based on different age groups. **Source:** Reprinted from Hirshkowitz et al. (2015). Copyright © 2015 National Sleep Foundation. Published by Elsevier Inc.

function of retrieval may occur both consciously and unconsciously. Despite the fact that the stages of encoding and retrieval take place during wakefulness, the stage of consolidation occurs during sleep via the reinforcement of the neuronal synapses, which participate in the shaping of memories. The way sleep affects this process remains unknown, but it is speculated that the distinct phases of sleep are characterized by distinct features of brainwaves, which are linked to the conformation of different classes of memory. Indeed, according to the two-stage memory system, memories are initially encoded into a fast-learning store (i.e., the hippocampus in the declarative memory system) and then gradually transferred to a slow-learning store for long-term storage (i.e., the neocortex). Still, memories are unstable and vulnerable to interference by newly encoded information. Over time, the information is progressively passed to the slowly learning long-term store without overwriting older memories.

Sleep and Disease Risk

Although sleep occurs in ordinary intervals and is homeostatically regulated, many people disregard these physiological signals, thus undergoing voluntary sleep restriction. Even though small alterations to usual sleep patterns can be tolerated in the short-term, when the sleep deficit increases, adverse health effects become obvious. Results from experimental studies investigating the relationship between sleep deprivation and the risk of developing degenerative diseases, such as cardiovascular diseases and metabolic syndrome, show major biological disturbances to sleep-deprived individuals. These clinical consequences derive

from the activation of various biological pathways, such as deregulation of the autonomic cardiovascular control, altered inflammatory and immune response, endothelial dysfunction, increased oxidative stress, deregulation of the leptin-ghrelin system, and decreased insulin sensitivity. Indeed, data from epidemiological studies assessing the habitual sleep hours and the presence of certain diseases using appropriate questionnaires support the notion that both insufficient and prolonged sleep is associated with increased likelihood or risk of developing obesity, hypertension, and T2DM.

A number of studies attempted to evaluate the effect of insufficient sleep on human metabolism. *Donga* and colleagues measured insulin sensitivity in healthy adults after just one night of sleep deprivation (4 hours of sleep). Using the hyperinsulinemic-euglycemic clamp, the gold standard method of assessing insulin sensitivity, the researchers detected a notable decrease in insulin sensitivity in the hepatic and peripheral tissues. Specifically, sleep shortage by only 4 hours led to 22% elevated hepatic glucose synthesis, which implies impaired insulin sensitivity in the liver. Furthermore, the delivery of glucose to various body tissues decreased by 20%, implying impaired insulin sensitivity in the muscles, adipose tissue, and other organs. In addition to the effects on glucose metabolism, one night of sleep restriction resulted in perturbations in fat metabolism; non-esterified fatty acids (NEFAs) in plasma increased by 19%, implying impaired insulin sensitivity in adipose tissue.

Another study, in which participants were subjected to either 5.5 or 8.5 hours of sleep, revealed that inadequate sleep led to increased glucose intolerance and insulin resistance. Additionally, the stress hormones epinephrine and

Key Point

Frequent incidence of sleep deprivation might impair glucose tolerance and trigger the development of T2DM.

norepinephrine increased by 20–25% in the short sleep trial. Given that these hormones, along with cortisol, are secreted when the sympathetic and hypothalamic–pituitary–adrenal axis are activated (i.e., during stress), it is possible that sleep deprivation may affect the function of the autonomous nervous system. Poor sleep quality has also been associated with increased HbA1c. Therefore, the available data suggest that frequent incidence of sleep deprivation might impair glucose tolerance and trigger the development of T2DM.

Several epidemiological studies have suggested a link between sleep deprivation and increased BMI or obesity. It is noteworthy that children and adolescents appear to be more susceptible to the development of obesity after long-term exposure to sleep deprivation, compared to adults. As for adults, younger ones seem to be more prone to the detrimental effects of sleep debt compared to older ones. After 6.5 years of follow-up, the Seguimiento Universidad de Navarra (SUN) study reported that the risk of becoming obese doubles for individuals sleeping less than 5 hours per night, compared to those sleeping 7–8 hours. Other studies demonstrated that sleep restriction impairs the weight loss effort of overweight adults. It was shown that, under conditions of reduces caloric intake, sleep debt accelerated the loss of lean body mass by 60% but inhibited the loss of adipose tissue by 55%. It was speculated that the loss of lean body mass served the process of gluconeogenesis to maintain the metabolic requirements of the alert brain and other glucose-consuming tissues.

Sleep-deprived children consume more calories (~100 kcal/day) compared to those who have adequate sleep. This small difference could potentially be of clinical significance in the long term. In a recent study, *Tambalis* et al. (2018) reported that insufficient sleep duration was associated with an unhealthy lifestyle profile (such as skipping breakfast, consumption of fast food, increased screen time, and being overweight/obese) among children and adolescents.

A possible mechanism by which sleep deprivation is linked to weight gain comes from epidemiological data. Reduced sleep duration is connected to enhanced energy intake, consumption of several snacks throughout the day, and a general unhealthy dietary pattern. Indeed, studies have shown that an 8-day sleep debt, i.e., sleeping only 75% of usual sleep duration, resulted in a noteworthy increase in food consumption (559 kcal/d). Leptin and ghrelin concentrations did not change, and energy expended during physical activity was similar between the two trials. In the long run, the reported increment in energy intake could theoretically result in increased body weight, assuming that physical activity remains constant. Similar deductions were drawn from an experimental 5-day sleep restriction study, indicating increased hunger and food consumption, mainly after the evening meal (supper), which led to approximately 1 kg of weight gain. Of note, the augmentation of food consumption occurred in the absence of changes

in appetite-related hormones, which could rationalize this enhanced intake. For this reason, it was hypothesized that the increase in food intake under conditions of sleep deprivation is due to a physiological need to maintain vigilance for more hours during the day, underscoring the important contribution of sleep to energy homeostasis.

Key Point

The increase in food intake under conditions of sleep deprivation is due to a physiological need to maintain vigilance for more hours during the day.

The increased energy intake during repeated partial sleep deprivation appears to be mainly in the form of snacks rather than regular meals. Since no alterations in physical activity and appetite-regulation hormones are observed in these studies, the investigators hypothesized that other physiological mechanisms, e.g., intrinsic reward systems, contributed to excessive food intake. This excess caloric intake from snacks comes mainly from carbohydrate-rich foods consumed usually between late evening and early morning. The researchers postulated that sleep deprivation may be a preventable obesity risk factor especially for men and those with increased body weight in the past.

Key Point

Sleep deprivation may be a preventable obesity risk factor.

Another mechanism proposed to explain the detrimental association between sleep deprivation and obesity involves the contribution of the nervous and endocrine systems in appetite regulation through modulation of the levels of leptin and ghrelin. Leptin is a hormone secreted by the adipocytes; its concentration in blood increases after meals and conveys a signal of satiety to the brain and, accordingly, the cessation of energy intake. Leptin levels are increased during sleep, possibly as a consequence of the energy intake during the day. On the other hand, ghrelin, secreted by the stomach, induces appetite, limits energy expenditure, enhances energy intake, inhibits fat oxidation, and triggers gluconeogenesis. When the body is sleep-deprived, the level of ghrelin spikes, while the level of leptin falls, leading to an increase in hunger. After only 6 days of 4-hour nocturnal sleep, leptin mean concentrations were decreased by 19%, its maximum concentrations by 26%, and the range of its diurnal variation by 20%. The authors of this study hypothesized that sleep deprivation may trigger appetite and meal consumption at the end of the day.

Key Point

Sleep deprivation may trigger appetite and meal consumption at the end of the day.

Figure 10.5 summarizes possible pathways via which sleep duration might affect the development of many degenerative diseases. Short sleep duration is associated with increased hunger, irregular eating habits, increased snacking between meals, lower levels of physical activity, and lower fruit and vegetable consumption. Moreover, sleep deprivation combined with energy restriction causes alterations in the activity of the

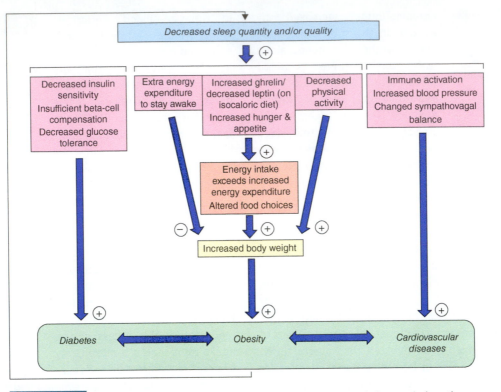

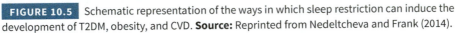

FIGURE 10.5   Schematic representation of the ways in which sleep restriction can induce the development of T2DM, obesity, and CVD. **Source:** Reprinted from Nedeltcheva and Frank (2014).

human neuroendocrine system, which can compromise the metabolic response to caloric deficiency and, as a consequence, interfere with weight loss efforts.

A systematic review of sleep habits of adolescents suggested that partial sleep deprivation (i.e., prolonged period of sleep deprivation with a limited amount of sleep) had small or no affect in adolescent cognitive functioning, while total sleep restriction resulted in impaired psychomotor vigilance tasks. Sufficient sleep was also shown to enhance the process of memory encoding in children and adolescents. Furthermore, prolonged sleep and better sleep quality appears to improve working memory, and sleeping right after a learning process appears to have a favorable effect on memory consolidation. Evidence suggests that sleeping is strongly and positively associated with cognitive functioning in terms of executive functions and school performance and with implementation of procedures requiring reasoning of higher level and complexity. Finally, a strong inverse correlation is found between sleeping hours and the manifestation of behavior-related problems.

In men over 60 years old, inadequate sleep is associated with 7 and 18% higher likelihood of all-cause and cardiovascular mortality, respectively. These findings may be reflective of the fact that older age is characterized by increased risk of a plethora of degenerative diseases, which in turn may affect the biological response to changes in the sleep pattern. However, it has been noted that even among youth, the number of sleeping hours appears to have a U-shaped relation to overall mortality, i.e., the risk increases when people sleep significantly less and significantly more than recommended for prolonged periods of time. Regarding the association of sleep duration

with hypertension, a meta-analysis of six prospective (n =9959) and 17 cross-sectional (n = 105,432) studies revealed that short sleep duration was associated with increased risk and incidence of hypertension among female subjects younger than 65 years, while long sleep duration was associated only with increased risk (not incidence) of hypertnesion.

Therefore, the scientific evidence suggests that sleep deprivation may cause a host of metabolic disturbances, resulting in chronic diseases such as T2DM, hypertension, obesity, and increased all-cause mortality. However, it should be noted that there is no consistency among studies in the definition of either short or long sleep duration. Moreover, solid evidence for rationalizing the involved mechanistic pathways is lacking, while results regarding those pathways are mainly derived from epidemiological studies that do not entail causality.

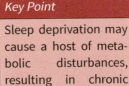

Key Point

Sleep deprivation may cause a host of metabolic disturbances, resulting in chronic diseases.

Impact of Siesta on Health

Sleep, delicious and profound, the very counterfeit of death.

Homer, *The Odyssey* (800–600 BCE)

Sleep, these little slices of death – how I loathe them.

Edgar Allan Poe

Studies conducted mainly in Mediterranean populations highlight the practice of daytime napping as a protective factor against all-cause and CVD mortality. Short (<40 minutes) daytime napping is associated with lower risk of cardiovascular disease, compared to non-nappers. In 2007, a large study in Greek adults investigated the association between siesta and the risk of CHD mortality. Afternoon napping, independently of its frequency and duration, was associated with significantly reduced likelihood of dying from CHD, in both genders. For the occasional nappers, the protective effect reached 12%, while for the systematic nappers it was estimated to be 37%, compared to the non-nappers. The reduced risk for CHD was evident only in individuals who were healthy at the beginning of the study. When persons with CHD, stroke, and cancer were included in the analysis, no inverse correlation between afternoon nap and CHD mortality was detected.

The results of the Ikaria study confirmed the finding that midday naps may have an advantageous health impact. Ikaria is a Greek island located in the Aegean Sea, one of the "Blue Zones" regions across the world where many of their inhabitants have substantially prolonged life expectancy, they remain physically active even after the age of 100 years, and they appear to share some behavioral commonalities. In the case of the Ikaria study, 13% of the study participants were men and women older than 80 years. The researchers demonstrated that in addition to other lifestyle habits that have been shown to positively affect health

> **Key Point**
>
> Midday naps may have an advantageous health impact.

(e.g., the adoption of a plant-based diet, regular physical activity, abstention from smoking, and active social life), the practice of napping was another longevity "secret" The majority of the participants stated that they napped on a regular basis, with men reporting greater engagement in this habit compared to women. All participants over 90 years old reported taking midday naps. These findings are in accordance with those of *Naska* and colleagues who reported lower CHD mortality rates among nappers, possibly because of the stress relief. Furthermore, the Ikaria study showed that frequent nappers had considerably lower depression rates, estimated by the Geriatric Depression Scale (GDS). Thus, the researchers speculated that napping may be one of the modifiable behavioral risk factors, which, in combination with other lifestyle factors, may affect life expectancy.

> **Key Point**
>
> Napping may be one of the modifiable behavioral risk factors, which, in combination with other lifestyle factors, may affect life expectancy.

However, not all studies agree with the notion that midday napping is good for your health. For example, a prospective study with 10 years of follow-up did not find any correlation between afternoon napping and overall mortality in men. Interestingly, afternoon sleep lasting over 2 hours was significantly correlated with increased risk of total and CVD mortality in males. *Wu* and colleagues observed that in middle-aged and older women, nap duration of over 1.5 hours was correlated with 17% increased risk for developing MetS, whereas no such association was found for males. Furthermore, the Guangzhou Biobank Cohort Study demonstrated that older adults who nap regularly have elevated levels of fasting glucose and higher risk for developing T2DM.

Participants in the EPIC–Norfolk study had 14% higher risk of overall mortality when their daily siesta lasted under 1 hour and 32% for siesta of longer length. These estimates were more evident for people under 65 years of age. *Naska* and colleagues also detected a 14% increase in all-cause mortality for individuals napping more than 2 hours, in the Greek cohort of the EPIC study. Compared to people who do not nap, those who slept for up to 1 hour had a 40% increased risk for mortality due to respiratory diseases, whereas people who slept for more than 1-hour midday had more than twice the risk of dying because of respiratory diseases. Finally, *Da Silva* and colleagues reported that elderly individuals who sleep more than recommended had 33% higher mortality rates and 43% higher risk of cardiovascular mortality compared to the control group.

The harmful impact of prolonged sleep on health might stem from underlying pathologies and deteriorating health, i.e., we cannot establish whether napping causes health problems or that people with health problems tend to nap more. It is also rather obvious that the increase in sleeping duration during the last weeks or months of life is most probably the result and not the cause of a disease. Nevertheless, there are data suggesting that prolonged sleep is associated with adverse health effects even in healthy individuals. Therefore, it has been suggested that apart from underlying diseases, long sleep duration might independently have a harmful effect on health. The exact mechanisms are not clear, but it has been proposed that alteration in the concentration of several cytokines, the decreased quotient of daylight to darkness, the activation of the sympathetic compartment of the nervous system, and the fragmentation of sleep may mediate the adverse effects of prolonged sleep on health.

> **Key Point**
>
> A short siesta helps some but not all individuals: people should respect the needs of their bodies, sleep well during the night, and nap or just rest midday if they feel tired.

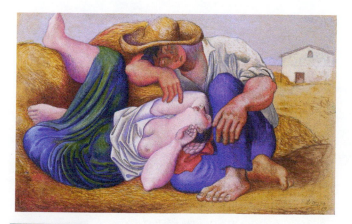

FIGURE 10.6 *Sleeping Peasants*, Pablo Picasso, 1919, Museum of Modern Art.

In summary it appears that a short siesta may have certain beneficial health effects in some but not all individuals. Hence, It is wise for people to respect the needs of their bodies, sleep well during the night, and nap or just rest midday if they feel tired.

The Effect of Shift Work on Sleep Patterns and Health

Long-term shift work or frequent changes in day vs. night employment (e.g., pilots and airline crews, hospital personnel, first responders) has been associated with an increased risk of heart disease, gastrointestinal problems, depression, certain cancers, T2DM, and obesity. Studies have shown that shift workers usually have irregular eating habits, unhealthy diets, and present with high triglyceride levels and insulin resistance. The mechanisms responsible for the detrimental effects of shift work on health may be related to decreased amount of sleep and the disruption of the body's circadian rhythms, especially as they relate to mealtimes and effects on appetite, as previously covered in detail in this chapter.

Apart from the risk in developing chronic diseases, shift work may also decrease productivity and increase the risk for accidents and on-the-job injuries. The risk for accidents increases when workers start their jobs in the evenings, and when their shifts last longer than 10 hours.

Take-Home Messages

- Sleep is not just the absence of wakefulness. It is considered a physiologically active state in which specific processes and metabolic pathways occur that are essential for the regulation of daytime functioning and overall well-being.
- Sleep is very important to the learning process, memory function, and neurodevelopment.
- Sleep can be separated into two phases; REM (rapid eye movement, also known as desynchronized sleep or active sleep, associated mostly with dreaming), and NREM (also known as synchronized sleep).
- The NREM sleep stages are quiet and stable, compared to REM sleep.
- Afternoon napping or siesta is common in many populations in the Mediterranean region, other countries in Southern Europe, South America, the Philippines, and mainland China.
- Siestas should last under 40 minutes; siestas longer than 60 minutes result in transitioning to the stage of deep sleep from which it is more difficult to awake.
- The amount and quality of sleep play a critical role in the process of learning and memory stabilization. The mechanistic pathways through which learning and memory occur are not fully understood, but they probably transpire via encoding, consolidation, and information retrieval.
- Sleep deprivation is associated with increased risk of metabolic syndrome, obesity, T2DM, CVD, and mortality.
- Daytime napping is considered a protective factor against all-cause and CVD mortality, following a J-curve relation. Short (below 40 minutes) daytime napping is associated with lower risk for cardiovascular disease, whereas long daytime napping (above 60 minutes) with higher risk, compared to non-nappers.

Self-Assessment Questions

1. Complete the sentence: Sleep is considered a physiologically active state in which _____.
2. What are the main theories explaining the need for sleep?
3. Choose the correct statement:
   a. The rapid-eye-movement phase (REM) is associated mostly with active muscle tone.
   b. The REM and NREM phases rotate following a cyclical pattern of 100–130 minutes.
   c. The REM and NREM phases rotate following a cyclical pattern of 70–120 minutes.
   d. REM sleep episodes last from less than 1 to 60 minutes or more.
4. State the physiological changes that occur during sleep.
5. Is sleep a significant component of the Mediterranean lifestyle? Please justify your answer.
6. What does the word siesta refer to?
7. How long should a siesta last?
8. According to the 2011 NSF recommendations for sleep, how long should adults sleep per day?
9. Briefly discuss how inadequate sleep can affect dietary habits.
10. How is shift work related to health?

Bibliography

Astill, R.G., Van der Heijden, K.B., Van Ijzendoorn, M.H., and Van Someren, E.J. (2012). Sleep, cognition, and behavioral problems in school-age children: a century of research meta-analyzed. *Psychol. Bull.* 138 (6): 1109–1138.

Banks, S. and Dinges, D.F. (2007). Behavioral and physiological consequences of sleep restriction. *J. Clin. Sleep Med.* 3 (5): 519–528.

Bateman, R.M., Sharpe, M.D., Jagger, J.E. et al. (2016). 36th International Symposium on Intensive Care and Emergency Medicine. *Critical Care* 20 (2): 13–182.

Bayon, V., Leger, D., Gomez-Merino, D. et al. (2014). Sleep debt and obesity. *Ann. Med.* 46 (5): 264–272.

Broussard, J.L., Ehrmann, D.A., Van Cauter, E. et al. (2012). Impaired insulin signaling in human adipocytes after experimental sleep restriction: a randomized, crossover study. *Ann. Intern. Med.* 157 (8): 549–557.

Burazeri, G., Gofin, J., and Kark, J.D. (2003). Siesta and mortality in a Mediterranean population: a community study in Jerusalem. *Sleep* 26 (5): 578–584.

Calvin, A.D., Carter, R.E., Adachi, T. et al. (2013). Effects of experimental sleep restriction on caloric intake and activity energy expenditure. *Chest* 144 (1): 79–86.

Carley, D.W. and Farabi, S.S. (2016). Physiology of sleep. *Diabetes Spectr.* 29 (1): 5–9.

Carskadon, M. and Dement, W. (2005). Normal human sleep: an overview. In: Kryger, M.H., Roth, T., Dement, W.C. (Eds.), *Principles and Practice of Sleep Medicine*, 4e, 13–23. Philadelphia, PA: Elsevier Saunders.

Chien, K.L., Chen, P.C., Hsu, H.C. et al. (2010). Habitual sleep duration and insomnia and the risk of cardiovascular events and all-cause death: report from a community-based cohort. *Sleep* 33 (2): 177–184.

Colten, H.R. and Altevogt, B.M. (eds.) (2006). *Sleep Disorders and Sleep Deprivation: An Unmet Public Health Problem.* Washington, DC: National Academies Press.

Cooper, C.B., Neufeld, E.V., Dolezal, B.A., and Martin, J.L. (2018). Sleep deprivation and obesity in adults: a brief narrative review. *BMJ Open Sport Exerc. Med.* 4 (1): e000392.

da Silva, A.A., de Mello, R.G., Schaan, C.W., Fuchs, F.D., Redline, S., and Fuchs, S.C. (2016). Sleep duration and mortality in the elderly: a systematic review with meta-analysis. *BMJ Open* 6 (2): e008119. https://doi.org/10.1136/bmjopen-2015-008119.

Dement, W.C. (1998). The study of human sleep: a historical perspective. *Thorax* 53: S2–S7.

Donga, E., van Dijk, M., van Dijk, J.G. et al. (2010). A single night of partial sleep deprivation induces insulin resistance in multiple metabolic pathways in healthy subjects. *J. Clin. Endocrinol. Metab.* 95 (6): 2963–2968.

Ford, E.S., Cunningham, T.J., and Croft, J.B. (2015). Trends in self-reported sleep duration among US adults from 1985 to 2012. *Sleep* 38 (5): 829–832.

Frank, M.G. (2011). Sleep and developmental plasticity not just for kids. *Prog. Brain Res.* 193: 221–232.

Frank, M.G. (2019). Sleep and brain plasticity. In: *Sleep, Memory and Synaptic Plasticity*, 107–124. New York: Springer.

Frost, P., Kolstad, H.A., and Bonde, J.P. (2009). Shift work and the risk of ischemic heart disease – a systematic review of the epidemiologic evidence. *Scand. J. Work Environ. Health* 35 (3): 163–179.

Gooley, J.J., Chamberlain, K., Smith, K.A. et al. (2011). Exposure to room light before bedtime suppresses melatonin onset and shortens melatonin duration in humans. *J. Clin. Endocrinol. Metab.* 96 (3): E463–E472.

Halberg, F., Cornelissen, G., Katinas, G. et al. (2003). Transdisciplinary unifying implications of circadian findings in the 1950s. *J. Circadian Rhythms* 1 (1): 2.

Hart, C.N., Carskadon, M.A., Considine, R.V. et al. (2013). Changes in children's sleep duration on food intake, weight, and leptin. *Pediatrics* 132 (6): e1473–e1480.

Hirshkowitz, M., Whiton, K., Albert, S.A. et al. (2015). National Sleep Foundation's sleep time duration recommendations: methodology and results summary. *Sleep Health* 1 (1): 40–43.

Iskra-Golec, I., Barnes-Farrell, J., and Bohle, P. (2016). Introduction to problems of shift work. In: *Social and Family Issues in Shift Work and Non Standard Working Hours*, 19–35. New York: Springer.

Klinzing, J.G., Niethard, N., and Born, J. (2019). Mechanisms of systems memory consolidation during sleep. *Nat. Neurosci.* 22 (10): 1598–1610.

Konopka, R.J. and Benzer, S. (1971). Clock mutants of Drosophila melanogaster. *Proc. Natl. Acad. Sci.* 68: 2112–2116.

Lam, K.B., Jiang, C.Q., Thomas, G.N. et al. (2010). Napping is associated with increased risk of type 2 diabetes: the Guangzhou biobank cohort study. *Sleep* 33 (3): 402–407.

Lee, K.A., Beyene, Y., Paparrigopoulos, T.J. et al. (2007). Circadian rhythms and sleep patterns in urban Greek couples. *Biol. Res. Nurs.* 9 (1): 42–48.

Lee, S.W.H., Ng, K.Y., and Chin, W.K. (2017). The impact of sleep amount and sleep quality on glycemic control in type 2 diabetes: a systematic review and meta-analysis. *Sleep Med. Rev.* 31: 91–101.

Leng, Y., Wainwright, N.W., Cappuccio, F.P. et al. (2014). Daytime napping and the risk of all-cause and cause-specific mortality: a 13-year follow-up of a British population. *Am. J. Epidemiol.* 179 (9): 1115–1124.

Liu, X., Zhang, Q., and Shang, X. (2015). Meta-analysis of self-reported daytime napping and risk of cardiovascular or all-cause mortality. *Med. Sci. Monit.* 21: 1269–1275.

Mantua, J. and Spencer, R.M.C. (2017). Exploring the nap paradox: are mid-day sleep bouts a friend or foe? *Sleep Med.* 37: 88–97.

Markwald, R.R., Melanson, E.L., Smith, M.R. et al. (2013). Impact of insufficient sleep on total daily energy expenditure, food intake, and weight gain. *Proc. Natl. Acad. Sci. U. S. A.* 110 (14): 5695–5700.

Matricciani, L., Dumuid, D., Paquet, C. et al. (2021). Sleep and cardiometabolic health in children and adults: examining sleep as a component of the 24-h day. *Sleep Med.* 78: 63–74. doi: 10.1016/j.sleep.2020.12.001.

Matricciani, L., Paquet, C., Fraysse, F. et al. (2021). Sleep and cardiometabolic risk: a cluster analysis of actigraphy-derived sleep profiles in adults and children. *Sleep* 44 (7): zsab014. doi: 10.1093/sleep/zsab014.

Moore, R.Y. (2007). Suprachiasmatic nucleus in sleep-wake regulation. *Sleep Med.* 8 (Suppl 3): 27–33.

Mukherjee, S., Patel, S.R., Kales, S.N. et al. (2015). An official American Thoracic Society statement: the importance of healthy sleep. Recommendations and future priorities. *Am. J. Respir. Crit. Care Med.* 191 (12): 1450–1458.

Naska, A., Oikonomou, E., Trichopoulou, A. et al. (2007). Siesta in healthy adults and coronary mortality in the general population. *Arch. Intern. Med.* 167 (3): 296–301.

National Sleep Foundation. (2011). How much sleep do we really need? https://www.sleepfoundation.org/how-sleep-works/how-much-sleep-do-we-really-need.

Nedeltcheva, A. and Frank, S. (2014). Metabolic effects of sleep disruption, links to obesity and diabetes. *Curr. Opin. Endocrinol. Diabetes Obes.* 21 (4): 293.

Nedeltcheva, A.V., Kessler, L., Imperial, J., and Penev, P.D. (2009). Exposure to recurrent sleep restriction in the setting of high caloric intake and physical inactivity results in increased insulin resistance and reduced glucose tolerance. *J. Clin. Endocrinol. Metab.* 94 (9): 3242–3250.

Nedeltcheva, A.V., Kilkus, J.M., Imperial, J. et al. (2010). Insufficient sleep undermines dietary efforts to reduce adiposity. *Ann. Intern. Med.* 153 (7): 435–441.

Panagiotakos, D.B., Chrysohoou, C., Siasos, G. et al. (2011). Sociodemographic and lifestyle statistics of oldest old people (>80 years) living in Ikaria island: the Ikaria study. *Cardiol. Res. Pract.* 2011: 679187.

Pièron, H. (1913). *Le probleme physiologique du sommeil.* Paris: Masson.

Presser, H.B. (2004). The economy that never sleeps. *Contexts* 3: 42–49.

Rasch, B. and Born, J. (2013). About sleep's role in memory. *Physiol. Rev.* 93 (2): 681–766.

Reutrakul, S. and Van Cauter, E. (2018). Sleep influences on obesity, insulin resistance, and risk of type 2 diabetes. *Metabolism* 84: 56–66.

Sayon-Orea, C., Bes-Rastrollo, M., Carlos, S. et al. (2013). Association between sleeping hours and siesta and the risk of obesity: the SUN Mediterranean cohort. *Obes. Facts* 6 (4): 337–347.

Shan, Z., Ma, H., Xie, M. et al. (2015). Sleep duration and risk of type 2 diabetes: a meta-analysis of prospective studies. *Diabetes Care* 38 (3): 529–537.

Siegel, J. (2001). A tribute to Nathaniel Kleitman. *Arch. Ital. Biol.* 139: 3–10.

Siegel, J.M. (2005). Clues to the functions of mammalian sleep. *Nature* 437 (7063): 1264–1271.

Siegel, J.M. (2009). Sleep viewed as a state of adaptive inactivity. *Nat. Rev. Neurosci.* 10 (10): 747–753.

Spaeth, A.M., Dinges, D.F., and Goel, N. (2013). Effects of experimental sleep restriction on weight gain, caloric intake, and meal timing in healthy adults. *Sleep* 36 (7): 981–990. doi: 10.5665/sleep.2792. PMID: 23814334; PMCID: PMC3669080.

Spiegel, K., Leproult, R., L'Hermite-Baleriaux, M. et al. (2004). Leptin levels are dependent on sleep duration: relationships with sympathovagal balance, carbohydrate regulation, cortisol, and thyrotropin. *J. Clin. Endocrinol. Metab.* 89 (11): 5762–5771.

Strohmaier, S., Devore, E.E., Zhang, Y., and Schernhammer, E.S. (2018). A review of data of findings on night shift work and the development of DM and CVD events: a synthesis of the proposed molecular mechanisms. *Curr. Diab. Rep.* 18 (12): 132.

Tambalis, K.D., Panagiotakos, D.B., Psarra, G., and Sidossis, L.S. (2018). Insufficient sleep duration is associated with dietary habits, screen time, and obesity in children. *J. Clin. Sleep Med.* 14 (10): 1689–1696.

Theorell-Haglow, J. and Lindberg, E. (2016). Sleep duration and obesity in adults: what are the connections? *Curr. Obes. Rep.* 5 (3): 333–343.

Tobaldini, E., Costantino, G., Solbiati, M. et al. (2017). Sleep, sleep deprivation, autonomic nervous system and cardiovascular diseases. *Neurosci. Biobehav. Rev.* 74 (Pt B): 321–329.

Wang, Y., Mei, H., Jiang, Y.R. et al. (2015). Relationship between duration of sleep and hypertension in adults: a meta-analysis. *J. Clin. Sleep Med.* 11 (9): 1047–1056.

Wu, J., Xu, G., Shen, L., Zhang, Y., Song, L., Yang, S., Yang, H., Liang, Y., Wu, T., and Wang, Y. (2015). Daily sleep duration and risk of metabolic syndrome among middle-aged and older Chinese adults: cross-sectional evidence from the Dongfeng-Tongji cohort study. *BMC Public Health* 15: 178. https://doi.org/10.1186/s12889-015-1521-z.

Yamada, T., Hara, K., Shojima, N. et al. (2015). Daytime napping and the risk of cardiovascular disease and all-cause mortality: a prospective study and dose-response meta-analysis. *Sleep* 38 (12): 1945–1953.

Zhong, G., Wang, Y., Tao, T. et al. (2015). Daytime napping and mortality from all causes, cardiovascular disease, and cancer: a meta-analysis of prospective cohort studies. *Sleep Med.* 16 (7): 811–819.

CHAPTER 11

Social Life, Spirituality, and Stress Management

In times of need, it's better to have a friend rather than money.

Greek proverb

Active social life and deep spirituality are important characteristics of the Mediterranean lifestyle. Both active social life and spirituality have been implicated in the "stress-free" or "relaxed" attitude that (used to) characterize the populations living in the Mediterranean region. There are many stress-reduction approaches to achieve relaxation: sleeping, socializing, exercising, listening to music, reading books, and many more. Physical activity and sleep have been thoroughly discussed previously in this book as integral components of the Mediterranean lifestyle. In this chapter, emphasis will be given to other ways of achieving relaxation that people in the Mediterranean region have used for thousands of years.

> **Key Point**
>
> Active social life and deep spirituality are important characteristics of the Mediterranean lifestyle.

Sociability and Social Ties

Human beings are by nature sociable; they tend to organize in communities whose structure embodies social interaction as an integral part of their lives. Social ties are defined as connections among people that are used for sharing information, knowledge, feelings, and experiences. Social ties can be weak, strong, or latent, based on the extent of exchanges and interactions between people. The Mediterranean populations are renowned for their openness and extroversion, character traits that are believed to have an advantageous impact on their health. Even though there is limited data on the prevalence of stress and the effects of relaxation in the Mediterranean people, it has long been hypothesized that their social character influences these factors and therefore their health. It is noteworthy that this predisposition of associating with other people and being in the company of others is an inherent behavioral trait of the populations bordering the Mediterranean basin. This disposition and attitude toward sociability is not taught but constitutes a natural consequence of the whole way of living in the Mediterranean countries.

> **Key Point**
>
> Social ties are defined as connections among people that are used for sharing information, knowledge, feelings, and experiences.

Social ties are often so strong that they turn into family ties, by coupling with matrimony or by baptizing a friend's offspring. The general sense in this part of the world is that establishing social ties is very significant; people who avoid interaction with others are seen with suspicion. Farming, which oftentimes demanded help from other fellow villagers, tends to strengthen social ties. This has resulted in the development of a sense of solidarity, i.e., a feeling of unity and mutual support within a group of individuals with a common interest.

Of note, the building of these bonds and practices had its own contribution to the occurrence of convivial meals, which were common during the breaks of agrarian activities. Furthermore, religion also played a critical role in the development of social ties in the past, when people were more religious and church attendance or participation in religious activities and festivals were widespread.

The positive and harmonious interactions and bonding with other persons – not only in the context of relatives and friends but also in the workplace – played a critical role in what is conceived to be social wellness. *Social wellness* may be defined as maintaining healthy relationships, enjoying being with others, developing friendships and intimate relations, caring about and being cared for by others, and contributing to the needs of a community. Importantly, this positive interaction can also contribute to emotional wellness, i.e., it assists in the understanding and expression of people's inner feelings, values, and attitudes, regardless of whether they are positive or negative.

Social Interaction, Quality of Social Ties, and Health Impact

Data from large longitudinal studies suggest that positive social interactions are predictive of better health in people of all ages. There is now strong scientific evidence supporting the notion that the nature of social interactions constitutes a reliable factor associated with morbidity and mortality. On the other hand, negative social interactions are often correlated with deteriorated health status for all age groups.

> **Key Point**
>
> The nature of social interactions constitutes a reliable factor associated with morbidity and mortality.

The nature of social relations affects cardiovascular responsiveness and the risk for developing CHD. Conversation about unpleasant personal experiences with ambivalent friends may cause blood pressure levels to rise. When similar stressful events are discussed in the company of beloved friends, no such adverse cardiovascular response is recorded. Furthermore, during and after a stress event, heart rate, blood pressure, and anxiety are substantially higher among individuals who are in the presence of ambivalent friends compared to trusted friends. There is now convincing scientific evidence to support the notion that unfriendliness and animosity can increase the risk for CHD. People whose intimate relationships are characterized by negativity have a 30% higher risk to develop CHD. Positive social interactions have been associated with decreased risk for developing visceral adiposity and low-grade inflammation in adolescents. It is well established that the presence of obesity and inflammation at a young age increases the risk for the subsequent development of insulin resistance, T2DM, and eventually CVD.

Telomere length is regarded as a marker for the biological age of a person. Telomeres are protective caps at the ends of chromosomes that become shorter with each cell division. If they become too short, the genes they protect could be damaged and the cell stops dividing and renewing. This mechanism is one of many that have been proposed to determine the rate of the aging process. For two people of the same chronological age, the person with shorter telomeres has an increased risk of developing age-related diseases such as Alzheimer's or cancer, and even a shorter life expectancy. People who reported having many contradictory social relations had shortened telomeres, independent of the presence of other factors (e.g., positive relations, age, health-related behaviors, etc.). Women were shown to be more vulnerable than men to these ambivalent social bonds in terms of telomere shortening; the association between telomere length and social ambivalence was mainly mediated by the relationships with parents, friends, and associates in other social networks.

> **Key Point**
>
> Telomere length is regarded as a marker for the biological age of a person.

Middle-aged and older adults seem to be especially susceptible to stressors such as negative social relationships. Contradictory and unfriendly feelings may have negative effects on the person's physical and psychological health. Interestingly, inconsistency of social relations is associated with greater implications on physical health than totally negative relations. Furthermore, unpleasant interchange with people belonging to what is conceived as a "bad" social networks has been found to be associated with a decline in the intention for reconciliation, firmer and prolonged unpleasant sentiments, and reduced ability to cope with these negative interactions. On the other hand, pleasant social relationships can counteract the potential harmful influence of the unpleasant ones on mental health.

> **Key Point**
>
> Middle-aged and older adults seem to be especially susceptible to stressors such as negative social relationships.

As we age, we tend to pursue social relationships that give us only positive feelings, i.e., we avoid associating with negative people or persons for whom we have uncertain feelings. Common social activities among the elderly are characterized by altruism (giving, supporting, sharing, making others happy), creativity (painting, singing, being in nature, knitting/crocheting, traveling), games, and motion. This population group states that the principal incentive for these activities is the sense of belonging, relaxation, stimulation, and enjoyment. The engagement in these activities may also strengthen cognition. In home-dwelling patients with early stage dementia, participation in person-centered physical and social activities has been shown to offer a sense of belonging. Findings from the Dancing Mind Randomized Controlled Trial indicated that, among healthy and active community-dwelling elderly persons, social dancing tended to ameliorate cognitive functions, such as delayed verbal and visuospatial recall.

> **Key Point**
>
> As we age, we tend to pursue social relationships that offer us only positive feelings.

People who have positive and rewarding relationships with family and friends tend to have better mental health. On the other hand,

> **Key Point**
>
> People who have positive and rewarding relationships with family and friends tend to have better mental health.

when people of any age experience many negative social relationships/events, they are more likely to experience impaired psychological function. Contradictory social interactions increase the risk for developing depressive symptoms in older adults. In summary, negative social interactions constitute a risk factor for adverse health outcomes in individuals of all ages.

Mechanisms Connecting Social Interaction and Health

There are seven proposed mechanisms by which social relationships and social integration may affect a person's health: social influence and/or comparison, social control, meaning of life based on social roles, self-esteem, sense of control, belonging and companionship, and perceived support availability.

People tend to alter their behavior in order to assimilate in social groups they are related to, especially when they regard them to be significant. In this sense, the attitude of peers toward health can affect an individual's perspective about health. The use of substances (e.g., tobacco, alcohol, and drugs), the adherence to diet or medical prescriptions, health checks conducted in the frame of prevention, but also behaviors with beneficial or adverse health impacts are often adopted because of *social influence*.

Social control is another dimension of the aforementioned mechanisms, pertaining to the endeavor of social associates to intervene in the adoption of specific health practices that they consider to be advantageous for a person they are associated with. These attempts can prevent unhealthy behaviors, but they can also trigger unhealthy choices when the counseling is deemed to constitute a breach of privacy, and cause resistance to change for health improvement. Social control might affect psychological and physical functioning, as social partners can probably recognize mood disturbances that can be linked to sleep deprivation, aberrant appetite, and tobacco or alcohol abuse, and offer advice in order to help.

Social roles refers to the special position a person possesses within society. Dipole relationships are common in social structure., e.g., parent and child, professor and student, husband and wife. Within these relationships the right of one part is the obligation of the other part. In the context of these interactions, pressure can be applied between pairs in order to choose or reject specific health practices. Whether people respond or not to behavioral guidance is a matter of acceptance of their social position and whether they recognize this position as an element of their social identity.

High *self-esteem* is positively associated with decreased levels of anxiety, distress, and depressive symptoms; it increases the feelings of happiness and life satisfaction, contributing this way to better psychological status. The feeling of adequacy in the various roles that people are engaged in influences their mental condition. Additionally, the *sense of control* over life derives from the adequacy people display in their social roles. A sense of mastery over life and assertiveness leads to decreased anxiety and depression symptoms and reduced response to stressful factors.

The *sense of belonging* that social interaction bestows may also constitute a defense against health stressors. *Belongingness* (i.e., the human emotional need to be an accepted member of a group) is a corollary of the recognition and acknowledgment of a person's competencies by their social environment, but it is neither guaranteed nor secured. Therefore, when people enjoy the acceptance of their associates and the sense of being part of a group, the sense of companionship follows, due to the fact that the members of a group share the same interests and tasks. Hence, fellowship has the potential to reinforce psychological and physical functioning. On the other hand, people who do not enjoy companionship have been shown to experience symptoms of anxiety, depression, and fragile health and to follow unhealthy practices.

The seventh mechanistic pathway through which social interaction may beneficially affect health status is the support a person perceives from *social relationships*. This support may be emotional, informational, or instrumental. Perceived emotional support is strongly associated with favorable physical and psychological health outcomes but also prolonged lifespan. Finally, social support is believed to be advantageous independently of the presence of stressors met in the everyday life or major stress-provoking circumstances that are experienced in high frequency.

The Spiritual Dimension of Relaxation in the Mediterranean Lifestyle

People in the Mediterranean region use various methods to relax from life stressors. Religious attendance holds a prominent position among these methods, especially in previous decades when attending religious services was more common. The sense of being spiritually connected with a superior power and the faith of the existence of this power defined to a great extent the attitude to life, as well as the state of inner balance and peaceful mind that Mediterranean natives used to have. Interestingly, the frequent participation in ecclesiastical rituals, the personal engagement in religious practices like praying, and the dependence on one's religious beliefs as a source of strength may have had a unique contribution to the health status of people in the Mediterranean region.

Achieving and maintaining a peaceful and harmonic status in all aspects of life play a critical role in the attainment of spiritual wellness. This should be consistent with one's values and perspectives in order to be combined efficiently and constructively to reach one's goals. Furthermore, spiritual wellness is closely related to and interacts with intellectual and emotional wellness. Releasing the mind from constraints and prejudices allows for encountering new challenges and perspectives that can lead to increased effectiveness of future decision-making processes and social interface. Comprehending and being in contact with one's inner self – confronting and managing life adversities but also expressing constructively oneself in terms of emotions – contributes to the accomplishment of emotional well-being.

The Effect of Spirituality and Stress Management on Health

Even though it has been suggested that spiritualism is related to better health functioning and outcomes, there is no consistent way to determine it. Indeed, the definition of spirituality seems to be elusive, as each person may perceive it in a different way. In 2022, Coyle sought to compose a conceptual framework of the approaches employed to determine spiritualism. This included transcendence, as a sense of connectedness with God, no matter what the term "God" represents for each person. This approach may offer people a spiritual viewpoint predisposing them toward the adoption of healthy behaviors, but it may also enhance serenity and equanimity, even in the presence of negative events. Even when the transcendent approach is not experienced as connectedness with God but with a person's inner being, it can strengthen self-confidence and constitute a standard benchmark and recourse.

Religious individuals may derive social support via their engagement in ecclesiastical rituals and activities, and therefore, they may be more likely to conform to sound habits. Robust value systems allow people to consciously accept what happens to them and constructively manage any adverse situations. Nevertheless, the extent to which value systems reinforce health status is highly contingent on the attributes of the values each person holds. Therefore, spirituality is approached both as a feature of pietism and strong faith in a particular ideology.

Irrespective of whether people strongly believe in God, altruism, themselves, human relationships, or whatever else, these beliefs could comprise lifelong guiding principles capable of affecting their health. This notion can be rationalized by the fact that firmly held values and principles, religious or not, have the potential to bestow incentives, abilities, power, and hope, and in this way, they can help people to confront disease states. Especially among persons with chronic disease and during late adulthood, spirituality has been shown to amplify adaptation in difficult circumstances. Moreover, it has been proposed that finding meaning and having a purpose in life

may create a positive attitude toward it, which, in turn, can predispose toward more sound health practices, resulting in better health. It has been suggested that people prepossessed by a sense of purpose and meaning through their engagement in a religious community had fewer chances to adopt unhealthy habits, such as heavy drinking and drug use. Additionally, even when they do form unhealthy habits, they may not experience the same adverse health effects as do people who do not have a strong sense of purpose and meaning for their lives.

Engagement in religious communities may have the potential to prevent disease development through peace of mind and the self-assurance it creates. For instance, it has been suggested that blood pressure may be higher among nonpious smokers compared to religious ones. Of note, epidemiological findings have shown that social engagement in the context of an ecclesiastical community is strongly associated with increased life expectancy, while social support seems to account for only about 25% of the observed trend. This may be due to the fact that religious service attendance likely affects health not simply because of social support but also because it potentially shapes so much of one's outlook, behavior, beliefs, diet, and sense of life's meaning and purpose. In general, it has been suggested that when people believe in God and His/Her intentions, they can more easily accept a negative condition, like an illness, because they are convinced that whatever they undergo has a certain reason and serves a higher purpose.

Meditation and Health Status

Many around the world engage in the practice of meditation in attempts to gain health benefits. People who meditate state that this mental training bestows on them a sense of balance, self-control, and consciousness and also helps them to relax. Meditation has recently been approved as a complementary practice in the health sector or as a major element of more holistic health approaches. Meditation practices stem primarily from Eastern cultures in which mental training was incorporated within the medical practice.

The effects of meditation on health seem to be real and significant. Buddhist meditation has been shown to have positive effects on reducing stress, increasing mindfulness, and improving blood pressure and vascular endothelial function. It appears that the benefits derive from the effects on chronic inflammation and psychological distress, which are thought to be mediators of high blood pressure and cardiovascular diseases. Numerous studies have also demonstrated the role of mindfulness-based stress reduction in T2DM, showing modest improvements in body weight regulation and glycemic control. Even though these studies are of short duration and with small sample sizes, mindfulness meditation-based interventions seem to affect all domains of holistic care, biological, psychological, and social. "Buddhist walking meditation" has been shown to have favorable health effects and is perhaps superior to traditional walking programs as a treatment protocol for T2DM patients. Patients participating in Buddhist walking meditation groups appear to have decreased arterial stiffness and lower HbA1c, systolic and diastolic blood pressure, and blood cortisol.

Yoga is practiced in religions like Buddhism and Hinduism; it incorporates physical, mental, and spiritual features. Even a short-term engagement in yoga can improve CVD and T2DM risk factors among high-risk populations. Yoga-based lifestyle interventions in obese individuals may lower body weight, BMI waist and hip circumference, waist to hip ratio, and systolic and diastolic blood pressure. Furthermore, improvements in blood glucose levels, fasting insulin, IL-6, HOMA-IR, and lipid profile have also been documented. Practicing yoga is useful in improving quality of life among overweight/obese individuals.

In Western cultures, meditation is primarily connected to religiosity. As mentioned above, meditation is largely influenced by Eastern traditions, but this does not mean that they necessarily assimilate the religious dimension of the practice. People who meditate seek ways to make their living sounder and to improve behavioral norms with a positive impact on their psychological and overall health functioning.

There are many different ways to meditate, with some practices being fused within religion, others aiming at experiencing spirituality irrespective of the religious element, and others focused solely on meditation as a mental training separated from any kind of spirituality. Nonetheless, all of these practices share the same methodology: they concentrate attention on a certain topic by insulating the mind from exterior stimuli and by voiding the mind of anything associated with the exterior world. In this way, those who meditate master their attention, owing to the fact that they learn to tranquilize and coordinate their thoughts and judgments. Three main types of meditation are found in the literature: concentration meditation, in which a particular object is the center of attention until silencing of thoughts is achieved; mindfulness meditation, which aims at widening the objective perception of whatever surfaces in the mind without reacting to this; and contemplative meditation, constituting a combination of the two former types. It has been proposed that both self-possession and control over composure, attained via the various types of meditating, alter the way of thinking, improve behavioral standards, and induce consciousness, but they also contribute to the harmonization of body functioning and metabolism.

Meditation has been shown to decrease oxygen consumption, heart rate, and sympathetic nervous system activity, enhance the activity of the parasympathetic nervous system, and increase the electrical resistance of the skin, which decreases due to emotional stress. The observed alterations in human physiology were associated with a decrease in stress and anxiety and an enhanced sense of relaxation, factors that are known to have favorable health impact. Moreover, meditation has been linked to increased blood flow to the brain, mainly to the left-side anterior cortex and the insula, areas of the brain associated with mood improvement. The mastery over attention achieved by meditation can improve cerebral functioning and possibly constitute a protective shield against brain disturbances. Furthermore, when compared with relaxation training, meditation training was found to be superior in terms of attention maintenance and self-control.

> **Key Point**
> Meditation has been linked to increased blood flow to the brain.

Given that brain dynamics appear to be altered during meditation, it is possible that the perception and management of external stressors is altered in a way that facilitates the adoption of healthier behaviors. It has been speculated that mental predisposition has the potential to affect the functions of the body and play a role in the development of diseases via its effect on the equilibrium of hormonal release. Another way through which meditation may improve health is by enhancing immune function. Subjects who practiced mindfulness meditation for 8 weeks had higher concentrations of antibodies against the influenza virus. The investigators attributed this effect to significant increases in left-sided anterior activation, a pattern previously associated with positive affects on immune function.

Individuals experiencing chronic medical conditions can also benefit from mindfulness meditation in alleviating depressive symptoms, anxiety, and anguish, in the frame of cognitive behavioral therapy. Meditation can lead to a modest relief of psychological stress, mainly through attenuation of pain, anxiety, and depression. Therefore, mindfulness meditation is recommended for persons with psychological/psychiatric conditions such as panic and prolonged duress stress disorder. Finally, even among healthy people, those who meditate regularly experience less resentful thoughts and feelings, anxiety, and stress and have enhanced feelings of understanding and self-compassion. Nonetheless, meditation is not panacea, and despite the favorable effects it may have on health, its practice is contradicted whenever there are concerns regarding reality testing, ego boundaries, lack of empathy, or rigid overcontrol.

> **Key Point**
> Meditation can lead to a modest relief of psychological stress, mainly through attenuation of pain, anxiety, and depression.

Take-Home Messages

- Conviviality and stress relief are important components of the Mediterranean lifestyle.
- The Mediterranean populations are characterized by openness and extroversion, which are believed to have an advantageous impact on their health.
- Positive interactions with others and the establishment of firm bonds play a critical role in achieving physical, social, and emotional wellness. On the other hand, negative interactions and ambivalent bonds constitute a risk factor for adverse health outcomes.
- Spiritual practices, such as the frequent presence in ecclesiastical rituals, praying to a higher power, and the dependence on one's religious beliefs as a recourse and as a source of strength, are believed to have had a unique contribution to the health status of the Mediterranean populations.

- Spirituality is a lifelong guiding principle that may exert a positive impact on health. Firmly held values and principles have the potential to enhance incentives, abilities, and hope, and in this way, they can help people to confront disease states.
- Finding meaning and having a purpose in life can create a positive attitude toward health, which, in turn, can predispose to balanced health practices but also coping better with high-stress situations, including medical problems.
- Meditation is an ancient form of stress relief that has recently been accepted as a complementary practice in modern medical science. It results in alterations in human physiology associated with a decrease in stress and anxiety and has been associated with improvements in mental health in healthy and chronically ill individuals.

Self-Assessment Questions

1. Choose the correct statement:
   a. Conversation about unpleasant personal experiences with ambivalent friends may cause blood pressure levels to rise.
   b. Social wellness is defined as having many rich friends.
   c. Mediterranean populations are renowned for their openness and extroversion, character traits that are believed to have a negative impact on their health.
   d. Telomere length is regarded as a marker for the biological height of a person.
2. What are the proposed mechanisms for the favorable effect of social relationships and social integration on people's health?
3. Complete the sentences:
   a. Social control may affect _____.
   b. Within a dipole relationship, the right of one part is _____.
   c. High self-esteem is positively associated with _____.
   d. Perceived emotional support is strongly associated with _____.

4. Can a positive attitude help people improve their health?
5. What is meditation?
6. How is spirituality related to health?
7. Briefly discuss the conviviality aspect of the MedL.
8. Characterize the following statements as true (T) or false (F).
   a. As people age, they tend to be related to negative people or persons for whom they have uncertain feelings ( ).
   b. Human beings are by nature sociable; they tend to organize in communities whose structure embodies social interaction as an integral part of their lives ( ).
   c. Spiritual wellness is closely related to and interacts with intellectual and emotional wellness ( ).
   d. The sense of belonging that social interaction bestows may constitute a defense against health stressors ( ).
   e. Robust value systems allow people to consciously accept what happens to them and constructively manage adverse situations ( ).

Bibliography

Bruce, M.A., Norris, K.C., and Thorpe, R.J. Jr. (2020). Religious service attendance and despair among health professionals – a catalyst for new avenues of inquiry. *JAMA Psychiatry* 77 (7): 670–671.

Chen, Y., Koh, H.K., Kawachi, I. et al. (2020). Religious service attendance and deaths related to drugs, alcohol, and suicide among US health care professionals. *JAMA Psychiatry* 77 (7): 737–744.

Coyle, J. (2002). Spirituality and health: towards a framework for exploring the relationship between spirituality and health. *J. Adv. Nurs.* 37 (6): 589–597.

Cramer, H., Ward, L., Saper, R. et al. (2015). The safety of yoga: a systematic review and meta-analysis of randomized controlled trials. *Am. J. Epidemiol.* 182 (4): 281–293. doi: 10.1093/aje/kwv071

De Vogli, R., Chandola, T., and Marmot, M.G. (2007). Negative aspects of close relationships and heart disease. *Arch. Intern. Med.* 167 (18): 1951–1957.

Fiori, K.L., Windsor, T.D., Pearson, E.L., and Crisp, D.A. (2013). Can positive social exchanges buffer the detrimental effects of negative social exchanges? Age and gender differences. *Gerontology* 59 (1): 40–52.

Flatt, J.D., Hughes, T.F., Documet, P.I. et al. (2015). A qualitative study on the types and purposes of social activities in late life. *Act. Adapt. Aging* 39 (2): 109–132.

Goyal, M., Singh, S., Sibinga, E.M. et al. (2014). Meditation programs for psychological stress and well-being: a systematic review and meta-analysis. *JAMA Intern. Med.* 174 (3): 357–368.

Holt-Lunstad, J. and Clark, B.D. (2014). Social stressors and cardiovascular response: influence of ambivalent relationships and behavioral ambivalence. *Int. J. Psychophysiol.* 93 (3): 381–389.

Holt-Lunstad, J., Smith, T.W., and Uchino, B.N. (2008). Can hostility interfere with the health benefits of giving and receiving social support? The impact of cynical hostility on cardiovascular reactivity during social support interactions among friends. *Ann. Behav. Med.* 35 (3): 319–330.

Merom, D., Grunseit, A., Eramudugolla, R. et al. (2016). Cognitive benefits of social dancing and walking in old age: the dancing mind randomized controlled trial. *Front. Aging Neurosci.* 8: 26.

Pawlikowski, J., Bialowolski, P., Weziak-Bialowolska, D., and VanderWeele, T.J. (2019). Religious service attendance, health behaviors and well-being – an outcome-wide longitudinal analysis. *Eur. J. Public Health* 29 (6): 1177–1183.

Quilty, M.T., Saper, R.B., Goldstein, R. et al. (2013). Yoga in the real world: perceptions, motivators, barriers, and patterns of use. *Glob Adv Health Med*, 2(1), 44-49. doi: 10.7453/gahmj.2013.2.1.008

Sampaio, C.V., Lima, M.G., and Ladeia, A.M. (2017). Meditation, health and scientific investigations: review of the literature. *J. Relig. Health.* 56 (2): 411–427.

Saper, R.B. (2015). Minding the mat: moving the yoga field forward. *Glob. Adv. Health Med.* 4 (3): 5–6. doi: 10.7453/gahmj.2015.054.

Saper, R.B., Lemaster, C., Delitto, A. et al. Yoga, physical therapy, or education for chronic low back pain: a randomized noninferiority trial. *Ann. Intern. Med.* 167 (2): 85–94. doi: 10.7326/M16-2579.

Schneider, R.H., Grim, C.E., Rainforth, M.V. et al. (2012). Stress reduction in the secondary prevention of cardiovascular disease: randomized, controlled trial of transcendental meditation and health education in blacks. *Circ. Cardiovasc. Qual. Outcomes.* 5 (6): 750–758.

Sessanna, L., Finnell, D., and Jezewski, M.A. (2007). Spirituality in nursing and health-related literature: a concept analysis. *J. Holist. Nurs.* 25 (4): 252–262; discussion 263–264.

Spence, N.D., Farvid, M.S., Warner, E.T. et al. (2020). Religious service attendance, religious coping, and risk of hypertension in women participating in the Nurses' Health Study II. *Am. J. Epidemiol.* 189 (3): 193–203.

Stoewen, D.L. (2017). Dimensions of wellness: change your habits, change your life. *Can. Vet. J.* 58 (8): 861–862.

Thoits, P.A. (2011). Mechanisms linking social ties and support to physical and mental health. *J. Health Soc. Behav.* 52 (2): 145–161.

Uchino, B.N., Cawthon, R.M., Smith, T.W. et al. (2012). Social relationships and health: is feeling positive, negative, or both (ambivalent) about your social ties related to telomeres? *Health Psychol.* 31 (6): 789–796.

Uchino, B.N., Smith, T.W., Carlisle, M. et al. (2013). The quality of spouses' social networks contributes to each other's cardiovascular risk. *PLoS One* 8 (8): e71881.

Yang, Y.C., Boen, C., Gerken, K. et al. (2016). Social relationships and physiological determinants of longevity across the human life span. *Proc. Natl. Acad. Sci. U. S. A.* 113 (3): 578–583.

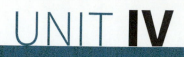

Mediterranean Lifestyle in Clinical Practice

UNIT IV

Mediterranean Lifestyle and Timeless
Recipes

Use of the Mediterranean Lifestyle Paradigm in the Prevention and Treatment of the Metabolic Syndrome

Definition and Health Burden of the Metabolic Syndrome

The metabolic syndrome (MetS) is a constellation of interconnected physiological, biochemical, clinical, and metabolic factors that directly increase the risk of several adverse health outcomes related to other NCDs. These factors include impaired glucose metabolism, hypertension, dyslipidemia, and obesity (particularly central or visceral adiposity) (Alberti et al. 2009). Results from epidemiological, experimental, and clinical studies suggest that these metabolic disorders, combined with insulin resistance, low-grade inflammation, and chronic oxidative stress, are involved in the pathogenesis of most, if not all, major modern chronic diseases, and their management is crucial for disease prevention. The associations, risk-factor clustering, and health implications of these individual disorders have been extensively studied for decades. Nowadays, it

> **Key Point**
>
> The metabolic syndrome (MetS) is a constellation of interconnected physiological, biochemical, clinical, and metabolic factors that directly increase the risk of several adverse health outcomes related to other NCDs.

> **Key Point**
>
> The MetS is a perilous condition with a rising prevalence worldwide, related to obesity, unhealthy diet, and sedentary lifestyle.

is widely accepted that the MetS is a perilous condition with a rising prevalence worldwide, related to obesity, unhealthy diet, and sedentary lifestyle.

Even though there is general agreement on the MetS as an important chronic condition that predisposes to various cardiometabolic diseases, disagreement still exists regarding the ideal diagnostic criteria or cutoffs for each metabolic component. Several definitions of the MetS have been proposed; in 1998 by a consultation group on the definition of diabetes for the WHO (Alberti and Zimmet 1998); in 2001 by the National Cholesterol Education Program Adult Treatment Panel III (National Cholesterol Education Program Expert Panel on Detection, Evaluation, and Treatment of High Blood Cholesterol in Adults, 2002); and in 2005 by the International Diabetes Federation (Alberti et al. 2005) and the American Heart Association/National Heart, Lung, and Blood Institute (Grundy et al. 2005). Finally, in 2009, six major health organizations, i.e., the International Diabetes Federation Task Force on Epidemiology and Prevention, the National Heart, Lung, and Blood Institute, the American Heart Association, the World Heart Federation, the International Atherosclerosis Society, and the International Association for the Study of Obesity, published a joint statement with updated criteria for the MetS to serve as universal tool for its diagnosis in clinical practice, public health, and research (Table 12.1) (Alberti et al. 2009).

According to the latest criteria, the presence of the MetS is defined as the coexistence of three or more of the five following components: (i) increased waist circumference, indicative of central obesity; (ii) increased fasting glucose levels, i.e., ≥100 mg/dl

Textbook of Lifestyle Medicine, First Edition. Labros S. Sidossis and Stefanos N. Kales.
© 2022 John Wiley & Sons Ltd. Published 2022 by John Wiley & Sons Ltd.

TABLE 12.1   Criteria for clinical diagnosis of the metabolic syndrome.

Measure	Categorical cut points
Elevated waist circumference[a]	Population- and country-specific definitions (Table 12.2)
Elevated TG (Drug treatment for elevated TG is an alternate indicator.[b])	≥150 mg/dL (1.7 mmol/L)
Reduced HDLC (Drug treatment for reduced HDLC is an alternate indicator.[b])	≤40 mg/dL (1.0 mmol/L) in males; ≤50 mg/dL (1.3 mmol/L) in females
Elevated blood pressure (Antihypertensive drug treatment in a patient with a history of hypertension is an alternate indicator.)	Systolic ≥130 and/or diastolic ≥85 mmHg
Elevated fasting glucose[c] (Drug treatment of elevated glucose is an alternate indicator.)	≥100 mg/dL (5.6 mmol/L)

HDLC, high-density lipoprotein cholesterol; TG, triglycerides.

[a] It is recommended that the International Diabetes Federation cut points be used for non-Europeans and either the International Diabetes Federation or American Heart Association/National Heart, Lung, and Blood Institute cut points be used for people of European origin until more data are available (see Table 12.2).

[b] The most commonly used drugs for elevated TG and reduced HDLC are fibrates and nicotinic acid. A patient taking one of these drugs can be presumed to have high TG and low HDLC. High-dose n-3 fatty acids presumes high TG.

[c] Most patients with type 2 diabetes mellitus will have the metabolic syndrome by the proposed criteria.

Source: Reprinted with permission from Alberti et al. (2009).

(≥5.6 mmol/l), use of antidiabetic medication, or presence of diabetes mellitus; (iii) decreased HDLC levels, i.e., ≤40 mg/dl (≤1.0 mmol/l) for males and ≤50 mg/dl (≤1.3 mmol/l) for females, or use of relevant medication; (iv) increased triglyceride levels, i.e., ≥150 mg/dl (≥1.7 mmol/l), or use of lipid-lowering medication; (v) hypertension, i.e., systolic/diastolic blood pressure ≥130/85 mmHg or use of antihypertensive medication. For all MetS components, a single set of cut points is used except waist circumference, for which population-specific cut points are recommended (Table 12.2) (Alberti et al. 2009).

Lifestyle Medicine in Chronic Disease Management

Given the close association between the MetS and NCDs, lifestyle interventions for the management of the MetS and its components are currently the subject of intense research and scientific debate, as well as one of the main goals of health policy in every country in the world (Castro-Barquero et al. 2020). Although genetics play a crucial role in almost all NCDs, important modifiable risk factors for the development of NCDs include lifestyle habits, such as tobacco use, physical inactivity, unhealthy diet, excess consumption of alcohol, and stress. It has been estimated that ~6 million deaths every year are attributed to tobacco use (including the effects of exposure to secondhand smoke), ~3 million to sedentariness, ~2 million to excessive drinking, and ~2 million to excess salt intake (Lim et al. 2012; Lozano et al. 2012; Mozaffarian et al. 2014; Murray and Lopez 2013). Hypertension, impaired glucose metabolism, hypercholesterolemia, and obesity – all important and intrerrelated components of the MetS – mediate much of the relationship between these lifestyle risk factors and the incidence of NCDs.

In the past, physicians often ignored patients' lifestyle choices, and medication was often the only suggested treatment. Only recently have clinicians started to evaluate basic lifestyle choices and prescribe lifestyle changes or refer their patients to other health professionals, such as dietitians-nutritionists, exercise specialists, psychologists, sleep experts, etc. The term *lifestyle medicine* has appeared in the scientific literature to describe the use of whole food, plant-predominant dietary patterns, regular physical activity, restorative sleep, stress management, avoidance of risky substances, and positive social connection as a primary therapeutic modality for the prevention, treatment, and reversal of chronic disease, in conjunction with available drug therapies and surgical procedures when indicated.

Since no one is specialized in all aspects of a person's life, treatment within the context of *lifestyle medicine* is usually provided by a multidisciplinary team of health professionals from many fields: medicine, nutrition, exercise, psychology, sleep, and others. In lifestyle medicine,

> **Key Point**
>
> Lifestyle interventions for the management of the MetS and its components are currently the subject of intense research and scientific debate.

> **Key Point**
>
> Important modifiable risk factors for the development of NCDs include lifestyle habits, such as tobacco use, physical inactivity, unhealthy diet, excess consumption of alcohol, and stress.

> **Key Point**
>
> The term *lifestyle medicine* has appeared in the scientific literature to describe the use of whole food, plant-predominant dietary patterns, regular physical activity, restorative sleep, stress management, avoidance of risky substances, and positive social connection as a primary therapeutic modality for the prevention, treatment, and reversal of chronic disease.

> **Key Point**
>
> In lifestyle medicine, patients are no longer a passive recipient of care but active partners who make decisions and assume responsibility for the changes that need to take place in their life to improve their health and wellness.

TABLE 12.2 Recommended waist circumference thresholds.

Population	Organization (reference)	Recommended waist circumference threshold for abdominal obesity (cm)	
		Men	**Women**
European	IDF (Grundy et al. 2005)	≥94	≥80
Caucasian	WHO (WHO 2000)	≥94 (increased risk) ≥102 (even higher risk)	≥80 (increased risk) ≥88 (even higher risk)
United States	AHA/NHLBI (ATP III[a]) (National Institutes of Health 1998)	≥102	≥88
Canada	Health Canada (Douketis et al. 2005; Khan et al. 2006)	≥102	≥88
European	European Cardiovascular Societies (Graham et al. 2007)	≥102	≥88
Asian (including Japanese)	IDF (Grundy et al. 2005)	≥90	≥80
Asian	WHO (Hara et al. 2006)	≥90	≥80
Japanese	Japanese Obesity Society (Examination Committee of Criteria for 'Obesity Disease' in Japan, Japan Society for the Study of Obesity 2002; Oka et al. 2008)	≥85	≥80
China	Cooperative Task Force (Zhou and Cooperative Meta-Analysis Group of the Working Group on Obesity in China 2002)	≥85	≥80
Middle East, Mediterranean	IDF (Grundy et al. 2005)	≥94	≥80
Sub-Saharan African	IDF (Grundy et al. 2005)	≥94	≥80
Ethnic Central and South American	IDF (Grundy et al. 2005)	≥90	≥80

AHA, American Heart Association; ATP, Adult Treatment Panel; IDF, International Diabetes Federation; NHLBI, National Heart, Lung, and Blood Institute; WHO, World Health Organization.

[a] Recent AHA/NHLBI guidelines for the metabolic syndrome recognize an increased risk for cardiovascular diseases and diabetes at waist circumference thresholds of ≥94 cm in men and ≥80 cm in women and identify these as optional cut points for individuals or populations with increased insulin resistance.

Source: Reprinted with permission from Alberti et al. (2009).

TABLE 12.3   Differences between conventional and lifestyle medicine approaches.

Conventional medicine	Lifestyle medicine
Treats individual risk factors.	Addresses poor lifestyle choices.
Patient is a passive recipient of care.	Patient is an active partner in care.
Patient is not required to make big changes.	Patient is required to make big changes.
Treatment is often short term.	Treatment is always long term.
Responsibility is on the clinician.	Responsibility is also on the patient.
Medication is often the "end" treatment.	Medication may be needed, but the emphasis is on lifestyle changes.
Emphasizes diagnosis and prescription.	Emphasizes motivation and compliance.
Goal is disease management.	Goal is primary/secondary/tertiary prevention and disease management.
Little consideration of environment.	Increased consideration of environment.
Side effects are balanced by the benefits.	Side effects are not common but require greater attention.
Involves other medical specialists.	Involves allied health professionals in addition to other medical specialists.
Doctor generally operates independently.	Doctor is part of a team.

Source: Adapted with permission from Egger et al. (2010).

patients are no longer passive recipients of care but active partners who make decisions and assume responsibility for the changes that need to take place in their life to improve their health and wellness. This can be achieved through a patient/client-centered counseling style, focused on increasing motivation, health efficacy, and health literacy, at a user-friendly practice environment with team care involvement (Phillips et al. 2020; Katz et al. 2018; Kent et al. 2016; Birrell et al. 2021). Table 12.3 lists the main differences between conventional medicine and lifestyle medicine (Egger et al. 2010).

In this unit, we will present examples of managing clinical conditions that belong to the MetS disease cluster using lifestyle medicine approaches. We will use the Mediterranean lifestyle paradigm, one of the most successful and studied healthy lifestyle patterns. The various components of the MetS will be presented as cases, providing a step-by-step description of the methods a clinician should use to evaluate all aspects of a patient's lifestyle. Following, we will provide comprehensive treatment protocols using lifestyle modifications pertinent to specific disorders. We hope that this will become a useful tool in the hands of clinicians when managing patients using lifestyle medicine as the first, and possibly most important, line of defense against NCDs, along with available medical, drug, and surgical treatments.

Take-Home Messages

- The MetS is a perilous condition that increases the risk of several adverse health outcomes related to NCDs and has a rising prevalence worldwide, related to obesity, unhealthy diet, and sedentary lifestyle.
- Although genetics play a crucial role in almost all NCDs, important modifiable risk factors also include lifestyle habits, such as tobacco use, physical inactivity, and unhealthy diet.
- Lifestyle interventions for the management of the MetS and its components are currently the subject of intense research and scientific debate.

- Conventional/traditional medicine emphasizes diagnosis, uses medications as the core treatment for diseases, and treats the patient as a passive recipient of care.
- Lifestyle medicine emphasizes beneficial lifestyle changes as a means to prevent and treat diseases, promotes patients' motivation and compliance, and is provided by a multidisciplinary team of health professionals, with the patient being an active partner.

Self-Assessment Questions

1. Describe the MetS and its relationship with NCDs.
2. What are the criteria for the diagnosis of the MetS?
3. Provide the definition of lifestyle medicine.
4. Discuss the differences between conventional and lifestyle medicine.

Bibliography

Alberti, K.G., Eckel, R.H., Grundy, S.M. et al. (2009). Harmonizing the metabolic syndrome: a joint interim statement of the International Diabetes Federation Task Force on Epidemiology and Prevention; National Heart, Lung, and Blood Institute; American Heart Association; World Heart Federation; International Atherosclerosis Society; and International Association for the Study of Obesity. *Circulation* 120 (16): 1640–1645. https://doi.org/10.1161/CIRCULATIONAHA.109.192644.

Alberti, K.G. and Zimmet, P.Z. (1998). Definition, diagnosis and classification of diabetes mellitus and its complications. Part 1: diagnosis and classification of diabetes mellitus provisional report of a WHO consultation. *Diabet. Med.* 15 (7): 539–553. https://doi.org/10.1002/(SICI)1096-9136(199807)15:7<539::AID-DIA668>3.0.CO;2-S.

Alberti, K.G., Zimmet, P., Shaw, J., and Group IDFETFC. (2005). The metabolic syndrome – a new worldwide definition. *Lancet* 366 (9491): 1059–1062. https://doi.org/10.1016/S0140-6736(05)67402-8.

Birrell, F.N., Pinder, R.J., and Lawson, R.J. (2021). Lifestyle medicine is no Trojan horse: it is an inclusive, evidence-based, and patient-focused movement. *Br. J. Gen. Pract.* 71 (708): 300. doi: 10.3399/bjgp21X716201.

Castro-Barquero, S., Ruiz-Leon, A.M., Sierra-Perez, M., Estruch, R., and Casas, R. (2020). Dietary strategies for metabolic syndrome: a comprehensive review. *Nutrients* 12 (10): 2983. doi: 10.3390/nu12102983

Douketis, J.D., Paradis, G., Keller, H., and Martineau, C. (2005). Canadian guidelines for body weight classification in adults: application in clinical practice to screen for overweight and obesity and to assess disease risk. *CMAJ* 172 (8): 995–998. https://doi.org/10.1503/cmaj.045170.

Egger, G., Binns, A., and Rossner, S. (2010). *Managing Diseases of Lifestyle in the 21st Century*. New York: McGraw-Hill.

Examination Committee of Criteria for "Obesity Disease" in Japan, Japan Society for the Study of Obesity. (2002). New criteria for "obesity disease" in Japan. *Circ. J.* 66 (11): 987–992. https://doi.org/10.1253/circj.66.987.

Graham, I., Atar, D., Borch-Johnsen, K. et al. (2007). European guidelines on cardiovascular disease prevention in clinical practice: executive summary. *Atherosclerosis* 194 (1): 1–45. https://doi.org/10.1016/j.atherosclerosis.2007.08.024.

Grundy, S.M., Cleeman, J.I., Daniels, S.R. et al. (2005). Diagnosis and management of the metabolic syndrome: an American Heart Association/National Heart, Lung, and Blood Institute scientific statement. *Circulation* 112 (17): 2735–2752. https://doi.org/10.1161/CIRCULATIONAHA.105.169404.

Hara, K., Matsushita, Y., Horikoshi, M. et al. (2006). A proposal for the cutoff point of waist circumference for the diagnosis of metabolic syndrome in the Japanese population. *Diabetes Care* 29 (5): 1123–1124. https://doi.org/10.2337/diacare.2951123.

Katz, D.L., Frates, E.P., Bonnet, J.P., Gupta, S.K., Vartiainen, E., and Carmona, R.H. (2018). Lifestyle as medicine: the case for a true health initiative. *Am. J. Health Promot.* 32 (6): 1452–1458. doi: 10.1177/0890117117705949

Kent, K., Johnson, J.D., Simeon, K., and Frates, E.P. (2016). Case series in lifestyle medicine: a team approach to behavior changes. *Am. J. Lifestyle Med.* 10 (6): 388–397. doi: 10.1177/1559827616638288.

Khan, N.A., McAlister, F.A., Rabkin, S.W. et al. (2006). The 2006 Canadian Hypertension Education Program recommendations for the management of hypertension: part II – therapy. *Can. J. Cardiol.* 22 (7): 583–593. https://doi.org/10.1016/s0828-282x(06)70280-x.

Lim, S.S., Vos, T., Flaxman, A.D. et al. (2012). A comparative risk assessment of burden of disease and injury attributable to 67 risk factors and risk factor clusters in 21 regions, 1990-2010: a systematic analysis for the Global Burden of Disease Study 2010. *Lancet* 380 (9859): 2224–2260. https://doi.org/10.1016/S0140-6736(12)61766-8.

Lozano, R., Naghavi, M., Foreman, K. et al. (2012). Global and regional mortality from 235 causes of death for 20 age groups in 1990 and 2010: a systematic analysis for the Global Burden of Disease Study 2010. *Lancet* 380 (9859): 2095–2128. https://doi.org/10.1016/S0140-6736(12)61728-0.

Mozaffarian, D., Fahimi, S., Singh, G.M. et al. (2014). Global sodium consumption and death from cardiovascular causes. *N. Engl. J. Med.* 371 (7): 624–634. https://doi.org/10.1056/NEJMoa1304127.

Murray, C.J. and Lopez, A.D. (2013). Measuring the global burden of disease. *N. Engl. J. Med.* 369 (5): 448–457. https://doi.org/10.1056/NEJMra1201534.

National Cholesterol Education Program Expert Panel on Detection, Evaluation, and Treatment of High Blood Cholesterol in Adults. (2002). Third report of the National Cholesterol Education Program (NCEP) expert panel on detection, evaluation, and treatment of high blood cholesterol in adults (adult treatment panel III) final report. *Circulation* 106 (25): 3143–3421.

National Institutes of Health. (1998). Clinical guidelines on the identification, evaluation, and treatment of overweight and obesity in adults – the evidence report. *Obes. Res.* 6 (Suppl 2): 51S–209S.

Oka, R., Kobayashi, J., Yagi, K. et al. (2008). Reassessment of the cutoff values of waist circumference and visceral fat area for identifying Japanese subjects at risk for the metabolic syndrome. *Diabetes Res. Clin. Pract.* 79 (3): 474–481. https://doi.org/10.1016/j.diabres.2007.10.016.

Phillips, E.M., Frates, E.P., and Park, D.J. (2020). Lifestyle medicine. *Phys. Med. Rehabil. Clin. N. Am.* 31 (4): 515–526. doi: 10.1016/j.pmr.2020.07.006.

World Health Organization. (2000). *Obesity: Preventing and Managing the Global Epidemic*, vol. 894: i–xii, 1–253. Geneva: Report of a WHO Consultation. World Health Organ Tech Rep Ser.

Zhou, B.F. and Cooperative Meta-Analysis Group of the Working Group on Obesity in China. (2002). Predictive values of body mass index and waist circumference for risk factors of certain related diseases in Chinese adults – study on optimal cut-off points of body mass index and waist circumference in Chinese adults. *Biomed. Environ. Sci.* 15 (1): 83–96.

CHAPTER 13

Obesity Case Study

Mrs. CK is a 52-year-old perimenopausal woman who recently visited her primary care physician (PCP) for an annual checkup; she was referred to you for lifestyle evaluation and consultation. She is married, she has a 16-year-old son and a 7-year-old daughter, and she works as a secretary for a law firm. Mrs. CK had no prior history of chronic disease and was found healthy at her last medical evaluation. However, she has been complaining of knee pain for the past 12 months, and her PCP advised her to "lose some weight." She has a family history of T2DM and hypertension. Mrs. CK has a sedentary lifestyle, does not smoke, and drinks small amounts of alcohol on special occasions. Her current body weight is 95.3 kg, height 1.67 m, waist circumference 97.5 cm, and blood pressure 128/86 mmHg.

Assessment

Assessment of Anthropometry

According to the WHO, obesity is defined as a chronic disease involving the excessive accumulation of fat in the body, which poses health risks and leads to a reduced life expectancy (WHO 2000). In clinical practice, the diagnosis of obesity is based on simple anthropometric measurements, i.e., body weight and height, which should be part of almost all medical and health encounters, especially routine health examinations and assessments of chronic disease. Accurate body weight and height measurements are crucial for the assessment of an overweight/ obese patient and can be performed as follows: body weight should be measured to the nearest 100 g with a digital scale placed on a hard, flat surface, with the patients standing on the center of the scale without support, wearing light clothing and being barefoot, with their arms hanging loosely by their sides, head facing forward, and weight distributed evenly on both feet. Although dry body weight (morning body weight after an overnight fast) is the most accurate measurement, this cannot always be achieved in clinical practice. In this case, measuring a patient's body weight under similar conditions is important when repeated measurements are obtained. Height can be measured with a stadiometer to the nearest 0.5 cm at the end of normal expiration, with the patient's weight equally distributed on both feet; head, upper back, buttocks, calves, and heels on the vertical line of the stadiometer; and head placed in the Frankfort horizontal plane, i.e., the position of the head when the upper margin of the ear openings and the lower margin of the eye orbit are horizontal and parallel to the ground.

Based on weight and height measurements, the BMI of a patient can be calculated as (weight [kg] ÷ height^2 [m^2]). BMI is an easy, quick, and practical estimate of adiposity in adults, which correlates well with both body fat and health risks (morbidity and mortality risk). BMI is widely used in clinical practice to provide a rough assessment of body composition status, based on which a clinical decision for body weight change can be made. The official classification of BMI values according to the WHO is presented in Table 13.1 (Stegenga et al. 2014). BMI values ≥25 kg/m^2 and ≥30 kg/m^2 classify an individual in the category of overweight and obesity, respectively. It is also worth noting that in addition to the assessment of body weight status, BMI provides an estimate of the morbidity risk associated with excessive body weight; it is the main index used in clinical practice and epidemiology for anthropometric evaluation. As shown in Table 13.1, the risk of morbidity increases gradually, as the values of the BMI increase beyond their normal range, with individuals classified as obese class III, i.e., with BMI values ≥40 kg/m^2, being at extremely high risk of health complications associated with excessive body weight compared to normal-weight individuals (Stegenga et al. 2014).

> **Key Point**
>
> Obesity is defined as a chronic disease involving the excessive accumulation of fat in the body, which poses health risks and leads to a reduced life expectancy.

> **Key Point**
>
> BMI is an easy, quick, and practical estimate of adiposity in adults, which correlates well with both body fat and health risks.

TABLE 13.1 **Classification of BMI values in adults.**

Classification	BMI (kg/m²)	Morbidity risk[a]
Underweight	<18.5	Increased
Healthy	18.5–24.9	Reference category
Overweight	25.0–29.9	Maybe increased for BMI > 28
Obesity I	30.0–34.9	Increased – high
Obesity II	35.0–39.9	Very high
Obesity III	≥40.0	Extremely high

[a] Compared to the healthy weight group.
Source: Adapted with permission from Stegenga et al. (2014).

Mrs. CK currently weighs 95.3 kg and her height is 1.67 m. Her BMI is 95.3 kg ÷ (1.67 m)² = 34.17 kg/m². According to the classification of BMI values, she is considered obese class I and has a high risk of morbidity associated with excessive body weight.

Although BMI-defined obesity is accurate in detecting excess adiposity and predicting adverse health outcomes in most cases, BMI should be interpreted with caution because it is not a direct measure of adiposity; i.e., it cannot distinguish whether a patient has increased body weight due to increased fat mass or increased lean (bone and muscle) mass. This limitation makes its use problematic in some population groups, such as athletes, who may be mistakenly classified as overweight or obese due to increased muscle mass. For example, two people with the same height and weight, and therefore same BMI, may have very different phenotypes; one may be a weight lifter with high amounts of muscle mass and the other a sedentary obese person with high amounts of fat mass. Other groups of the population in which BMI should be used with caution are patients with liver, heart, or kidney diseases who may present a fictitiously increased body mass due to fluid retention; the elderly, who often present with reduced lean body mass due to a phenomenon called sarcopenia (involuntary decrease in muscle mass and strength); and people with very short stature. Moreover, in some groups of patients, such as those with heart failure and chronic kidney disease, BMI and mortality rate appear to have a U-shaped relationship. In these diseases, which are accompanied by a malnutrition state, a low BMI may reflect a severely reduced lean body mass; in these cases, BMI values in the categories of overweight and obesity class I are associated with lower mortality rates.

Given the limitations of BMI, the anthropometric evaluation of obese patients should also include the measurement of waist circumference (WC), as it provides a rough estimate of the body's abdominal fat stores. This is very important because central fat accumulation (abdominal adiposity) is a significant risk factor for cardiovascular and metabolic diseases and can

> **Key Point**
>
> BMI should be interpreted with caution because it is not a direct measure of adiposity.

better predict health risk compared to total body fat. WC should ideally be measured to the nearest 0.1 cm between the lowest rib and the superior border of the iliac crest at the end of normal expiration, using an inelastic measuring tape positioned parallel to the floor and with the patient standing. When the abovementioned anatomic points are hard to distinguish, the maximum WC in the abdomen can be measured instead. According to the guidelines of the WHO for Caucasians, WC values >94 cm (men) and >80 cm (women) are considered high, while values >102 cm (men) and >88 cm (women) are considered very high. Although WC and BMI are strongly correlated, WC is an independent predictor of morbidity risk. Table 13.2 shows the risk of morbidity of an individual based on the combined use of BMI and WC values (Stegenga et al. 2014). WC measurements are particularly useful in individuals who are categorized as overweight or obese class I based on their BMI; in these individuals, increased WC values are associated with increased cardiometabolic risk. As shown in Table 13.2, a patient who according to BMI is classified as obese class I is at increased risk of morbidity when WC is within desired levels, high risk when WC is high, and very high risk when WC is very high. However, for patients classified as obese class II or higher, i.e., BMI values of ≥35 kg/m², WC does not

> **Key Point**
>
> The anthropometric evaluation of obese patients should also include the measurement of waist circumference, as it provides a rough estimate of the body's abdominal fat stores.

> **Key Point**
>
> Central fat accumulation (abdominal adiposity) is a significant risk factor for cardiovascular and metabolic diseases and can better predict health risk compared to total body fat.

> **Key Point**
>
> Although WC and BMI are strongly correlated, WC is an independent predictor of morbidity risk.

TABLE 13.2 **Morbidity risk according to BMI and WC values.**

BMI category	Morbidity risk		
	Low WC[a]	High WC[a]	Very high WC[a]
Overweight	Not increased	Increased	High
Obesity I	Increased	High	Very high
Obesity II	Very high	Very high	Very high
Obesity III	Extremely high	Extremely high	Extremely high

BMI, body mass index; WC, waist circumference.
[a] For men, WC <94 cm is considered normal, 94–102 cm is considered high, and >102 cm is considered very high. For women, WC <80 cm is considered normal, 80–88 cm is considered high, and >88 cm is considered very high.
Source: Reprinted with permission from Stegenga et al. (2014).

add to morbidity risk, and its measurement is not expected to provide important additional information beyond those attained by measuring only the BMI (Stegenga et al. 2014).

Mrs. CK has a WC of 97.5 cm, which is considered very high. According to the combined evaluation of her BMI (obesity class I) and WC values, she is at a very high morbidity risk.

Once the diagnosis of obesity is established, a history describing the fluctuations of the patient's body weight over time is also important. Obtaining body weight history allows for the exploration of the causes of the increased weight and leads to better, individualized treatment plans that are more in line with the patient's needs. The body weight history should record the minimum and maximum body weight in adulthood, the identification of critical periods and events that led to overweight, and a history of previous weight-loss efforts (Seagle et al. 2009). An easy way to get all of the necessary information is to ask the patient to draw a graph of important changes in body weight during adulthood and note the facts/events that correlate with increases or decreases in body weight, which are usually accompanied by significant changes in lifestyle habits. Figure 13.1 shows a common body weight fluctuation pattern associated with life events (Kushner 2012). In many patients, weight gain is triggered or accelerated by smoking cessation, starting a medication, or a stressful event, such as a change in marital or occupational status, the death of a loved one, and the diagnosis of a disease. For women, events that increase the risk of excess weight gain also include pregnancy and menopause. Accordingly, decreases in body weight of an overweight/obese patient usually indicate past weight-loss

> **Key Point**
>
> Obtaining body weight history allows for the exploration of the causes of increased weight and leads to better, individualized treatment plans that are more in line with the patient's needs.

efforts; in this case, it is important to evaluate the means by which weight loss was achieved (e.g., diet, exercise, medication, collaboration with a health professional, etc.) and the degree of weight-loss maintenance (successful maintenance or weight regain).

After discussing the body weight history with Mrs. CK, you recorded the following information: Mrs. CK weighed 62–65 kg as a young adult, and her weight fluctuated only during holidays when she usually gained a few kg but then easily returned to her pre-holiday weight within 1–2 weeks. She got married when she was 30 years old and gradually started gaining some weight due to long working hours until the age of 36, when she had her first child. However, after the pregnancy, she was unable to lose 10 kg out of a total of 15 kg that she gained during pregnancy. At the age of 40, she weighed ~80 kg and at the age of 45 she got pregnant again, gained a total of 18 kg, and was able to lose only 5 kg postpartum. Ever since, her usual body weight is ~90 kg and she has been struggling with weight-loss diets that she follows without medical supervision. At the time of evaluation, Mrs. CK reported gaining 4 kg during the last 2 months after quitting a fad very-low-carbohydrate diet that she found on the internet and followed for ~1 month.

Body Composition Assessment

Based on the definition of obesity, it is clear that it is the excess body fat, usually ≥25% of total weight in men and ≥32% in women, rather than an overall increased body mass that is associated with negative health effects. Given that BMI is an estimate of the total body mass, body composition analysis can be used to assess specific components of the human body (e.g., body fat, lean body mass, and muscle mass). Several methods of body composition analysis are available, which are continuously being modified in order to optimize the accuracy, validity, and repeatability of body fat assessment. The most commonly used methods are bioelectrical impedance analysis (BIA) and the latest multi-frequency bioelectrical spectroscopy (BIS) mode, techniques based on isotope dilution, hydrodensitometry or underwater weighing, air displacement plethysmography (ADP), dual-energy X-ray absorptiometry (DEXA), computed tomography (CT), magnetic resonance imaging (MRI), magnetic resonance spectroscopy (MRS), and some advanced forms of 3D photon scanning. Table 13.3 provides a brief overview of the available body composition assessment methods. Overall, depending on the method, body composition analysis allows the estimation or the calculation of total lean body mass, muscle mass, bone tissue, total body water, extracellular and intracellular water, total body fat mass and its individual compartments, such as the subcutaneous, visceral,

> **Key Point**
>
> Body composition analysis can be used to assess specific components of the human body (e.g., increased body fat, suboptimal muscle mass).

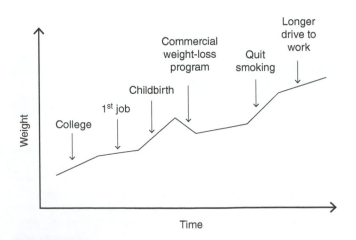

FIGURE 13.1 Lifestyle events–body weight graph. Patients are asked to mark life events that have contributed to current weight. This patient has experienced a progressive weight gain that has recently been accelerated by smoking cessation and longer driving to work. **Source:** Adapted with permission from Kushner (2012).

TABLE 13.3 Overview of body composition assessment methods.

Method	Measurements	Advantages	Disadvantages
Bioelectrical impedance/spectroscopy	Total, extracellular, and intracellular water	↓ cost, portable, simple, quick, safe	Depends on population-specific equations, ↓ precision
Isotope dilution techniques	Total and extracellular water	Applicable in all ages, easy provision of isotopes	↓ precision in some diseases, expensive equipment, ↑ analyses burden
Hydrodensitometry/underwater weighing	Body weight, body density, residual lung volume	Relatively ↑ precision, relatively ↓ cost	Difficult application (especially in obese individuals)
Air displacement plethysmography	Total body volume, total water	Wide age range, relatively ↑ precision, quick	↓ precision in some diseases, expensive, massive equipment
Dual-energy X-ray absorptiometry	Total/segmental fat and lean body mass, bone mass and density	↓ radiation, valid assessment of fat and lean mass of extremities	↑ error (obesity), expensive equipment, specialized personnel
Computed tomography	Segmental fat mass	↑ precision and repeatability	↑ cost, ↑ radiation
Magnetic resonance imaging/spectroscopy	Total/segmental fat body mass, muscle mass, liver fat	↑ precision and repeatability for total and segmental body fat mass	↑ cost, ↑ assessment time

Source: Adapted with permission from Lee and Gallagher (2008).

and intramuscular adipose tissue, as well as the fat deposited in or around various organs, such as the liver or the kidneys (Duren et al. 2008; Ellis 2000; Lee and Gallagher 2008).

All body composition analysis methods are characterized by limitations, most notably high cost and requirements for specialized medical facilities, due to the need for special equipment and experienced personnel. With the exception of BIA, which is affordable and simple to use, these limitations make the use of other methods unrealistic in daily clinical practice. In addition, almost all available methods are characterized by additional limitations in obese patients. For example, all methods have used assumptions about the density of body tissues and their water and electrolyte content. However, these assumptions may not apply to obese and other types of patients, in whom various metabolic and hormonal disorders alter the distribution and ratio of water and electrolytes in the various tissues of the body; therefore, the validity of the methods based on such assumptions, such as BIA and isotope dilution techniques, is limited. Moreover, estimating body composition is difficult in obese individuals due to their increased body volume, which may exceed the permissible limits of the available equipment, such as DEXA, CT, and MRI, or make it difficult for patients to undergo the assessment, as is the case with hydrodensitometry and ADP. Finally, to date, there are no formal criteria that correlate the results of body composition

assessment with health risks, or formal recommendations that suggest specific treatment protocols based on them. Therefore, body composition assessment is used primarily for research purposes and not as part of the routine evaluation and follow-up of an obese patient in clinical practice (Duren et al. 2008; Ellis 2000; Lee and Gallagher 2008). Out of all available techniques, BIA is the most convenient, as it is portable, has a relatively low cost, and offers important information on body composition in certain groups of patients, e.g., those with both high body and muscle mass and those who are classified as overweight according to their BMI but have a proportionally high fat mass due to low muscle mass. BIA is also clinically useful for helping patients to focus on changes in lean body mass and fat mass instead of total body weight.

> **Key Point**
> All body composition analysis methods are characterized by limitations, most notably high cost and requirements for specialized medical facilities.

> **Key Point**
> From all available techniques, BIA is the most convenient, as it is portable, has a relatively low cost, and offers important information on body composition in certain groups of patients.

Clinical Assessment and Physical Examination

Obese patients are at an increased risk to develop a plethora of diseases, including insulin resistance and T2DM, hypertension, dyslipidemia, cardiovascular disease (coronary heart disease and left ventricular hypertrophy/cardiomegaly), stroke, some types of cancer, obstructive sleep apnea, gallbladder disease, hyperuricemia and gout, and osteoarthritis. A thorough medical history, a review of symptoms, and a physical examination represent a rough, albeit easy and inexpensive way to screen for medical conditions, and should be performed in all obese individuals before any kind of intervention is designed and implemented. Table 13.4 presents a review of common clinical and physical examination findings (Barlow and Expert 2007).

History and physical examination alone cannot effectively screen for many conditions, such as dyslipidemia and T2DM. Therefore, these conditions must be identified with appropriate laboratory tests. Table 13.5 summarizes typical laboratory assessments performed on overweight/obese patients (Krebs et al. 2007). The results of the history, physical examination, and laboratory tests may suggest the need for additional diagnostic tests.

Drug-induced weight gain should always be considered when there is a change in body weight coincident with starting a new medication. Medications that are associated with weight gain include neuroleptics (thioridazine, haloperidol, olanzapine, quetiapine, risperidone, and clozapine), antidepressants (amitriptyline, nortriptyline, imipramine, doxepin, phenelzine, paroxetine, and mirtazapine), anticonvulsants (valproate, carbamazepine, and gabapentin), antidiabetic drugs (insulin, sulfonylureas, and thiazolidinediones), antihistamines (cyproheptadine), β- and α-adrenergic blockers (propranolol and doxazosin), and steroid hormones (contraceptives, glucocorticoids, and progestational steroids) (Kushner and Ryan 2014).

TABLE 13.4 Findings on clinical/physical assessment and possible causes/explanations.

	Findings	Possible causes
Symptoms	Anxiety, social isolation, insomnia	Depression
	Shortness of breath, exercise intolerance	Asthma, lack of physical conditioning, body habitus
	Snoring, daytime sleepiness and fatigue	Obstructive sleep apnea, obesity hypoventilation syndrome
	Abdominal pain	Gastroesophageal reflux disease, constipation, gallbladder disease, nonalcoholic fatty liver disease
	Hip pain, knee pain, walking pain	Slipped capital femoral epiphysis, musculoskeletal stress from weight (may be barrier to physical activity)
	Irregular menses	Polycystic ovary syndrome
	Polyphagia, polyuria, polydipsia	Type 2 diabetes mellitus
Signs	Elevated blood pressure	Hypertension
	Acanthosis nigricans	Common in obese individuals, especially when skin is dark; insulin resistance
	Excessive acne, hirsutism	Polycystic ovary syndrome
	Skin irritation, inflammation	Consequence of severe obesity
	Tonsillar hypertrophy	Obstructive sleep apnea
	Goiter	Hypothyroidism
	Wheezing	Asthma (may explain or contribute to exercise intolerance)
	Abdominal tenderness	Gastroesophageal reflux disorder, gallbladder disease, nonalcoholic fatty liver disease
	Hepatomegaly	Nonalcoholic fatty liver disease

Source: Adapted with permission from Barlow and Expert (2007).

TABLE 13.5 Laboratory assessments to be considered in obese patients.

Disease/disorder	Assessments
Dyslipidemia	Lipidemic profile (total cholesterol, low-density lipoprotein cholesterol, high-density lipoprotein cholesterol and triglycerides)
Cardiac disease	Electro/echocardiography; high-sensitivity C-reactive protein
Hypertension	24-h ambulatory blood pressure monitoring, echocardiography
Nonalcoholic fatty liver disease	Liver enzymes, liver ultrasonography
Hypothyroidism	Serum thyroid-stimulating hormone
Diabetes mellitus	Fasting glucose, glycated hemoglobin and urinary microalbumin or microalbumin/creatinine ratio
Sleep apnea	Polysomnography (home or in-lab sleep study), resting oxygen saturation
Orthopedic disease	Radiographs as indicated by history and physical examination
Hirsutism and oligomenorrhea	Plasma 17-hydroxyprogesterone, plasma dehydroepiandrosterone, androstenedione, testosterone, and free testosterone, luteinizing hormone and follicle stimulation hormone measurements

Source: Adapted with permission from Barlow and Expert (2007).

Mrs. CK has no history of chronic disease and was found otherwise healthy during the medical check-up a month ago. For the past year, she has been complaining of knee pain, possibly due to musculoskeletal stress from excess weight; her PCP referred her to you for lifestyle modification. For the last 6 months, she has also been experiencing hot flashes, night sweats, and mood changes, possibly related to menopause. In her latest blood work, the following assessments were performed: glucose 88 mg/dl, total cholesterol 198 mg/dl, HDL-cholesterol 38 mg/dl, LDL-cholesterol 141 mg/dl, and triglycerides 92 mg/dl. All values were within or close to the normal range. Her echocardiogram and upper abdominal ultrasound were normal. Mrs. CK has taken paroxetine on a daily basis since the age of 45 due to postpartum depression that persists to date. Paroxetine is a commonly prescribed antidepressant associated with weight gain. Substitution with a weight-neutral/lowering medication, e.g., fluoxetine, should be considered.

Dietary Assessment

Dietary assessment is a fundamental part of the assessment of every obese patient. Dietary assessment can be performed using a variety of tools, depending on the level of information that the health professional wants to obtain. An overview of the available tools for dietary assessment at an individual level is presented in Table 13.6 (Shim et al. 2014; Thompson and Byers 1994).

> **Key Point**
>
> Dietary assessment is a fundamental part of the assessment of every obese patient.

When choosing a dietary assessment method, a health professional must answer the following questions: Do I need information about nutrients, foods, food groups, other food constituents, or specific dietary behaviors? Is a qualitative or quantitative dietary assessment needed? What level of accuracy is desirable? What is the time period of interest? What are the constraints in terms of time and respondent characteristics? All available dietary assessment tools are characterized by strengths and weaknesses, as summarized in Table 13.7 (Thompson and Subar 2013). The 24-hour recall (provided in Appendix D.1) and the food record provide detailed information about the foods and beverages consumed and the patient's eating habits. However, 24-hour recalls are largely based on the patient's short-term memory and are therefore characterized by recall errors, especially in older individuals with impaired cognitive function. On the other hand, food records have a high burden for patients (require measurements and calculations) and can lead to changes in dietary behavior, as patients tend to present a more balanced diet, a fact that limits the ability to assess the actual dietary intake. Food frequency questionnaires (provided in Appendix D.2) are mostly used in research and have a limited value in clinical practice, because they are time-consuming and assess long-term dietary habits in a qualitative or a semiquantitative way; in most cases, a short diet history or a brief tool is preferable for the assessment of long-term dietary habits and diet quality.

In clinical practice, a short diet history can assess long-term dietary habits of a patient and identify behaviors that are linked to specific dietary problems. The short diet history should focus on the frequency of consumption of basic food groups (e.g., fruits, vegetables, legumes, grains, fish, white and red meat, fats and oils),

> **Key Point**
>
> A short diet history can assess long-term dietary habits of a patient and identify behaviors that are linked to specific dietary problems.

TABLE 13.6   Overview of dietary assessment methods.

Diet history	Dietary history is any dietary assessment that asks the respondent to report about past diet. It can vary in content and structure and usually refers to dietary assessment methods that ascertain a person's usual food intake. Details about characteristics of commonly consumed foods are assessed in addition to the frequency and amount of food consumed.
24-h dietary recall	The respondent is asked to remember and report all the meals consumed in the past 24 hours, the location and conditions for each meal, and exact quantities and cooking methods for each food/beverage. The recall is typically conducted by a personal interview, either in print or in a computer-assisted form. For the evaluation of typical dietary habits ≥2 recalls are needed. A model 24-h dietary recall is provided in Appendix D.1.
Dietary record	The respondent records the foods/beverages and the amount of each consumed over a period of several days. The amounts consumed may be measured with a food scale or household measuring devices (such as cups, tablespoons, etc.) or estimated, using models or pictures. Typically, the consumption of foods/beverages over 3–4 consecutive days is recorded.
Food frequency questionnaire	The respondent is asked to report the usual frequency of consumption of each food from a list of foods for a specific period (usually ≥1 month). Only information on frequency and sometimes quantity from a list of foods is collected, with little detail on other characteristics of the foods, such as cooking methods or the combinations of foods in meals. A validated 69-item food frequency questionnaire (Bountziouka et al. 2012) is provided in Appendix D.2.
Brief tools	They are useful in cases that do not require either assessment of the total diet or quantitative accuracy in dietary estimates. Such methods can be simplified food frequency questionnaires that assess the quality of the diet, e.g., tools that evaluate adherence to the healthy Mediterranean diet, or may focus on specific eating behaviors and dietary characteristics (e.g., calcium intake). Two validated tools to assess adherence to the Mediterranean diet, i.e., the Mediterranean Diet Score (Panagiotakos et al. 2006) and the 14-item Mediterranean Diet Adherence Screener (Martinez-Gonzalez et al. 2004; Schroder et al. 2011), are provided in Appendices D.3 and D.4.

TABLE 13.7   Characteristics of dietary assessment methods.

		24-h dietary recall	Food record	Food frequency questionnaire	Diet history	Brief instruments
Type of information	Food description	x	x	x	x	x
	Meal information	x	x		x	
Dietary approach	Total diet	x (>1 day)	x	x	x	
	Specific components					x
Time interval	Short-term	x	x		x	
	Long-term			x	x	x
Cognitive requirements	Measurement and recording		x			
	Memory (short-term)	x			x	
	Ability of generalization in the past			x	x	x
Potential for reactivity (change in dietary behavior)			x			
Assessment time	<15 mins	x			x	x
	>15 mins		x	x	x	

Source: Adapted with permission from Thompson and Subar (2013).

typical meal patterns (e.g., breakfast consumption, number of meals per day, snacks throughout the day, nibbling, etc.), food preferences, allergies and intolerances, as well as the use of dietary supplements. Other dietary behaviors and characteristics that are linked to obesity and can potentially be targets to dietary intervention (consumption of energy-dense foods, such as sweets, salty snacks, sugar-sweetened beverages and fast food, water intake, alcohol consumption, emotional eating, typical portion sizes, meal conditions, etc.) should also be evaluated.

After interviewing Mrs. CK about her dietary habits, you recorded the following information: Mrs. CK tries to cook as healthy as possible at home for her family, but she spends too much time at the office. For breakfast, she usually has a cup of coffee at work, along with any snack available at the office, such as cookies, pretzels, or breadsticks. For lunch, she consumes whatever she can find at a canteen near her work, and although she tries to make healthy choices, she admits consuming baked goods and pastries on most days of the week. The only meal she eats at home is dinner; she usually cooks chicken 2 times/week, red meat (usually pork) 2 times/week, fish 1 time/week, and pasta 2 times/week. For cooking she uses butter or margarine, depending on the recipe. After dinner she always has an urge for dessert; she particularly enjoys commercial sweets with chocolate. Fruits are not part of her daily diet, and she reports consuming ~3–4 fruits/week, usually as a snack at the office. She is not fond of whole grains and legumes and avoids certain types of vegetables, such as eggplants, peas, and cabbage, because she believes that they cause her abdominal bloating and distension. She usually drinks 2 cups of coffee with sugar per day and avoids sugar-sweetened beverages, such as packaged fruit juices and regular soda. She does not report any food allergies.

In addition to the diet history, a representative 24-hour dietary recall (provided in Appendix D.1) is also a useful tool for the estimation of daily meal patterns, energy intake, and macronutrient and micronutrient intake using algorithms or specialized nutrition software. The dietary recall can be obtained using the three-pass approach (Jonnalagadda et al. 2000). The patient is first asked to provide a quick list of all foods and beverages consumed during the past 24 hours (first pass). Then, starting with the first food item, the interviewer probes for details on all of the foods consumed, including the exact types, amounts, additions/toppings, preparation methods and meal conditions, such as place of consumption, eating alone or with company, and parallel activities (second pass). The final pass of the interview includes a review of all foods, giving the patient and the interviewer the opportunity to correct any information that is inaccurate or to add data that were previously ignored (third pass). To facilitate an accurate portion size evaluation, patients can be asked to report quantities of individual foods and beverages consumed using typical household objects as measuring devices (e.g., teaspoons, tablespoons, tea cups, etc.) and other commonly known items and size approximations (e.g., matchbox, cell phone, card deck, hand palm, etc.).

> **Key Point**
>
> A representative 24-hour dietary recall is also a useful tool for the estimation of daily meal patterns, energy intake, and macronutrient and micronutrient intake.

It must be noted that underreporting of dietary intake is common among obese patients. The term *underreporting* refers to the tendency of some people to report a lower dietary intake compared to the actual one. This phenomenon is apparent in ~25% of the general population; however, it is much more common in obese people, and especially women, the elderly, and individuals of low socioeconomic status. Most people usually underreport snacks consumed between main meals and foods and beverages that are high in carbohydrates (Braam et al. 1998; Murakami and Livingstone 2015).

In the context of the 24-hour dietary recall (Appendix D.1), Mrs. CK described the consumption of foods and beverages of the previous day as follows:
Breakfast: 1 cup of instant coffee with 2 teaspoons of sugar and 2–3 cinnamon cookies
Snack: 1 cup of instant coffee with 2 teaspoons of sugar and 1 banana
Lunch: 1 cheese pie and 1 chocolate croissant
Dinner: 200 g of roasted chicken with 1 cup of roasted potatoes, 1 cup of green salad with ~2 tablespoons of olive oil, 60 g of white cheese, and 2 slices of white bread
Late evening snack: 1 big slice of chocolate cake

Physical Activity Assessment

Physical activity assessment is a crucial part of the overall assessment of an obese patient. Low levels of physical activity, combined with a sedentary lifestyle, have been associated with both weight gain and regain after weight loss. Physical activity assessment can be performed using a variety of tools, depending on the level of information that the clinician needs to obtain. Typical tools include questionnaires, which assess the patient's physical activity habits; activity logs, in which the patient is asked to record all the activities he/she performs during the day for a certain number of days; and use of portable devices to evaluate parameters directly related to a patient's level of physical activity, such as pedometers, accelerometers, and heart rate monitors. All assessment methods are characterized by strengths and limitations, as shown in Table 13.8 (Strath et al. 2013; Warren et al. 2010). The choice of the appropriate method by the health professional depends on various factors, such as the type and characteristics of physical activity they want to emphasize, the time period of the evaluation, and the requirements of each method from the patient. For example, physical activity questionnaires are characterized by low cost and low burden on the patient, and they can assess the type, frequency, intensity, and duration of physical activity performed at home, at work, and during free time; however, they are often prone to recall bias, are accurate and valid only in

TABLE 13.8   Overview of physical activity assessment methods.

Method	Strengths	Limitations
Questionnaire	↓ cost & patient burden, assessment of frequency, intensity, and duration of all kinds of physical activity	↑ recall bias, population-specific, ↓ validity for occasional physical activity
Log	↓ cost, detailed assessment of frequency, intensity, and duration of all kinds of physical activity, ↓ recall bias	↑ patient burden, ↑ burden for analyses, population-specific, potential for change in behavior
Pedometer	↓ cost and patient burden, easy data processing, easy use in all populations, can be used for motivation	↓ precision, inability to assess frequency, intensity, and duration of physical activities
Accelerometer	↓ cost, detailed assessment of frequency, intensity, and duration of all kinds of physical activity, patient record	Failure to detect activities, such as stair climbing and weight lifting, ↑ burden for analyses
Heart rate monitor	↓ patient burden (for ↓ time interval), ↑ correlation with medium- and high-intensity physical activity	Can be affected by emotions, medications, caffeine, etc., ↓ correlation with low-intensity physical activity

Source: Adapted with permission from Strath et al. (2013).

populations for which they have been validated, and do not detect occasional physical activity that can vary from day to day. On the other hand, pedometers have low cost, do not impose a burden on the patient (measurements are done automatically), can detect even occasional/spontaneous physical activity, and are not population-specific; however, they cannot record the type, frequency, intensity, and duration of physical activity but only provide a rough estimate of the quantity of walking (number of steps) during the day.

> **Key Point**
>
> Low levels of physical activity, combined with a sedentary lifestyle, have been associated with weight gain and regain after weight loss.

In clinical practice, important information about physical activity can be obtained through short physical activity questionnaires or a detailed description of activities performed during the previous day (physical activity recall) or a typical day. Two commonly used questionnaires to assess physical activity levels, i.e., the International Physical Activity Questionnaire (IPAQ) (Craig et al. 2003) and the Athens Physical Activity Questionnaire (APAQ) (Kavouras et al. 2016), are provided in Appendices D.5 and D.6. The assessment of physical activity of an obese patient should focus on the daily activities performed at home, at work and during leisure time, with emphasis on walking, as most obese patients do not usually perform organized exercise or engage in sports. In addition, it is useful to evaluate the time spent on moderate-intensity activities, such as brisk walking, dancing, and swimming, as well as the time spent on sedentary activities, such as watching TV and using a P/C, mobile phone, or other electronic device. This information can be used to determine whether the obese patient meets the recommendations for at least 30 minutes of moderate-intensity physical activity per day (or most days of a week) and for engaging in sedentary

> **Key Point**
>
> Important information about physical activity can be obtained through short physical activity questionnaires.

activities for a maximum of 2 hours/day. A pedometer can additionally be provided to patients to evaluate their daily walking habits and to motivate them to self-monitor and gradually increase daily steps to the desired amount through goalsetting.

After interviewing Mrs. CK about her physical activity habits, you recorded the following information: Mrs. CK recognizes the benefits of exercise and she has been trying to stay as active as possible during her adulthood by participating in organized group activities, such as modern dance and aerobic classes. However, since she had her daughter 7 years ago, she has limited free time to exercise due to long working hours and increased responsibilities at home. At the time of the evaluation, she is completely sedentary, and the only type of physical activity she performs is housework. Her daily routine includes driving her daughter to school and then driving to work, a sedentary job with ~8 hours/day in front of a P/C, and then another drive back home late in the afternoon. When she reaches home, she has dinner with her family, she cooks for the next day, and then she relaxes in front of the TV for a couple of hours before going to bed. During weekends, she tries to walk for recreation. However, during the past year the pain in her knees has impaired her walking ability. After providing a pedometer to Mrs. CK for 1 week, you record the following: day 1, 2323 steps; day 2, 1897 steps; day 3, 2177 steps; day 4, 1526 steps; day 5, 1653 steps; day 6, 3226 steps; day 7, 1981 steps.

Sleep Assessment

Sleep habits affect body weight and the person's overall health and well-being. Sleep plays an important role in maintaining metabolic homeostasis; on the other hand, sleep deprivation, even short-term, has been shown to cause a variety of physiological, metabolic, and hormonal abnormalities. These abnormalities can lead to increased appetite and increased sensitivity to stimuli for food intake. Furthermore, the feeling of fatigue and exhaustion, caused by insufficient sleep, may lead to low functionality and reduced physical activity during the day. Increased energy intake and reduced levels of physical activity may result in positive energy balance and eventually weight gain (Beccuti and Pannain 2011; Leger et al. 2015).

The assessment of sleep habits in clinical practice can be performed using simple questions, such as, "How many hours do you usually sleep at night?" or through a detailed description of the sleep pattern of a typical day or week. Moreover, the Pittsburgh Sleep Quality Index (PSQI) is a short and validated instrument to assess a patient's overall sleep quality (provided in Appendix D.7) (Buysse et al. 1989). Consisting of 10 items, the PSQI evaluates various aspects of sleep; seven component scores and one composite score can then be calculated. The component scores consist of subjective sleep quality, sleep latency (i.e., how long it takes to fall asleep), sleep duration, habitual sleep efficiency (i.e., the percentage of time in bed that one is asleep), sleep disturbances (e.g., arousals, apneas, and bad dreams), use of sleeping medication, and daytime dysfunction. Each item is weighted on a 0–3 interval scale. The global PSQI score is then calculated by summing the seven component scores, providing an overall score ranging from 0 to 21, where higher scores denote worse sleep quality.

The relationship between sleep habits and obesity is bidirectional. As mentioned before, insufficient or low-quality sleep can lead to weight gain; however, the presence of obesity is also a strong risk factor for the development of sleep disorders, mainly obstructive sleep apnea (OSA)

(Figure 13.2) (Dobrosielski et al. 2017). OSA is a sleep disorder characterized by recurrent complete or partial interruptions of breathing during sleep due to obstruction of the upper airways; it typically presents as snoring and leads to disturbances in gas exchange, hypoxia, and consequent arousals (Jordan et al. 2014). Beyond its adverse impact on sleep duration, sleep quality, and the functionality and cognitive function during the day (typical symptoms include fatigue, sleepiness, decreased reflexes, impaired memory, etc.), OSA is recognized as a major risk factor for morbidity and mortality. This is due to its strong association with cardiometabolic diseases, including the metabolic syndrome, T2DM, and cardiovascular disease (Jordan et al. 2014). In the adult population, the prevalence of OSA is estimated to be ~25%; in obese subjects the prevalence may be up to 50–90% (Romero-Corral et al. 2010). Therefore, if symptoms of snoring or daytime sleepiness are present, specific questionnaires, such as the Berlin questionnaire (provided in Appendix D.8) (Netzer et al. 1999) or the STOP-BANG questionnaire (provided in Appendix D.9) (Chung et al. 2008) and diagnostic sleep testing (e.g., a home or in-lab sleep study) can be used to evaluate the presence of OSA in obese patients.

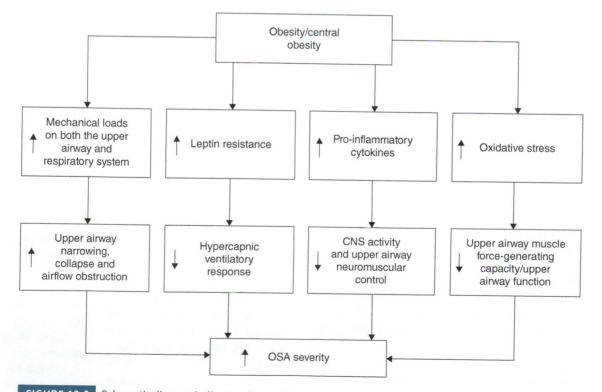

FIGURE 13.2 Schematic diagram indicating the possible mechanisms linking obesity/central obesity with the development of OSA. CNS, central nervous system. **Source:** Reprinted with permission from Dobrosielski et al. (2017).

After interviewing Mrs. CK about her sleep habits, you recorded the following information: During a typical working week, Mrs. CK wakes up around 7:00 A.M. to prepare her young daughter for school and then goes to work until 5:00 P.M. Due to long working hours she is never able to have a midday nap. At night, she cooks for the next day and does some household chores until 11:00 P.M. and then she always watches TV for a couple of hours and enjoys her chocolate dessert. As she stated, "This is the only time during the day that I can relax and find some time for myself." She usually goes to bed around 1:00 A.M. During weekends, she wakes up around 9:00 A.M., has a midday nap from 4:00–6:00 P.M., and goes to bed around 1:00 A.M., unless a social event keeps her awake until later. She does not report symptoms of daytime sleepiness, and her husband has never complained of snoring or witnessed pauses of breathing during her sleep. After completing the PSQI, Mrs. CK's total score was 15, suggesting a relatively low sleep quality.

Stress Assessment

Stress is a condition in which expectations, whether genetically programmed, established by prior learning, or deduced from circumstances, do not match current or anticipated perceptions of the internal or external environment (Goldstein 2010). This mismatch between what is observed or sensed and what is expected or programmed evokes patterned, compensatory mechanisms and reactions, known as the *stress response*. Within seconds after a perceived stressor, catecholamines, such as epinephrine and norepinephrine, are produced in the sympathetic nervous system and in the adrenal medulla, causing an increase in heart rate and constriction of blood vessels. Furthermore, epinephrine stimulates glycogenolysis in the liver, leading to higher serum glucose levels providing energy for a defensive reaction. Catecholamines are also linked to the hypothalamic–pituitary–adrenal (HPA) axis and stimulate the production of cortisol, which supports the action of catecholamines. The effects of these major stress mediators induced by acute stress, though essential for the survival of an organism, can also have negative effects, especially in the case of chronic exposure to stressful stimuli (Agorastos and Chrousos 2021; Gassen et al. 2017; Pervanidou and Chrousos 2018; Stefanaki et al. 2018).

Chronic activation of the sympathetic nervous system and the HPA axis contribute to chronically elevated cortisol levels and an anabolic state that promotes fat storage within visceral depots; this leads to increased risk of hypertension, dyslipidemia, impaired glucose metabolism, MetS, and cardiovascular disease. Stress can also enhance weight gain and fat deposition through changes in eating behavior, including alterations in the pattern of food intake, emotional eating, and increased susceptibility to the rewarding properties of foods (Scott et al. 2012; van der Valk et al. 2018). Therefore, chronic stress, often arising from poor interpersonal relationships, job or unemployment stress, poor self-esteem, and low socioeconomic status, is strongly linked to obesity, especially abdominal obesity, and associated comorbidities; its evaluation and management is considered crucial in the context of an efficient obesity treatment.

> **Key Point**
>
> Stress is a condition in which expectations do not match current or anticipated perceptions of the internal or external environment.

> **Key Point**
>
> Chronic stress is strongly linked to obesity, especially abdominal obesity, and associated comorbidities.

Although the evaluation of stress should ideally be performed by a trained specialist, several easy and fast tools can be used in clinical practice by health professionals to provide a rough assessment of a patient's stress levels. The Perceived Stress Scale (PSS) (provided in Appendix D.10) (Cohen et al. 1983) is one of the most widely used instruments for measuring the perception of stress. It is a measure of the degree to which situations in one's life are appraised as stressful. The PSS includes 10 questions that were designed to determine how unpredictable, uncontrollable, and overloaded respondents find their lives. The PSS score ranges from 0 to 40, with higher values indicating higher levels of perceived stress; scores ranging from 0 to 13 are indicative of low perceived stress, 14–26 are indicative of moderate perceived stress, and 27–40 are indicative of high perceived stress. The Zung Self-Rating Anxiety Scale (SAS) (provided in Appendix D.11) (Zung 1971) is another questionnaire designed to measure anxiety levels, based on scoring in four groups of manifestations: cognitive, autonomic, motor, and central nervous system symptoms. The total SAS raw score is 20–80 and is then converted to an "anxiety index" score (range: 25–100); higher values indicate higher levels of anxiety (20–44 normal range, 45–59 mild to moderate anxiety, 60–74 marked to severe anxiety, and ≥75 extreme anxiety).

Mrs. CK states that her demanding job coupled with her responsibilities as a mother and wife are a bit stressful and leave her only limited time to relax. Mrs. CK's PSS (Appendix D.10) score was 25, indicative of a moderate perceived stress.

Obesity Management

General Principles

Obesity is a multifactorial condition, caused by an interaction between predisposing genetic and metabolic factors and a rapidly changing way of living. In most animals, including humans, there is a strong selection bias in favor of regulatory systems that vigorously defend against decreases in body weight. As a result, maintaining a new, healthier weight after

> **Key Point**
>
> Obesity should be considered a chronic relapsing disease in which multiple modalities of treatment should be considered, including lifestyle counseling, pharmacotherapy, and surgery.

significant weight loss is very difficult for most overweight/obese patients. Therefore, obesity should be considered a chronic relapsing disease in which multiple modalities of treatment should be considered, including lifestyle counseling, pharmacotherapy, and surgery.

Managing obesity should have wider objectives than weight loss alone; it should primarily aim to manage comorbidities and improving the patient's quality of life and well-being. Appropriate management of complications should include management of dyslipidemia, optimizing glycemic control in diabetic patients, normalizing blood pressure in hypertension, effectively managing pulmonary disorders such as sleep apnea syndrome, improving pain management and mobility in osteoarthritis, managing of psychosocial disturbances including mood disorders, eating disorders, low self-esteem, and body image disturbance. It is widely accepted that significant clinical benefits may be achieved even by modest weight loss and lifestyle modification (improved nutritional content of the diet and modest increases in physical activity and fitness). Maintenance of weight loss and prevention and treatment of comorbidities are the two main criteria for success. Referral to an obesity specialist (or an obesity management team) should be considered if the patient fails to lose weight in response to the prescribed intervention. Moreover, weight cycling, defined by repeated loss and regain of body weight, is associated with increased risk for hypertension, dyslipidemia, gallbladder disease, and psychological distress and may require appropriate psychological care. Last but not least, obesity is a chronic disease; frequent follow-ups and continued supervision are necessary to prevent weight regain and to monitor disease risks.

> **Key Point**
>
> Managing obesity should have wider objectives than weight loss alone; it should aim to manage comorbidities and improve the patient's quality of life.

> **Key Point**
>
> Obesity is a chronic disease; frequent follow-ups and continued supervision are necessary to prevent weight regain and to monitor disease risks.

Intervention

Multicomponent interventions are the treatment of choice for obesity. A weight management program should start with behavior change strategies to reduce energy intake, improve quality of diet, increase physical activity level and decrease inactivity, and improve other lifestyle factors, e.g., sleep habits and stress levels. However, on an individual level, the exact nature of the ideal intervention can vary significantly between obese patients; health

> **Key Point**
>
> The exact nature of the ideal intervention can vary significantly between obese patients; health professionals should consider many factors when designing a treatment plan.

TABLE 13.9 Level of intervention based on BMI and WC values.

BMI category	WC category			Comorbidities
	Low	High	Very high	
Overweight	1	2	2	3
Obesity I	2	2	2	3
Obesity II	3	3	3	4
Obesity III	4	4	4	4
1	General advice on healthy weight and lifestyle			
2	Diet and physical activity			
3	Diet and physical activity; consider drugs			
4	Diet and physical activity; consider drugs; consider surgery			

BMI, body mass index; WC, waist circumference.
Source: Reprinted with permission from Stegenga et al. (2014).

professionals should consider a large number of factors when designing a treatment plan. For instance, what kind of intervention must be implemented? How intense should the intervention be? Is lifestyle modification enough or should medical therapies be considered?

A simple obesity classification system described in the 2014 National Institute for Health and Care Excellence (NICE) guidelines can serve as a tool for clinical decision-making on obesity treatment (Table 13.9) (Stegenga et al. 2014). The system is based on BMI and WC values, according to which obesity is classified into four categories; each category corresponds to a suggested level of intervention. The level of intervention increases as the patient's BMI and WC increase, is higher for patients with comorbidities, and must be adjusted as needed, depending on the patient's clinical needs and potential to benefit from weight loss.

Mrs. CK has obesity class I (BMI 34.17 kg/m²) and very high WC values (97.5 cm). Given that her medical history is free of comorbidities, based on the NICE system, the indicated level of intervention is 2, i.e., intervention should focus on lifestyle modification (diet, physical activity, sleep, stress management), while drugs and bariatric surgery are not yet necessary.

Although classifications based on anthropometric data continue to serve their function as surrogate measures for the magnitude of body fat and its distribution, and to assess progress in management, they lack sensitivity and specificity when applied to individuals. For instance, individuals with the same BMI can have an almost twofold difference in total body fat, whereas individuals with the same amount of total body fat can present with a wide range of WCs. Furthermore, there is large interindividual variation in the amount of visceral fat present in individuals with the same WC. Given the aforementioned limitations, anthropometric measurements alone are insufficient to guide clinical decision-making in overweight/obese individuals; disease- and functionality-related indices can provide valuable clinical information to guide and evaluate obesity treatment. The Edmonton obesity staging system is a system based on simple clinical assessments that include medical history, clinical and functional assessments, as well as simple routine diagnostic investigations, that are easily and widely available (Table 13.10). Rather than simply categorizing patients based on anthropometric measures, this staging system provides a measure for the presence and severity of obesity-related risk factors, comorbidities, and functional limitations that can serve as a guide for obesity management (Sharma and Kushner 2009). The rationale for a clinical staging system is based on the notion that patients with current, obesity-related health problems should be treated more aggressively. Furthermore, in the context of limited resources, a staging system can assist in the identification of patients who will most likely benefit from aggressive and resource-intensive weight loss.

Mrs. CK has no history of chronic diseases other than obesity. However, she has been complaining of pain in her knees for the last 12 months; further X-ray testing revealed no definite signs of degenerative joint disease (mild functional limitations, physical symptoms, and/or impairment of well-being). In addition, her systolic/diastolic blood pressure is 128/86 mmHg, which is classified as elevated (>120/80 mmHg) (i.e., presence of obesity-related subclinical risk factors). Based on the Edmonton system, Mrs. CK has obesity stage 1 that requires intense lifestyle interventions, including diet, exercise, stress management, and sleep pattern modification, to prevent further weight gain, along with monitoring of health status.*

Target Weight Loss

Defining a target weight loss for an obese patient is a challenging task. How much weight should an obese patient lose to achieve clinically significant improvements in health and wellness? What is the optimal weight-loss rate? Is there an ideal body weight value? Before initiating a weight-loss intervention it is also useful to address motivation for change: How important is weight loss for the patient, and how confident is the patient that he/she can lose weight and maintain the new weight? It is widely accepted that there is no ideal weight-loss target for all obese patients. The weight-loss goal must be set for each patient,

TABLE 13.10 **The Edmonton Obesity Staging System.**

Stage	Description	Management
0	No apparent obesity-related risk factors (e.g., blood pressure, serum lipids, fasting glucose, etc. within normal range), no physical symptoms, no psychopathology, no functional limitations and/or impairment of well-being.	Identification of factors contributing to increased body weight. Counseling to prevent further weight gain through lifestyle measures, including healthy eating and increased physical activity.
1	Presence of obesity-related subclinical risk factors (e.g., borderline hypertension, impaired fasting glucose, elevated liver enzymes, etc.), mild physical symptoms (e.g., dyspnea on moderate exertion, occasional aches and pains, fatigue, etc.), mild psychopathology, mild functional limitations and/or mild impairment of well-being.	Investigation for other (non–weight related) contributors to risk factors. More intense lifestyle interventions, including diet and exercise, to prevent further weight gain and promote weight loss. Monitoring of risk factors and health status.
2	Presence of established obesity-related chronic disease (e.g., hypertension, type 2 diabetes mellitus, sleep apnea, osteoarthritis, reflux disease, polycystic ovary syndrome, anxiety disorder, etc.), moderate limitations in activities of daily living, and/or well-being.	Initiation of obesity treatment including considerations of all behavioral, pharmacological, and surgical treatment options. Close monitoring and management of comorbidities as indicated.
3	Established end-organ damage such as myocardial infarction, heart failure, diabetic complications, incapacitating osteoarthritis, significant psychopathology, significant functional limitations, and decreased sense of well-being.	More intensive obesity treatment, including consideration of all behavioral, pharmacological, and surgical treatment options. Aggressive management of comorbidities as indicated.
4	Severe (potentially end-stage) disabilities from obesity-related chronic diseases, severe disabling psychopathology, severe functional limitations and/or severe impairment of well-being.	Aggressive obesity management as deemed feasible. Palliative measures, including pain management, occupational therapy, and psychosocial support.

Source: Reprinted with permission from Sharma and Kushner (2009).

Key Point

A 5–10% weight-loss goal over a period of 6 months is realistic and of proven health benefit, but even a loss of 3–5% is beneficial, especially for obese patients with high cardiovascular risk or obesity-related disorders.

based on the person's health status, desires, and motivation, and must be realistic, specific, and measurable. In general, a 5–10% weight-loss goal over a period of 6 months is realistic and of proven benefit. An even greater (≥10%) weight loss may be considered for patients with higher degrees of obesity (BMI ≥ 35 kg/m²); however, even a mild weight loss of 3–5% is beneficial, especially for obese patients with high cardiovascular risk or established obesity-related disorders (Jensen et al. 2014; Yumuk et al. 2015). This is very important, given that many overweight/obese individuals have unrealistically high weight-loss goals, which are difficult to achieve and even more difficult to maintain and often lead to frustration, disappointment, and discontinuation of weight-loss efforts.

Mrs. CK currently weighs 95.3 kg. Based on her body weight history, her weight has not been lower than 80.0 kg during the last 10 years and has been gradually increasing after her second pregnancy. Now she feels confident that she can lose weight, and she is motivated by the fact that weight loss will help her alleviate the pain in her knees, will make her more active, and will improve her mood and body image. She states that when her weight was 80.0 kg, she was happier with her body, and this is what she hopes to achieve with your help, i.e., a weight loss of 15 kg. A more realistic and with a better chance to sustain goal for Mrs. CK would be a 5–10% weight loss; although she would still be overweight, this initial weight loss could lead to significant improvements in blood pressure and the knee pain. If this initial goal is achieved and maintained for at least 1 year, then another 5–10% weight loss could be considered.

Dietary Modification

The optimal diet for weight loss has been a topic for debate in the scientific literature for many years. Past research has focused on the effect of diet's macronutrient manipulation on body weight, and several types of diets with different macronutrient composition, such as low-fat, high-protein, or low-carbohydrate diets, have been tested and compared as tools for obesity management. The findings of this research suggest that balanced hypocaloric diets result in similar, clinically significant weight loss and health benefits, regardless of which macronutrients they emphasize. In general, many types of hypocaloric diets have beneficial effects on reducing risk factors for obesity-related disorders and on promoting adherence,

Key Point

Balanced hypocaloric diets result in similar, clinically significant weight loss and health benefits, regardless of which macronutrients they emphasize.

diet acceptability and sustainability, satiety and satisfaction. Balanced hypocaloric diets can be tailored to individual patients on the basis of their personal and cultural preferences and may have the best chance for long-term success. Therefore, caloric restriction, achieved through reduced intake of either fat or carbohydrate or a combination of the two, is fundamental for weight loss (Sacks et al. 2009; Shai et al. 2008; Gow et al. 2014; Tobias et al. 2015.). According to the Guidelines for the Management of Overweight and Obesity in Adults published in *Circulation* in 2014 (Jensen et al. 2014), all of the dietary approaches (listed in alphabetical order) in Table 13.11 are associated with weight loss if reductions in dietary energy intake are achieved. Among these dietary approaches, a Mediterranean calorie-restricted diet has been shown to be superior in terms of weight-loss maintenance, compared to a low-fat calorie-restricted diet or a low-carbohydrate diet without calorie restriction, and can be a useful tool for the long-term dietary management of obesity (Schwarzfuchs et al. 2012).

Energy restriction should be individualized and take into account the patient's nutritional habits, physical activity level, comorbidities, and previous dieting attempts. Energy restriction can be achieved by three major approaches. The first requires the estimation of the patient's energy requirements and prescription of an energy deficit ranging between 500 kcal/d and 750 kcal/d or 30% of usual caloric intake (Jensen et al. 2014; Yumuk et al. 2015). Although indirect calorimetry is the gold standard method for estimating energy requirements, by measuring basal metabolic rate (BMR), in clinical practice patients' energy requirements are typically calculated with the use of equations that predict BMR, taking into account the patient's gender, age, and current body weight, e.g., the Schofield (Schofield 1985) or Mifflin-St. Jeor (Mifflin et al. 1990) equations. The Schofield equations have been adapted by the WHO and are most commonly used for the estimation of energy needs in clinical practice (Table 13.12). The result is then multiplied by a physical activity factor to adjust for energy expenditure due to exercise; 1.2–1.4 for sedentary, 1.4–1.6 for mildly active, 1.6–1.8 for moderately active, and >1.8 for very active individuals. A 500-kcal daily deficit will produce an average weight loss of approximately 0.5 kg weekly, which should be the desired weight-loss target for most obese patients. Alternatively, an easy rule of

Key Point

Caloric restriction, achieved through reduced intake of either fat or carbohydrate or a combination of the two, is fundamental for weight loss.

Key Point

A Mediterranean calorie-restricted diet has been shown to be superior in terms of weight-loss maintenance.

Key Point

Energy restriction should be individualized and take into account the patient's nutritional habits, physical activity level, comorbidities and previous dieting attempts.

Dietary approaches that can produce weight loss in obese adults.

A diet from the European Association for the Study of Diabetes Guidelines, which focuses on targeting food groups, rather than prescribed energy restriction, while still achieving an energy deficit.

High-protein diet (25% of total calories from protein, 30% from fat, and 45% from carbohydrate), with provision of foods in quantities to produce an energy deficit.

High-protein Zone™-type diet (5 meals/d, each with 40% of total calories from carbohydrate, 30% from protein, and 30% from fat) without a formally prescribed energy restriction plan but with an energy deficit.

Lacto-ovo-vegetarian-style diet with prescribed energy restriction.

Low-calorie diet with prescribed energy restriction.

Low-carbohydrate diet (initially <20 g/d carbohydrate) without a formally prescribed energy restriction plan but with an energy deficit.

Low-fat diet (20% of total calories from fat) without a formally prescribed energy restriction plan but with an energy deficit.

Low-fat vegan-style diet (10–25% of total calories from fat) without a formally prescribed energy restriction plan but with an energy deficit.

Low-glycemic-load diet, either with formally prescribed energy restriction or without a formally prescribed energy restriction plan, but with an energy deficit.

Lower-fat (≤30% fat), high-dairy (4 servings/d) diets with or without increased fiber and/or low-glycemic-index (low-glycemic-load) foods with prescribed energy restriction.

Macronutrient-targeted diets (15 or 25% of total calories from protein; 20 or 40% from fat; 35, 45, 55, or 65% from carbohydrate) with prescribed energy restriction.

Mediterranean-style diet with prescribed energy restriction.

Moderate-protein diet (12% of total calories from protein, 58% from carbohydrate, and 30% from fat) with provision of foods that achieve an energy deficit.

Provision of high-glycemic-load or low-glycemic-load meals with prescribed energy restriction.

The American Heart Association-style Step 1 diet (prescribed energy restriction of 1500–1800 kcal/d, <30% of total calories from fat, <10% from saturated fat).

Source: Adapted with permission from Jensen et al. (2014).

TABLE 13.12 **The Schofield equations for the estimation of BMR.**

Age (years)	Men (kcal/d)	Women (kcal/d)
<3	$(59.5 \times BW) - 30$	$(58.3 \times BW) - 31$
3–10	$(22.7 \times BW) + 504$	$(20.3 \times BW) + 486$
10–18	$(17.7 \times BW) + 658$	$(13.4 \times BW) + 693$
18–30	$(15.1 \times BW) + 692$	$(14.8 \times BW) + 487$
30–60	$(11.5 \times BW) + 873$	$(8.1 \times BW) + 846$
>60	$(11.7 \times BW) + 588$	$(9.1 \times BW) + 658$

BMR, basal metabolic rate; BW, body weight in kg.

an obese patient is the gold standard approach, in clinical practice, standard low-calorie diets (LCDs) and very-low-calorie diets (VLCDs) are routinely used by health professionals and prescribed for the dietary management of obesity. LCDs, consisting of normal meals and partial meal replacements, have an energy content between 800 and 1500 kcal/d and are considered safe and efficient for weight loss in the majority of obese patients. VLCDs usually provide less than 800 kcal/d and may be used only as part of a comprehensive program under the supervision of a trained physician, when rapid weight loss is required (e.g., in the case of a surgery that requires a pre-op weight loss). The administration of VLCDs should be limited to specific patients and for short periods of time, given that their long-term use can result in nutritional deficits and various undesirable side effects, such as micronutrient imbalance, loss of lean muscle and bone mass, nonalcoholic fatty liver disease, gallbladder disease, constipation, and symptoms of dizziness, fatigue, and headaches. VLCDs are unsuitable as a sole source of nutrition for children and adolescents, pregnant or lactating women, and the elderly. Meal replacement diets, i.e., diets in which one or two daily meal portions are substituted by standard VLCD meals, can also contribute to a nutritionally well-balanced diet and weight-loss maintenance (Dubnov-Raz and Berry 2008; Greenwald 2006; Tsai and Wadden 2006; Andela et al. 2019.).

The third approach is the ad libitum approach, in which a formal energy deficit target is not prescribed to the patient but

> **Key Point**
>
> In clinical practice, standard low-calorie diets (LCDs) and very-low-calorie diets (VLCDs) are routinely used by health professionals and prescribed for the dietary management of obesity.

> **Key Point**
>
> The administration of VLCDs should be limited to specific patients and for short periods of time, given that their long-term use can result in nutritional deficits and undesirable side effects.

thumb is a daily energy requirement of 20–25 kcal/kg for either gender but, for the same body weight, this creates a greater energy deficit in men.

In the second approach, a target energy intake that is less than that required for energy balance is set, usually <1500 kcal/d for women and <1800 kcal/d for men. Although an individualized decision for the optimal energy intake for lower calorie intake is achieved by restriction or elimination of particular food groups or provision of prescribed foods. This approach focuses on dietary quality rather than quantity and aims at achieving energy deficit through healthier food choices and the substitution of energy-dense foods with lighter versions rather than through prescribing a specific daily energy intake to achieve a negative energy balance.

Mrs. CK is 52 years old and weighs 95.3 kg. Based on the Schofield equations for women aged 30–60 years old, her estimated BMR is $8.126 \times 95.3 + 845.6 = {\sim}1620$ kcal/day. Given that she is sedentary, multiplying her BMR with 1.3 leads to a total daily energy expenditure of ~2270 kcal. An energy deficit of 500–750 kcal would lead to a target daily energy intake of ~1520–1770 kcal to achieve the desired weight loss. Alternatively, 20–25 kcal/kg translates into a target energy intake of ~1910–2290 kcal/day, which is higher than that predicted by the Schofield equation but still sufficient to create a negative energy balance.

Besides caloric restriction through a prescribed dietary plan, dietary advice should encourage healthy dietary behaviors that can help reduce caloric intake and promote weight-loss dietary practices. Healthy eating counseling must emphasize the need to increase consumption of food groups such as fruits, vegetables, legumes, whole grains, and fish, and the need to keep the consumption of processed meat products, ultraprocessed foods that contain added sugars, solid fats and salt, sugar-sweetened beverages, and alcohol-containing beverages within a reasonable frequency. Even if a patient is unable to substantially limit his/her caloric intake, adherence to a balanced diet can greatly reduce health risks and even promote a modest weight loss through the substitution of processed energy-dense foods with health-promoting foods high in dietary fiber and micronutrients.

It must be noted that there are no single nutrients, foods, or food groups that can promote or hinder weight loss. A balanced diet that encompasses foods from all major food groups in moderation, poses no strict restrictions, and ensures an adequate intake of all of the important nutrients on a weekly basis is the cornerstone of a healthy lifestyle. Such a diet should be encouraged for all obese patients, unless medical conditions that require specific dietary modifications are present. Other advice toward weight loss includes: frequent and nutritionally complete meals (three main meals: breakfast, lunch, and dinner plus healthy snacks throughout the day if necessary); correct identification of hunger and satiety (avoidance of comfort foods, emotional eating, eating due to stimuli and social overeating, low eating

> **Key Point**
>
> Dietary advice should encourage healthy dietary behaviors that can help reduce caloric intake and promote weight-loss dietary practices.

> **Key Point**
>
> There are no single nutrients, foods, or food groups that can promote or hinder weight loss.

speed, etc.); portion control (use of smaller plates, use of personal utensils, use of individual/small packages for packaged foods, etc.); and proper meal conditions (quiet environment, sitting at the table, family or social meals, eating without parallel activities like TV, etc.).

According to Mrs. CK's dietary assessment, individualized dietary counseling toward weight loss and a healthy diet should focus on:

- *Portion control. Mrs. CK has one big main meal per day (dinner) at home, and a restriction of her typical portion size would create a significant energy deficit. Ways to achieve this portion decline include:*

  a. *Cutting down on the usual dinner portion size by about a quarter.*

  b. *Consumption of an abundant portion of seasonal salad with dinner. Vegetables are rich in dietary fiber and can promote satiety. Vegetables can be consumed at the start of the meal as a means to limit the intake of other more energy-dense foods.*

  c. *Use of smaller plates for serving. Smaller plates can make a small food portion seem larger. This can ameliorate the psychological stress associated with dieting.*

  d. *Education on hunger and satiety. Mrs. CK should be advised to eat her dinner slowly to better recognize the feeling of satiety, and stop eating before she gets too full.*

- *Moderation in the consumption of sweets. Given her daily sweet consumption, a realistic goal would be to reduce the frequency of consumption to two to three portions per week and reduce portion size (e.g., one thin slice of chocolate cake). Other less energy-dense choices should be considered, such as sweets based on milk/yogurt, fruit preserves, nuts with honey, etc.*

- *Adoption of a healthy dietary pattern, such as the Mediterranean diet. Specific advice for Mrs. CK to adapt a Mediterranean-style diet includes:*

  a. *Increase consumption of fruits (gradual increase to two to three fruits/day with emphasis on a variety of fresh, whole, seasonal fruits).*

  b. *Increase consumption of vegetables (a seasonal salad, preferably eaten before the main course, with emphasis on a variety of fresh seasonal raw/cooked vegetables).*

  c. *Consume whole grains (whole-grain bread or pasta) instead of refined ones.*

  d. *Increase consumption of legumes and fish instead of pasta or meat-based meals.*

  e. *Substitute margarine and butter with extra-virgin olive oil in cooking.*

- *Balanced meal pattern. Advise on daily breakfast consumption preferably at home (e.g., yogurt with fruits, milk with oatmeal, etc.); consumption of healthy snacks, such as fruits, nuts, and dairy products, at the office; consumption of a light, healthy lunch at the office (e.g., a chicken salad or a whole-grain cheese sandwich) or a packed lunch from home (whatever is cooked on the previous night) to avoid energy-dense fast-food choices.*

Physical Activity Modification

Physical activity should be an integral component of any weight-reduction program. Numerous studies have reported additive benefits of combining exercise with caloric restriction on reducing body weight and body fat and preserving fat-free mass, as compared to diet alone (Geliebter et al. 2014; Poirier and Despres 2001; Willis et al. 2012). Aerobic-type activities (walking, swimming, cycling) are the optimal mode of exercise for reducing fat mass, while resistance training limits loss of lean mass during weight loss. Current guidelines recommend at least 150 min/week of moderate aerobic exercise along with a few weekly sessions of resistance exercise to preserve lean body mass and increase muscle strength. Table 13.13 provides an overview of the WHO global recommendations on physical activity for adults aged 18–64 years old (WHO 2010).

> **Key Point**
>
> Physical activity should be an integral component of any weight-reduction program.

> **Key Point**
>
> Aerobic-type activities are the optimal mode of exercise for reducing fat mass, while resistance training limits loss of lean mass during weight loss.

Increasing activity to ≥150 minutes of moderate-intensity aerobic activity per week is fundamental for all obese patients and can reduce intra-abdominal fat while preserving lean mass, attenuate the weight-loss-induced decline of resting energy expenditure, reduce blood pressure, improve glucose tolerance, insulin sensitivity, lipid profile, and physical fitness, have a positive influence on the long-term weight maintenance, improve feelings of well-being and self-esteem, and reduce anxiety and depression (Kay and Fiatarone Singh 2006; Lee et al. 1985; Ross et al. 2004). Further objectives should be to reduce sedentary behavior (e.g., television viewing and computer or cell phone use) and increase daily lifestyle activities (e.g., walking or cycling instead of using a car, climbing stairs instead of using elevators). Most importantly, exercise advice must be tailored to the patient's ability and health status and focus on a gradual increase toward higher but safe levels.

> **Key Point**
>
> Exercise advice must be tailored to the patient's ability and health status and focus on a gradual increase toward higher but safe levels.

TABLE 13.13 **Physical activity guidelines for adults 18–64 years.**[a]

Adults aged 18–64 should accumulate ≥150 minutes of moderate-intensity aerobic physical activity each week or perform ≥75 minutes of vigorous-intensity aerobic physical activity per week or an equivalent combination of moderate- and vigorous-intensity activity.

Aerobic activity should be performed in bouts of ≥10 minutes duration.

For additional health benefits, adults should increase moderate-intensity aerobic physical activity to 300 minutes/week, or engage in 150 minutes of vigorous-intensity aerobic physical activity/ week, or an equivalent combination of moderate- and vigorous-intensity activity.

Muscle-strengthening activities involving major muscle groups should be performed in addition to aerobic training on 2 or more days a week.

In adults aged 18–64, physical activity should include leisure-time physical activity (e.g., walking, dancing, gardening, hiking, swimming), transportation (e.g., walking or cycling), occupational (i.e., work), household chores, play, games, sports, or planned exercise, in the context of daily, family, and community activities.

[a] Inactive adults or adults with disease limitations will achieve significant health benefits if they move from the category of "no activity" to "some level" of activity, even if they do not meet the current guidelines. Adults who currently do not meet the recommendations for physical activity should aim to a gradual increase in duration, frequency, and finally intensity as a target to achieving the guidelines. (WHO 2010).

Mrs. CK was completely sedentary at the time of your evaluation, and any increase in her physical activity level would be beneficial. Walking is the easiest and more sustainable form of physical activity, and a realistic goal would be to aim for a 20-minute walk on 2–3 days per week, with a gradual increase to a 30-minute walk on most days of the week. A pedometer can help to set weekly goals of physical activity and self-monitor physical activity level. Other advice to achieve an increase in physical activity should focus on parking farther away from entrances, using stairs instead of elevators, taking a short walk after lunch break at the office, walking for daily shopping, as well as family activities during weekends that involve physical activity (swimming, walking, recreational cycling, or low-intensity hiking, etc.) or any kind of sports that she enjoys.

Sleep Modification

Sleep modification must focus on sleep quantity and sleep quality. According to the Joint Consensus Statement of the American Academy of Sleep Medicine and the Sleep Research Society, adults should sleep for 7 hours or more per night on a regular basis to promote optimal health. Sleeping less than 7 hours per night on a regular basis is considered in-adequate

Key Point

Adults should sleep for 7 hours or more per night on a regular basis to promote optimal health.

Key Point

Sleeping more than 9 hours per night might be indicative of the presence of an underlying psychological or sleep disorder.

and is associated with adverse health outcomes, including weight gain and obesity, diabetes mellitus, hypertension, heart disease and stroke, depression, impaired immune function, increased pain, impaired performance, increased errors, greater risk of accidents, and increased risk of death. On the other hand, sleeping more than 9 hours per night on a regular basis may be appropriate for young adults, individuals recovering from sleep debt, and individuals with illnesses. For others, sleeping more than 9 hours per night might be indicative of the presence of an underlying psychological or sleep disorder. People concerned that they are sleeping too little or too much should consult their health-care provider; further sleep testing might be required in case symptoms of sleep disorders, such as OSA, are present.

Key Point

Education on sleep hygiene should be part of a lifestyle intervention of an obese patient.

Sleep quality is another important parameter that can promote a healthy weight; therefore, education on sleep hygiene should be part of a lifestyle intervention of an obese patient. The National Sleep Foundation lists eight sleep hygiene practices:

1. Limit daytime naps to 30 minutes. Napping does not make up for inadequate night-time sleep; however, a short nap of 20–30 minutes can help to improve mood, alertness, and performance.

2. Avoid stimulants, such as caffeine and nicotine, 4–6 hours before bedtime.

3. Avoid alcohol before bedtime. While alcohol is well known to promote a sense of relaxation, excessive drinking can disrupt normal sleep patterns and architecture.

4. Avoid working out before bedtime. A short (10-minute) interval of aerobic exercise before sleep, such as walking, can improve night-time sleep quality; however, strenuous workouts before bedtime should be avoided.

5. Avoid foods that can disrupt sleep, such as fatty or fried meals, spicy dishes, and citrus fruits that can trigger gastrointestinal symptoms, such as gastroesophageal reflux.

6. Ensure adequate exposure to natural light. Exposure to sunlight during the day, as well as darkness at night, helps to maintain a healthy sleep–wake cycle.

7. Establish a regular relaxing bedtime routine. A regular nightly routine, such as taking a warm shower or bath, reading a book, or light stretches, helps the body recognize that it is bedtime.

8. Make sure that the sleep environment is pleasant. This includes comfortable mattress and pillows; a cool bedroom; avoidance of bright light from lamps; not using cell phones or watching TV; and ensuring a dark and quiet environment, such as with dark curtains, eye shades, ear plugs, or "white noise" machines.

According to Mrs. CK's sleep habits assessment, she suffers from chronic sleep deprivation (average daily sleep duration: 5–6 hours), which is a risk factor for morbidity and early mortality. In addition, her sleep quality is relatively low, as indicated by her score in the PSQI (Appendix D.7). Mrs. CK should be encouraged to gradually increase her daily sleep duration to 7 hours as recommended for adults and be educated on sleep hygiene. Other goals of the intervention plan, such as cutting down on dinner portions, increasing physical activity level, and losing weight, are also expected to gradually contribute to better sleep quality.

Stress Management

Given the strong link between stress and obesity, stress management is increasingly recognized as an important part of obesity management. Even when stress is not clearly present prior to weight loss, strict dieting approaches (e.g., strict hypocaloric diets) and patients' unrealistic weight-loss goals can contribute to stress and hinder lifestyle change efforts. In this context, nondieting approaches that do not involve preoccupation with food regimens or weight-loss goals and reduce dieting-induced feelings of guilt and deprivation can be useful for managing obesity. Such approaches contribute to alleviating the psychological distress caused by long-term dieting failure and focus on the improvement of health behaviors and psychological well-being.

Key Point

Nondieting approaches that do not involve preoccupation with food regimens or weight-loss goals and that reduce feelings of guilt and deprivation can be useful for managing obesity.

Stress-management techniques, such as progressive muscular relaxation, applied relaxation, diaphragmatic breathing, virtual reality, and imagination-based techniques, are key features of nondieting approaches for obesity management (Bradshaw et al. 2010; Katzer et al. 2008; Manzoni et al. 2009; Rosmond et al. 1996).

In addition, some flexibility and balance exercises have been shown to exert strong anti-stress effects and can be recommended as a means to reduce stress and increase physical activity. Tai chi and yoga, originating from China and India, respectively, are two of the most popular mind–body exercises, practiced by all age groups with different health conditions around the world, for health promotion and disease prevention. Compared to conventional exercises that usually focus on muscular strength and endurance, tai chi and yoga share similar elements; training involves mind–body cultivation through slow voluntary movements, full-body stretching and relaxation, diaphragmatic breathing practice, meditative state of mind, and mental concentration. Given that these practices are easy to learn, research has recently focused on the effects of mind–body exercise on health outcomes; the data support the notion that tai chi and yoga interventions yield significant improvements of self-reported outcomes of stress and objective physical function (Zou et al. 2018).

Counseling for Mrs. CK toward stress management should focus on the following:

- *Emphasis on beneficial lifestyle changes, i.e., adoption of a healthy diet, a physically active lifestyle, and optimal sleep patterns, rather than on specific weight-loss goals. Management of obesity should generally focus on health benefits rather than achieving and maintaining a perceived ideal body weight through strict dieting and deprivations.*
- *Flexibility and balance exercises, such as yoga and tai chi, could be recommended in addition to aerobic exercise to contribute to stress relief.*
- *If the symptoms of stress or anxiety are severe, Mrs. CK should be referred to a specialist for an in-depth assessment and individualized treatment.*

Behavior Change and Motivation

Lifestyle changes for the management of obesity require modifications in behaviors and practices that are difficult to achieve and maintain and require constant effort and frequent follow-up. Cognitive–behavioral therapy (CBT) is a blend of cognitive therapy and behavioral therapy that aims to help patients modify their insight and understanding of thoughts and beliefs

about health issues, including weight regulation, obesity, and its consequences. It also directly addresses behaviors that require change for health promotion, including successful weight loss and weight-loss maintenance. CBT involves several components, such as self-monitoring, techniques controlling the process of eating, stimulus control, and reinforcement. CBT elements should be part of a lifestyle management or, as a structured program, form the basis of specialized intervention. CBT can be provided not only by registered psychologists but also by other trained health professionals such as physicians, dieticians, exercise physiologists, or psychiatrists. An overview of cognitive–behavioral techniques that can be used in an obesity management intervention to facilitate

behavioral change is presented in Table 13.14 (Stuart 1996; Wadden et al. 2007, 2012; Wadden and Foster 2000; Frates and Bonnet 2016; Frates et al. 2017.).

Even though most obese patients recognize the health risks associated with obesity and are aware of the fundamental principles of a healthy lifestyle, they cannot change on their own or sustain beneficial changes long enough to produce significant results. For the successful management of obesity, it is important to encourage patients to believe that they are capable of change and establish a friendly environment with proper communication. Motivational interviewing (MI) is a technique originally used for managing substance abuse, in which the health professional becomes a helper in the change process and expresses acceptance of the patient. It is a way to interact with patients and help them resolve the ambivalence that prevents patients from realizing and achieving goals. The role of a health professional in MI is directive, with a goal of eliciting self-motivational statements and behavioral change from the patient. Essentially, MI activates the capacity for beneficial change that everyone possesses (Kelley et al. 2016).

MI is a counseling style based on the following assumptions:

- Ambivalence about change is normal and constitutes an important motivational obstacle.
- Ambivalence can be resolved by working with patients' intrinsic motivations and values.
- The alliance between the health professional and the patient is a collaborative partnership to which each brings important expertise.
- An empathic, supportive, yet directive counseling style provides conditions under which change can occur; on the other hand, direct argument and aggressive confrontation may tend to increase patients' defensiveness and reduce the likelihood of behavioral change.

The clinician should practice MI with five general principles in mind:

- Express empathy through reflective listening.
- Develop discrepancy between patients' goals or values and their current behavior.
- Avoid argument and direct confrontation.
- Adjust to patient resistance rather than opposing it directly.
- Support self-efficacy and optimism.

More resources on MI can be found at: www.ncbi.nlm.nih.gov/books/NBK64964.

TABLE 13.14   **Overview of techniques used to facilitate behavior change.**

Assessment of readiness for change. The process of change can be described in five stages:
1. Precontemplation – the person has no intention to change in the near future.
2. Contemplation – the person intends to change within the next 6 months.
3. Preparation – the person plans to change within the next month.
4. Action – the person has made significant modifications in behavior and way of life.
5. Maintenance – the person is working to prevent relapses and is confident of continuing to change.
Patients with low readiness for change should be motivated to take step-by-step actions toward a healthier lifestyle.

Assessment of self-efficacy for change. Perceived self-efficacy is defined as a person's belief in his/her ability to produce effects. Patients with low self-efficacy for lifestyle change can be assisted in identifying and empowering motives and positive powers (e.g., previous successful experiences, social support) that can facilitate behavior change and can be provided with suggestions and advice for overcoming perceived barriers for change.

Goal setting. Patients can be asked to set up practical, specific, and realistic goals (e.g., over the next 3 months I will consume 1 cup of seasonal salad with lunch and dinner on a daily basis). Goals can be broken into small steps, since success in meeting small goals helps to build confidence for continued success (e.g., for a person who weighs 120 kg, a 5–10% weight loss over 6 months can be translated into a weight loss of 0.5–1 kg every 2 weeks).

Self-monitoring. Self-monitoring is the process of observing and evaluating one's behavior. Patients can be asked to self-monitor specific lifestyle habits and record them in print diaries throughout the intervention, as a means to evaluate their success in meeting intervention goals. At the start of each session, self-monitoring data from the previous time interval can be reviewed by the health professional to evaluate adherence to the intervention, reward success, identify problems and barriers for behavior change, and provide solutions.

Problem solving. Problems in achieving goals must be identified through interview and addressed by the health professional with the goal of generating a solution plan. The solution plan must include: specifying the problem in relation to goal behaviors; brainstorming potential solutions for the problem, building on previously successful coping attempts; decision-making, i.e., discussing and anticipating the probable outcomes of different options; and implementation, i.e., trying out a plan and evaluating its effectiveness in the next session.

Stimulus control. Stimulus control is a term used to describe situations in which a behavior is triggered by the presence of some stimuli. Patients can be encouraged to identify stimuli for undesired lifestyle habits (e.g., food overconsumption) and to avoid or control them as a means to meet intervention goals. For example, if the presence of sweets on the kitchen table is a discriminating stimulus for consuming sweets, patients should be advised to avoid having sweets in the house or place them in a hidden spot to avoid frequent exposure.

Management of high-risk situations. High-risk situations are circumstances in which a stimulus can create a strong impulse for undesired lifestyle habits. The health professional can help patients identify personal high-risk situations for slips and lapses, and the group will practice coping with hypothetical high-risk situations during sessions. For example, patients can be given the hypothetical scenario of attending a social event with a buffet and asked to think of ways of coping with it without deviating from dietary intervention goals, or the scenario of a rainy day and asked to think of ways to remain physically active.

Relapse prevention. Relapse prevention is a strategy for reducing the likelihood and severity of relapse following the cessation or reduction of problematic behaviors. Patients in the maintenance stage of change for desired lifestyle habits must be motivated to attain the intervention goals and be reminded of the health benefits they acquire from adhering to the intervention and the risks from relapsing to their old undesired habits.

Take-Home Messages

- BMI is a useful index for excess weight and for predicting adverse health outcomes but should be interpreted with caution because it is not a direct measure of adiposity.
- WC should also be measured in obese patients as a means to evaluate central adiposity and cardiometabolic risk.
- Direct body composition assessment is used primarily for research purposes and is usually not part of the routine evaluation and follow-up of an obese patient in clinical practice.

- BIA devices are portable; they have a relatively low cost and are useful tools for body composition analysis in clinical practice.
- Body weight history, describing long-term fluctuations of body weight and the events that correlate with weight changes, is a useful tool to explore causes of overweight and design individualized treatment approaches for obese patients.
- Comprehensive lifestyle (dietary, physical activity, sleep, and stress) assessment is crucial for all obese patients

and can be performed using a variety of available tools. Emphasis must be placed on lifestyle behaviors that are linked to obesity and can be modified.

- Obesity is a chronic disease. Frequent follow-ups and continued supervision are necessary to prevent weight regain, to monitor disease risks, and to treat comorbidities.
- When planning a treatment for obesity, a health professional should take into account the patient's level of risk, based on anthropometric evaluation and the presence of comorbidities or functional limitations, the patient's individual preferences and social circumstances, as well as his/her experiences and outcomes of previous treatments.
- The purpose of lifestyle intervention for an obese patient goes beyond weight loss per se. Maintenance of weight loss and prevention and treatment of comorbidities should be the two main criteria for the success of a lifestyle intervention for the management of obesity.
- There is no specific weight-loss goal appropriate for all obese patients. Weight loss must be individualized based on the patient's health status, desires, and motivations.
- A 5–10% weight loss is realistic for most patients, although even a 3–5% weight loss can yield clinically significant health benefits.
- Balanced hypocaloric diets result in clinically meaningful weight loss and health benefits, regardless of which macronutrients they limit.

- A 500-kcal daily deficit will result in an average weight loss of about 0.5 kg/week in most obese patients, a desired and realistic weight-loss target.
- No nutrient or food can promote or hinder weight loss per se. A balanced diet that encompasses a variety of foods in moderation and ensures an adequate intake of all nutrients is the cornerstone of a healthy lifestyle and should be encouraged for all obese patients.
- Exercise is an important component of a weight-reduction program in conjunction with caloric reduction. Exercise advice must be tailored to the patient's ability and health and focus on a gradual increase to levels that are safe.
- Education on sleep quantity and sleep hygiene is important for all obese patients. If a sleep disorder is suspected, further sleep testing and referral to a sleep specialist is required.
- CBT techniques, such as self-monitoring, stimulus control, and reinforcement, can facilitate behavior change and should be part of a lifestyle program for obesity management.
- MI is a style of counseling that can help resolve the ambivalence that prevents obese patients from achieving lifestyle changes and health goals.

Self-Assessment Questions

1. Provide the definition of obesity.
2. Which of the following statements are true for obese patients?
   a. They sometimes set high and unrealistic weight-loss goals.
   b. They always provide an accurate report of their dietary intake.
   c. They may have little motivation to lose weight.
   d. Some are at high cardiometabolic risk compared to normal-weight individuals.
   e. They should not be treated unless they have comorbidities.
3. Discuss how sleep deprivation can result in weight gain.
4. What are the preferable tools for the estimation of body habitus in clinical practice?
   a. ADP or DEXA for a detailed assessment of body composition
   b. a detailed body weight history
   c. measurement of body weight and height, calculation of BMI, and measurement of WC to assess abdominal adiposity
   d. estimation of abdominal fat using magnetic resonance imaging/spectroscopy
   e. all of the above
5. A patient visiting your office states the following: "I am not sure if I can follow a specific diet or cut down on my meal portion sizes. Isn't there an easier way for me to lose some weight?" What is this patient's stage of change?
   a. precontemplation
   b. contemplation
   c. preparation
   d. action
   e. maintenance
6. What weight-loss goal would you set for an obese patient? Justify your answer.
7. Which of the following physical activity assessment methods provide information on the type, frequency, intensity, and duration of exercise?
   a. physical activity questionnaire
   b. accelerometer
   c. physical activity diary
   d. pedometer
8. Characterize the following statements as true (T) or false (F).
   a. Acanthosis nigricans is a possible sign of insulin resistance ( ).
   b. Low-carbohydrate diets are more effective for weight loss compared to low-fat diets ( ).
   c. Resistance training is the optimal mode of exercise for reducing fat mass ( ).
   d. A daily energy intake of 50–60 kcal/kg of body weight is suitable for weight loss in most obese people ( ).

e. Sleeping more than 9 hours a night might be indicative of the presence of an underlying psychological or sleep disorder ( ).

9. What kind of dietary advice would you provide to an obese patient in terms of diet quality and meal patterns?

10. What is cognitive–behavioral therapy?

11. Which of the following statements about BMI are true?
    a. It should be interpreted with caution in patients with fluid retention.
    b. It correlates negatively with body fat mass.
    c. It is not a direct measure of adiposity.
    d. It is calculated as body weight (in kg)/height (in m).
    e. All of the above

12. Briefly describe the three approaches to achieve energy restriction for weight loss.

13. Snoring and daytime sleepiness in obese patients are possible symptoms of:
    a. T2DM
    b. asthma
    c. OSA
    d. food allergies
    e. hypertension

14. Provide examples of diets that can produce weight loss in obese adults.

15. Characterize the following statements as true (T) or false (F).
    a. Pedometers have low cost and can assess the intensity of exercise ( ).
    b. Antioxidants play a key role in weight loss ( ).
    c. Inactive adults or those with disease limitations will have health benefits if they move from the category of "no activity" to "some level" of activity, even if they do not meet guidelines for physical activity ( ).
    d. In the context of a 24-hour dietary recall, the patient is required to measure and record all food and beverages consumed for a number of days ( ).
    e. Sleep deprivation can lead to various hormonal and metabolic disturbances that promote a positive energy balance and increase the risk of weight gain ( ).

16. A 42-year-old mildly active female patient visits your office. Her weight is 82.5 kg and her height 1.58 m. Calculate her BMR and recommend a target energy intake for weight loss.

17. Which of the following statements about VLCDs are true?
    a. They are the only dietary approach that has proven efficient for weight loss.
    b. Their administration should be limited for specific patients and for short periods of time, given that their long-term use can result in nutritional deficits.
    c. They are considered nutritionally complete, with the exception of some micronutrients, which may require supplementation.
    d. They may be used only as part of a comprehensive program under the supervision of a physician, when rapid weight loss is required.
    e. They usually provide less than 800 kcal/day.

18. What is motivational interviewing?

19. A Caucasian male patient weighs 102.8 kg, his height is 1.87 m, and his WC is 112.5 cm. Calculate his BMI and comment on his morbidity risk based on anthropometry.

20. How is stress related to obesity?

Bibliography

Agorastos, A. and Chrousos, G.P. (2021). The neuroendocrinology of stress: the stress-related continuum of chronic disease development. *Mol. Psychiatry*. doi: 10.1038/s41380-021-01224-9.

Andela, S., Burrows, T.L., Baur, L.A., Coyle, D.H., Collins, C.E., and Gow, M.L. (2019). Efficacy of very low-energy diet programs for weight loss: a systematic review with meta-analysis of intervention studies in children and adolescents with obesity. *Obes. Rev.* 20 (6): 871–882. doi: 10.1111/obr.12830.

Barlow, S.E. and Expert, C. (2007). Expert committee recommendations regarding the prevention, assessment, and treatment of child and adolescent overweight and obesity: summary report. *Pediatrics* 120 (Suppl 4): S164–S192. https://doi.org/10.1542/peds.2007-2329C.

Beccuti, G. and Pannain, S. (2011). Sleep and obesity. *Curr. Opin. Clin. Nutr. Metab. Care* 14 (4): 402–412. https://doi.org/10.1097/MCO.0b013e3283479109.

Bountziouka, V., Bathrellou, E., Giotopoulou, A. et al. (2012). Development, repeatability and validity regarding energy and macronutrient intake of a semi-quantitative food frequency questionnaire: methodological considerations. *Nutr. Metab. Cardiovasc. Dis.* 22 (8): 659–667. https://doi.org/10.1016/j.numecd.2010.10.015.

Braam, L.A., Ocke, M.C., Bueno-de-Mesquita, H.B., and Seidell, J.C. (1998). Determinants of obesity-related underreporting of energy intake. *Am. J. Epidemiol.* 147 (11): 1081–1086. https://doi.org/10.1093/oxfordjournals.aje.a009402.

Bradshaw, A.J., Horwath, C.C., Katzer, L., and Gray, A. (2010). Non-dieting group interventions for overweight and obese women: what predicts non-completion and does completion improve outcomes? *Public Health Nutr.* 13 (10): 1622–1628. https://doi.org/10.1017/S1368980009992977.

Buysse, D.J., Reynolds, C.F. 3rd, Monk, T.H. et al. (1989). The Pittsburgh Sleep Quality Index: a new instrument for psychiatric practice and research. *Psychiatry Res.* 28 (2): 193–213. https://doi.org/10.1016/0165-1781(89)90047-4.

Chung, F., Yegneswaran, B., Liao, P. et al. (2008). STOP questionnaire: a tool to screen patients for obstructive sleep apnea. *Anesthesiology* 108 (5): 812–821. https://doi.org/10.1097/ALN.0b013e31816d83e4.

Cohen, S., Kamarck, T., and Mermelstein, R. (1983). A global measure of perceived stress. *J. Health Soc. Behav.* 24 (4): 385–396.

Craig, C.L., Marshall, A.L., Sjostrom, M. et al. (2003). International Physical Activity Questionnaire: 12-country reliability and validity. *Med. Sci. Sports Exerc.* 35 (8): 1381–1395. https://doi.org/10.1249/01.MSS.0000078924.61453.FB.

Dobrosielski, D.A., Papandreou, C., Patil, S.P., and Salas-Salvado, J. (2017). Diet and exercise in the management of obstructive sleep apnoea and cardiovascular disease risk. *Eur. Respir. Rev.* 26 (144): 160110. https://doi.org/10.1183/16000617.0110-2016.

Dubnov-Raz, G. and Berry, E.M. (2008). The dietary treatment of obesity. *Endocrinol. Metab. Clin. North Am.* 37 (4): 873–886. https://doi.org/10.1016/j.ecl.2008.08.002.

Duren, D.L., Sherwood, R.J., Czerwinski, S.A. et al. (2008). Body composition methods: comparisons and interpretation. *J. Diabetes Sci. Technol.* 2 (6): 1139–1146. https://doi.org/10.1177/193229680800200623.

Ellis, K.J. (2000). Human body composition: in vivo methods. *Physiol. Rev.* 80 (2): 649–680. https://doi.org/10.1152/physrev.2000.80.2.649.

Frates, E.P., and Bonnet, J. (2016). Collaboration and negotiation: the key to therapeutic lifestyle change. *Am. J. Lifestyle Med.* 10 (5): 302–312. doi: 10.1177/1559827616638013.

Frates, E.P., Morris, E.C., Sannidhi, D., and Dysinger, W.S. (2017). The art and science of group visits in lifestyle medicine. *Am. J. Lifestyle Med.* 11 (5): 408–413. doi: 10.1177/1559827617698091.

Gassen, N.C., Chrousos, G.P., Binder, E.B., and Zannas, A.S. (2017). Life stress, glucocorticoid signaling, and the aging epigenome: implications for aging-related diseases. *Neurosci. Biobehav. Rev.* 74 (Pt B): 356–365. doi: 10.1016/j.neubiorev.2016.06.003.

Geliebter, A., Ochner, C.N., Dambkowski, C.L., and Hashim, S.A. (2014). Obesity-related hormones and metabolic risk factors: a randomized trial of diet plus either strength or aerobic training versus diet alone in overweight participants. *J. Diabetes Obes.* 1 (1): 1–7.

Goldstein, D.S. (2010). Adrenal responses to stress. *Cell. Mol. Neurobiol.* 30 (8): 1433–1440. https://doi.org/10.1007/s10571-010-9606-9.

Gow, M.L., Ho, M., Burrows, T.L., Baur, L.A., Stewart, L., Hutchesson, M.J., and Garnett, S.P. (2014). Impact of dietary macronutrient distribution on BMI and cardiometabolic outcomes in overweight and obese children and adolescents: a systematic review. *Nutr. Rev.* 72 (7): 453–470. doi: 10.1111/nure.12111.

Greenwald, A. (2006). Current nutritional treatments of obesity. *Adv. Psychosom. Med.* 27: 24–41. https://doi.org/10.1159/000090961.

Jensen, M.D., Ryan, D.H., Apovian, C.M. et al. (2014). 2013 AHA/ACC/TOS guideline for the management of overweight and obesity in adults: a report of the American College of Cardiology/American Heart Association Task Force on Practice Guidelines and the Obesity Society. *Circulation* 129 (25 Suppl 2): S102–S138. https://doi.org/10.1161/01.cir.0000437739.71477.ee.

Jonnalagadda, S.S., Mitchell, D.C., Smiciklas-Wright, H. et al. (2000). Accuracy of energy intake data estimated by a multiple-pass, 24-hour dietary recall technique. *J. Am. Diet. Assoc.* 100 (3): 303–308; quiz 9–11. https://doi.org/10.1016/s0002-8223(00)00095-x.

Jordan, A.S., McSharry, D.G., and Malhotra, A. (2014). Adult obstructive sleep apnoea. *Lancet* 383 (9918): 736–747. https://doi.org/10.1016/S0140-6736(13)60734-5.

Katzer, L., Bradshaw, A.J., Horwath, C.C. et al. (2008). Evaluation of a "nondieting" stress reduction program for overweight women: a randomized trial. *Am. J. Health Promot.* 22 (4): 264–274. https://doi.org/10.4278/060728113R1.1.

Kavouras, S.A., Maraki, M.I., Kollia, M. et al. (2016). Development, reliability and validity of a physical activity questionnaire for estimating energy expenditure in Greek adults. *Sci. Sports* 31 (3): e47–e53. https://doi.org/10.1016/j.scispo.2016.01.007.

Kay, S.J. and Fiatarone Singh, M.A. (2006). The influence of physical activity on abdominal fat: a systematic review of the literature. *Obes. Rev.* 7 (2): 183–200. https://doi.org/10.1111/j.1467-789X.2006.00250.x.

Kelley, C.P., Sbrocco, G., and Sbrocco, T. (2016). Behavioral

modification for the management of obesity. *Prim. Care* 43 (1): 159–175. https://doi.org/10.1016/j.pop.2015.10.004.

Krebs, N.F., Himes, J.H., Jacobson, D. et al. (2007). Assessment of child and adolescent overweight and obesity. *Pediatrics* 120 (Suppl 4): S193–S228. https://doi.org/10.1542/peds.2007-2329D.

Kushner, R.F. (2012). Clinical assessment and management of adult obesity. *Circulation* 126 (24): 2870–2877. https://doi.org/10.1161/CIRCULATIONAHA.111.075424.

Kushner, R.F. and Ryan, D.H. (2014). Assessment and lifestyle management of patients with obesity: clinical recommendations from systematic reviews. *JAMA* 312 (9): 943–952. https://doi.org/10.1001/jama.2014.10432.

Lee, S., Kuk, J.L., Davidson, L.E. et al. (2005). Exercise without weight loss is an effective strategy for obesity reduction in obese individuals with and without type 2 diabetes. *J. Appl. Physiol.* 99 (3): 1220–1225. https://doi.org/10.1152/japplphysiol.00053.2005.

Lee, S.Y. and Gallagher, D. (2008). Assessment methods in human body composition. *Curr. Opin. Clin. Nutr. Metab. Care* 11 (5): 566–572. https://doi.org/10.1097/MCO.0b013e32830b5f23.

Leger, D., Bayon, V., and de Sanctis, A. (2015). The role of sleep in the regulation of body weight. *Mol. Cell. Endocrinol.* 418 (Pt 2): 101–107. https://doi.org/10.1016/j.mce.2015.06.030.

Manzoni, G.M., Pagnini, F., Gorini, A. et al. (2009). Can relaxation training reduce emotional eating in women with obesity? An exploratory study with 3 months of follow-up. *J. Am. Diet. Assoc.* 109 (8): 1427–1432. https://doi.org/10.1016/j.jada.2009.05.004.

Martinez-Gonzalez, M.A., Fernandez-Jarne, E., Serrano-Martinez, M. et al. (2004). Development of a short dietary intake questionnaire for the quantitative estimation of adherence to a cardioprotective Mediterranean diet. *Eur. J. Clin. Nutr.* 58 (11): 1550–1552. https://doi.org/10.1038/sj.ejcn.1602004.

Mifflin, M.D., St. Jeor, S.T., Hill, L.A. et al. (1990). A new predictive equation for resting energy expenditure in healthy individuals. *Am. J. Clin. Nutr.* 51 (2): 241–247. https://doi.org/10.1093/ajcn/51.2.241.

Murakami, K. and Livingstone, M.B. (2015). Prevalence and characteristics of misreporting of energy intake in US adults: NHANES 2003-2012. *Br. J. Nutr.* 114 (8): 1294–1303. https://doi.org/10.1017/S0007114515002706.

Netzer, N.C., Stoohs, R.A., Netzer, C.M. et al. (1999). Using the Berlin questionnaire to identify patients at risk for the sleep apnea syndrome. *Ann. Intern. Med.* 131 (7): 485–491. https://doi.org/10.7326/0003-4819-131-7-199910050-00002.

Panagiotakos, D.B., Pitsavos, C., and Stefanadis, C. (2006). Dietary patterns: a Mediterranean diet score and its relation to clinical and biological markers of cardiovascular disease risk. *Nutr. Metab. Cardiovasc. Dis.* 16 (8): 559–568. https://doi.org/10.1016/j.numecd.2005.08.006.

Pervanidou, P. and Chrousos, G.P. (2018). Early-life stress: from neuroendocrine mechanisms to stress-related disorders. *Horm. Res. Paediatr.* 89 (5): 372–379. doi: 10.1159/000488468.

Poirier, P. and Despres, J.P. (2001). Exercise in weight management of obesity. *Cardiol. Clin.* 19 (3): 459–470. https://doi.org/10.1016/s0733-8651(05)70229-0.

Romero-Corral, A., Caples, S.M., Lopez-Jimenez, F., and Somers, V.K. (2010). Interactions between obesity and obstructive sleep apnea: implications for treatment. *Chest* 137 (3): 711–719. https://doi.org/10.1378/chest.09-0360.

Rosmond, R., Lapidus, L., Marin, P., and Bjorntorp, P. (1996). Mental distress, obesity and body fat distribution in middle-aged men. *Obes. Res.* 4 (3): 245–252. https://doi.org/10.1002/j.1550-8528.1996.tb00542.x.

Ross, R., Janssen, I., Dawson, J. et al. (2004). Exercise-induced reduction in obesity and insulin resistance in women: a randomized controlled trial. *Obes. Res.* 12 (5): 789–798. https://doi.org/10.1038/oby.2004.95.

Sacks, F.M., Bray, G.A., Carey, V.J. et al. (2009). Comparison of weight-loss diets with different compositions of fat, protein, and carbohydrates. *N. Engl. J. Med.* 360 (9): 859–873. https://doi.org/10.1056/NEJMoa0804748.

Schofield, W.N. (1985). Predicting basal metabolic rate, new standards and review of previous work. *Hum. Nutr. Clin. Nutr.* 39 (Suppl 1): 5–41.

Schroder, H., Fito, M., Estruch, R. et al. (2011). A short screener is valid for assessing Mediterranean diet adherence among older Spanish men and women. *J. Nutr.* 141 (6): 1140–1145. https://doi.org/10.3945/jn.110.135566.

Schwarzfuchs, D., Golan, R., and Shai, I. (2012). Four-year follow-up after two-year dietary interventions. *N. Engl. J. Med.* 367 (14): 1373–1374. https://doi.org/10.1056/NEJMc1204792.

Scott, K.A., Melhorn, S.J., and Sakai, R.R. (2012). Effects of chronic social stress on obesity. *Curr. Obes. Rep.* 1 (1): 16–25. https://doi.org/10.1007/s13679-011-0006-3.

Seagle, H.M., Strain, G.W., Makris, A. et al. (2009). Position of the American Dietetic Association: weight management. *J. Am. Diet. Assoc.* 109 (2): 330–346. https://doi.org/10.1016/j.jada.2008.11.041.

Shai, I., Schwarzfuchs, D., Henkin, Y. et al. (2008). Weight loss with a low-carbohydrate, Mediterranean, or low-fat diet. *N. Engl. J. Med.* 359 (3): 229–241. https://doi.org/10.1056/NEJMoa0708681.

Sharma, A.M. and Kushner, R.F. (2009). A proposed clinical staging system for obesity. *Int. J. Obes. (Lond)* 33 (3): 289–295. https://doi.org/10.1038/ijo.2009.2.

Shim, J.S., Oh, K., and Kim, H.C. (2014). Dietary assessment methods in epidemiologic studies. *Epidemiol. Health* 36: e2014009. https://doi.org/10.4178/epih/e2014009.

Stefanaki, C., Pervanidou, P., Boschiero, D., and Chrousos, G.P. (2018). Chronic stress and body composition disorders: implications for health and disease. *Hormones (Athens)* 17 (1): 33–43. doi: 10.1007/s42000-018-0023-7.

Stegenga, H., Haines, A., Jones, K. et al. (2014). Identification, assessment, and management of overweight and obesity: summary of updated NICE guidance. *Br. Med. J.* 349: g6608. https://doi.org/10.1136/bmj.g6608.

Strath, S.J., Kaminsky, L.A., Ainsworth, B.E. et al. (2013). Guide to the assessment of physical activity: clinical and research applications: a scientific statement from the American Heart Association. *Circulation* 128 (20): 2259–2279. https://doi.org/10.1161/01.cir.0000435708.67487.da.

Stuart, R.B. (1996). Behavioral control of overeating. 1967. *Obes. Res.* 4 (4): 411–417. https://doi.org/10.1002/j.1550-8528.1996.tb00249.x.

Thompson, F.E. and Byers, T. (1994). Dietary assessment resource manual. *J. Nutr.* 124 (11 Suppl): 2245S–2317S. https://doi.org/10.1093/jn/124.suppl_11.2245s.

Thompson, F.E. and Subar, A.F. (2013). Dietary assessment methodology. In: *Nutrition in the Prevention and Treatment of Disease*, 3e (eds. A.M. Coulston, C.J. Boushey, and M.G. Ferruzzi), 5–46. Cambridge, MA: Academic Press.

Tobias, D.K., Chen, M., Manson, J.E., Ludwig, D.S., Willett, W., and Hu, F.B. (2015). Effect of low-fat diet interventions versus other diet interventions on long-term weight change in adults: a systematic review and meta-analysis. *Lancet Diabetes Endocrinol.* 3 (12): 968–979. doi: 10.1016/S2213-8587(15)00367-8.

Tsai, A.G. and Wadden, T.A. (2006). The evolution of very-low-calorie diets: an update and meta-analysis. *Obesity (Silver Spring)* 14 (8): 1283–1293. https://doi.org/10.1038/oby.2006.146.

Tsigos, C., Kyrou, I., Kassi, E., and Chrousos, G.P. (2000). Stress: endocrine physiology and pathophysiology. In: K.R. Feingold, B. Anawalt, A. Boyce, G. Chrousos, W.W. de Herder, K. Dhatariya, K. Dungan, A. Grossman, J.M. Hershman, J. Hofland, S. Kalra, G. Kaltsas, C. Koch, P. Kopp, M. Korbonits, C.S. Kovacs, W. Kuohung, B. Laferrere, E.A. McGee, R. McLachlan, J.E. Morley, M. New, J. Purnell, R. Sahay, F. Singer, C.A. Stratakis, D.L. Trence & D.P. Wilson (Eds.), Endotext. South Dartmouth, MA: MDText.com, Inc.

van der Valk, E.S., Savas, M., and van Rossum, E.F.C. (2018). Stress and obesity: are there more susceptible individuals? *Curr. Obes. Rep.* 7 (2): 193–203. https://doi.org/10.1007/s13679-018-0306-y.

Wadden, T.A., Butryn, M.L., and Wilson, C. (2007). Lifestyle modification for the management of obesity. *Gastroenterology* 132 (6): 2226–2238. https://doi.org/10.1053/j.gastro.2007.03.051.

Wadden, T.A. and Foster, G.D. (2000). Behavioral treatment of obesity. *Med. Clin. North Am.* 84 (2): 441–461. https://doi.org/10.1016/s0025-7125(05)70230-3.

Wadden, T.A., Webb, V.L., Moran, C.H., and Bailer, B.A. (2012). Lifestyle modification for obesity: new developments in diet, physical activity, and behavior therapy. *Circulation* 125 (9): 1157–1170. https://doi.org/10.1161/CIRCULATIONAHA.111.039453.

Warren, J.M., Ekelund, U., Besson, H. et al. (2010). Assessment of physical activity – a review of methodologies with reference to epidemiological research: a report of the exercise physiology section of the European Association of Cardiovascular Prevention and Rehabilitation. *Eur. J. Cardiovasc. Prev. Rehabil.* 17 (2): 127–139. https://doi.org/10.1097/HJR.0b013e32832ed875.

Watson, N.F., Badr, M.S., Belensky, G. et al. (2015). Recommended amount of sleep for a healthy adult: a joint consensus statement of the American Academy of Sleep Medicine and Sleep Research Society. *J. Clin. Sleep Med.* 11 (6): 591–592. https://doi.org/10.5664/jcsm.4758.

Willis, L.H., Slentz, C.A., Bateman, L.A. et al. (2012). Effects of aerobic and/or resistance training on body mass and fat mass in overweight or obese adults. *J. Appl. Physiol.* 113 (12): 1831–1837. https://doi.org/10.1152/japplphysiol.01370.2011.

World Health Organization. (2000). *Obesity: Preventing and Managing the Global Epidemic*, vol. 894: i–xii, 1–253. Geneva: Report of a WHO Consultation. World Health Organ Tech Rep Ser.

World Health Organization. (2010). *Global Recommendations on Physical Activity for Health*. Geneva: WHO Guidelines Review Committee.

Yumuk, V., Tsigos, C., Fried, M. et al. (2015). European guidelines for obesity management in adults. *Obes. Facts* 8 (6): 402–424. https://doi.org/10.1159/000442721.

Zou, L., Sasaki, J.E., Wei, G.X. et al. (2018). Effects of mind–body exercises (tai chi/yoga) on heart rate variability parameters and perceived stress: a systematic review with meta-analysis of randomized controlled trials. *J. Clin. Med.* 7 (11). https://doi.org/10.3390/jcm7110404.

Zung, W.W. (1971). A rating instrument for anxiety disorders. *Psychosomatics* 12 (6): 371–379. https://doi.org/10.1016/S0033-3182(71)71479-0.

Type 2 Diabetes Mellitus Case Study

Mr. AM is a retired 65-year-old man who recently visited the ER with the following complaint: "I cut my foot over 2 months ago and it has not healed. I also need my eyes checked again because I have been having trouble reading the newspaper for the past few months." In addition to the unhealed wound and blurry vision, he reports frequent bladder infections and slight numbness in his feet. On admission to the hospital his blood glucose was 225 mg/dl, and after further testing he was diagnosed with type 2 diabetes mellitus (T2DM). His height is 1.72 m, weight is 89.5 kg, waist circumference is 108.5 cm, and blood pressure 130/77 mmHg. He is a widower, lives alone, and his two children visit him often. He has been smoking one pack of cigarettes/day for the last 30 years, he consumes alcohol on social occasions, and he has no other known illnesses. Upon hospital discharge, Mr. AM was prescribed metformin for blood glucose control and was referred to you for lifestyle evaluation and consultation.

Assessment

Clinical Assessment

Diabetes is a group of metabolic diseases characterized by hyperglycemia, resulting from defects in insulin production, insulin action, or both. The American Diabetes Association (2010) classifies diabetes into four general categories:

1. *Type 1 diabetes mellitus.* Also known as juvenile diabetes or insulin-dependent diabetes, type 1 diabetes results from autoimmune pancreatic β-cell destruction and usually leads to absolute insulin deficiency.

2. *Type 2 diabetes mellitus.* In T2DM, insulin resistance is the fundamental feature while the pancreas partly maintains its insulin production capacity.

3. *Gestational diabetes mellitus.* This is diagnosed in the second or third trimester of pregnancy, in the absence of diabetes mellitus prior to gestation.

4. *Other specific types of diabetes.* Various causes include monogenic diabetes syndromes and diseases of the exocrine pancreas.

Diabetes mellitus may be diagnosed based on plasma glucose criteria, either fasting plasma glucose (FPG) or 2-hour plasma glucose (2-h PG) during a 75-g oral glucose tolerance test (OGTT), or glycosylated hemoglobin (HbA1C) criteria (Table 14.1). In the absence of unequivocal hyperglycemia, diagnosis of diabetes mellitus requires two abnormal test results from the same sample or in two separate test samples (American Diabetes Association 2020b).

> **Key Point**
>
> Diabetes is a group of metabolic diseases characterized by hyperglycemia, resulting from defects in insulin production, insulin action, or both.

Mr. AM presented to the hospital with a random plasma glucose of 225 mg/dl and symptoms of hyperglycemia, including an unhealed foot wound, feet numbness, blurry vision, and history of bladder infections, fulfilling the criteria for the diagnosis of T2DM. Further testing revealed an FPG of 142 mg/dl and an A1C value of 8.2%, confirming the diagnosis.

T2DM is the most common form of diabetes. Globally, approximately 1 in 12 adults have the disease. In a healthy person in the postprandial state (i.e., for a few hours after consuming a meal), blood glucose concentration is increased. To maintain normoglycemia, the β-cells of the pancreas produce insulin, which blocks glucose output by the liver and increases glucose uptake by skeletal muscle and adipose tissue. In the presence of obesity and other disorders, such as inflammation and

Textbook of Lifestyle Medicine, First Edition. Labros S. Sidossis and Stefanos N. Kales.

TABLE 14.1   Criteria for the diagnosis of diabetes mellitus.

1. Fasting[a] plasma glucose ≥126 mg/dl (7.0 mmol/l)
2. 2-h plasma glucose ≥200 mg/dl (11.1 mmol/l) during an oral glucose tolerance test[b]
3. Glycated hemoglobin[c] ≥6.5% (48 mmol/mol)
4. In a patient with classic symptoms of hyperglycemia or hyperglycemic crisis, a random plasma glucose ≥200 mg/dl (11.1 mmol/l)

[a] Fasting is defined as no caloric intake for at least 8 hours.
[b] The glucose tolerance test measures the level of glucose in the blood in the fasting state and 2 hours after drinking a liquid containing a specific amount of glucose. The test is performed to assess the presence of diabetes, insulin resistance, impaired β-cell function, reactive hypoglycemia, or rare disorders of carbohydrate metabolism. In the most commonly performed version of the test, the oral glucose tolerance test (OGTT), a standard dose of glucose is ingested by mouth and blood levels are checked 2 hours later. Many variations of the test have been devised over the years for various purposes, with different standard doses of glucose, different routes of administration, different intervals and durations of sampling, and various substances measured in addition to blood glucose. For the diagnosis of T2DM, the test should be performed using a glucose load containing the equivalent of 75-g anhydrous glucose dissolved in water.
[c] The glycated hemoglobin test values reflect the patient's average blood glucose levels of the past 2–3 months. Specifically, the test measures what percentage of hemoglobin – a protein in red blood cells that carries oxygen – is coated with sugar (glycated). The higher the glycated hemoglobin level, the poorer the blood glucose control (the more severe the hyperglycemia) and the higher the risk of developing diabetes complications.
Source: Adapted with permission from American Diabetes Association (2020b).

oxidative stress, the action of insulin in insulin-sensitive tissues is diminished, a condition known as *insulin resistance*. Insulin resistance in muscle and adipose tissue results in reduced glucose clearance from the blood toward these tissues. In the liver, insulin resistance results in the suboptimal blockade of glycogenolysis and gluconeogenesis, after consuming a meal that contains carbohydrates; as a result, hepatic glucose enters the blood, when there is no need for it, as plenty of glucose is available from the gut, from the digestion and absorption of dietary carbohydrates. Finally, in T2DM the pancreas has diminished glucose-sensing ability in order to secrete insulin, a condition known as β-cell dysfunction. The above-mentioned abnormal conditions result in elevation of blood glucose levels leading to hyperglycemia (Figure 14.1) (Zheng et al. 2018).

> **Key Point**
>
> T2DM is the most common form of diabetes.

Once hyperglycemia occurs, patients with T2DM are at risk of developing complications that occur rapidly (acute) or over time (chronic) and may affect many organ systems. Acute complications include hyperglycemia, hyperosmolar state, hypoglycemia, and diabetic coma, all related to impaired glucose metabolism. Chronic complications include cardiovascular disease (coronary heart disease, cerebrovascular disease, and peripheral vascular disease), diabetic retinopathy (damage to

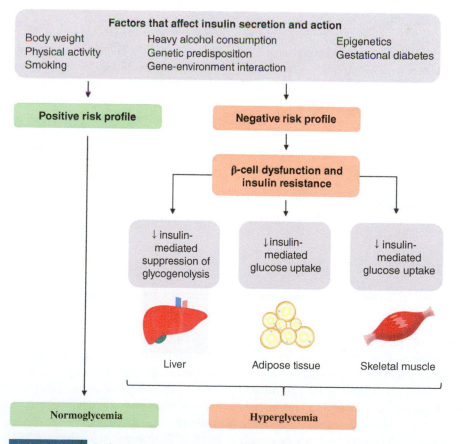

FIGURE 14.1 Pathophysiology of hyperglycemia in T2DM. Insulin secretion from the β-cells of the pancreas normally reduces glucose output by the liver and increases blood glucose uptake by skeletal muscle and adipose tissue. Hyperglycemia develops when there is β-cell dysfunction in the pancreas and/or there is resistance to the action of insulin.
Source: Adapted with permission from Zheng et al. (2018).

> **Key Point**
>
> Once hyperglycemia occurs, patients with T2DM are at risk of developing complications that occur rapidly (acute) or over time (chronic).

the retina, which can gradually lead to blindness), diabetic nephropathy (damage to the kidneys, which can lead to chronic kidney disease), and diabetic neuropathy (damage to the nerves; depending on the affected nerves, diabetic neuropathy symptoms can range from pain and numbness to a complete loss of sensation). All of the above-mentioned complications result from the devastating effects of increased blood glucose to the body's vessels and nerves (Faselis et al. 2020; Viigimaa et al. 2020). Infectious diseases are also a serious complication of T2DM, caused by the hyperglycemic environment that favors immune dysfunction, micro- and macro-angiopathies, and neuropathy. The most common form of infection is foot infection, which can lead to the so-called "diabetic foot" and, if left untreated, amputation (Boulton and Whitehouse 2000).

Anthropometric Assessment

Detailed instructions on how to perform anthropometric assessments have been presented in Chapter 13.

Mr. AM currently weighs 89.5 kg, and his height is 1.72 m. His body mass index (BMI) is 89.5 kg ÷ (1.72 m)² = 30.25 kg/m². According to the classification of BMI values, he is considered obese class I. In addition, his waist circumference is 108.5 cm, which is considered very high (indicative of abdominal adiposity), and combined with the high BMI classifies him to the "very high morbidity risk" category. After discussing with Mr. AM about his body weight history, you recorded the following information: Mr. AM has had a stable weight (~80–85 kg) for most of his adult life, but he gradually started gaining weight after the age of 60 years old when he lost his wife from a brain aneurysm and his daily routine changed dramatically. Ever since, his usual weight is 88–90 kg and he has never tried to lose weight.

Dietary Assessment

Detailed instructions on how to perform dietary assessments have been presented in Chapter 13.

After interviewing Mr. AM about his dietary habits, you recorded the following information: Mr. AM has always tried to eat as healthy as possible. However, since his wife passed away and his children moved out of the house, his dietary habits have changed dramatically. On most days of the week he cooks simple recipes for lunch, such as pasta, orzo, or rice with some kind of ready-made sauce. When his children visit him 2 times/week, he usually orders roasted chicken or pork and always buys some kind of chocolate dessert for his grandchildren, such as cake, chocolate bars, croissants, or cookies. For dinner he usually has either leftovers from lunch or a quick meal, such as sandwiches and salty

snacks. He is particularly fond of sugar-sweetened soda, which he consumes on a daily basis with the main meals. He rarely consumes legumes or fish and seafood, and fruits and vegetables are not part of his daily diet.

In the context of the 24-hour dietary recall (Appendix D.1), Mr. AM described the consumption of foods and beverages of the previous day as follows:

<u>Breakfast</u>: one cup of full-fat milk and one slice of white bread with one tablespoon of orange jam

<u>Morning snack</u>: one slice of cheese pie and one milk chocolate

<u>Lunch</u>: three cups of pasta carbonara with parmesan cheese, two slices of white bread, one cup of lettuce salad with two tablespoons of olive oil, and two glasses of regular Coca-Cola

<u>Afternoon snack</u>: one cup of coffee with three teaspoons of sugar and one milk chocolate

<u>Dinner</u>: one medium sandwich with ham, cheese, and mayonnaise, a handful of oregano potato chips, and two glasses of regular Coca-Cola

Physical Activity Assessment

Detailed instructions on how to perform physical activity assessments have been presented in Chapter 13.

After interviewing Mr. AM about his physical activity habits, you recorded the following information: Mr. AM was a military officer, and besides some short periods of military training including intense physical activity, his job was largely sedentary. When his wife was still alive, they used to walk almost on a daily basis for about 30 minutes in a park near their house. However, since he lost his wife 5 years ago, the only regular activity Mr. AM performs is a 10-minute walk for shopping at the local minimarket 3–4 times/week. At the time of your evaluation he is completely sedentary because his unhealed foot wound has limited his walking capacity, and the only type of physical activity he performs is light housework.

Sleep Assessment

Detailed instructions on how to perform sleep assessments have been presented in Chapter 13.

After interviewing Mr. AM about his sleep habits, you recorded the following information: During a typical day, he usually wakes up around 08:00, goes for shopping around 11:00 and has lunch around 15:00, after which he always has a siesta until 17:00. In the afternoon he does some housework, reads the newspaper, and talks on the phone with his kids. At night he usually watches TV from 20:00 to midnight and goes to bed around 00:30. During the last couple of months, Mr. AM reports having insomnia symptoms (increased time to fall asleep and frequent arousals during the night), as well as frequent headaches, increased sleepiness, and low functionality during the day. Using the Berlin questionnaire

(Appendix D.8), Mr. AM was categorized as at high risk for the presence of obstructive sleep apnea.

Stress Assessment

Detailed instructions on how to perform stress assessments are presented in Chapter 13.

Mr. AM is retired, and although he has a lot of free time, he has been less socially active since the death of his wife. As he stated, he is "rarely in the mood for social interactions other than with his children and grandchildren." Moreover, he frequently experiences fatigue, difficulty concentrating and sleeping, loss of interest in activities or hobbies, irritability and restlessness, all typical symptoms of stress, anxiety, and depression. Mr. AM's score in the Zung Self-Rating Anxiety Scale (Appendix D.11) was 65, indicative of marked to severe anxiety.

Type 2 Diabetes Mellitus Management

General Principles

A multidisciplinary team is considered essential for the efficient management of a patient with T2DM. The team's approach should be focused on integrated management with multiple treatment goals, including blood glucose, blood pressure and blood lipid control, weight control, lifestyle management, and regular follow-ups and screening for the prevention of diabetes comorbidities. While primary care physicians are the first point of contact and a source of continuous comprehensive care, their collaboration with other specialties, such as podiatrists, nurses, dietitians, exercise physiologists, optometrists, psychologists, and social workers, is considered crucial (McGill et al. 2017). With regard to pharmacotherapy, oral antidiabetic drugs are usually prescribed to patients with T2DM, to decrease the production of glucose by the liver and make muscle and adipose tissue more sensitive to insulin. Examples include biguanides (e.g., metformin), sulfonylureas (e.g., glimepiride), meglitinides (e.g., repaglinide), thiazolidinediones (e.g., pioglitazone), and α-glucosidase inhibitors (e.g., acarbose) (American Diabetes Association 2020a). In general, metformin is considered as the first-line drug treatment for T2DM.

> **Key Point**
>
> A multidisciplinary team is considered essential for the efficient management of a patient with T2DM.

> **Key Point**
>
> Oral antidiabetic drugs are usually prescribed to patients with T2DM, to decrease the production of glucose by the liver and make muscle and adipose tissue more sensitive to insulin.

Weight Control

Due to the strong relationship between adiposity and insulin resistance, weight loss has long been a recommended therapeutic strategy for obese adults with T2DM (American Diabetes Association 2020c). Reducing energy intake while maintaining a healthy eating pattern is the optimal approach to promote weight loss in diabetics. Energy restriction should be individualized and should take into account the patient's nutritional habits, physical activity level, comorbidities, and previous dieting attempts. There is not a specific weight-loss goal that suits all obese patients with T2DM; however, even modest weight loss (e.g., 3–5%) can yield significant clinical benefits (improved glycemia, blood pressure, and/or lipids) in some patients, especially those early in the disease process. Detailed instructions on weight-loss goals, how to estimate a patient's energy needs, and how to achieve energy restriction have been presented in Chapter 13.

> **Key Point**
>
> Reducing energy intake while maintaining a healthy eating pattern is the optimal approach to promote weight loss in diabetics.

> **Key Point**
>
> There is not a specific weight-loss goal that suits all obese patients with T2DM; however, even modest weight loss (e.g., 3–5%) can yield significant clinical benefits.

Mr. AM is 65 years old and weighs 89.5 kg. Based on the Schofield equations for men aged > 60 years old, his BMR is $11.711 \times 89.5 + 587.7 = {\sim}1640$ kcal. Given that he is sedentary, his BMR should be multiplied with a physical activity factor of 1.3, resulting in a total daily energy expenditure of ~2130 kcal. It must be noted that in older adults, aggressive weight loss is not recommended, given the possible presence of sarcopenia (a condition that occurs when muscle mass and quality decrease), the increased risk of fractures, and the positive association between low BMI values (<22.5 kg/m^2) and increased mortality (Goisser et al. 2020). Daily energy intake of 1800 kcal (producing a daily energy deficit of 300 kcal) seems appropriate for Mr. AM to achieve a gradual modest weight loss but also preserve a healthy nutritional state.

Dietary Modification

Nutrition therapy is recommended for all patients with T2DM. Due to the progressive nature of the disease, nutritional interventions alone are generally not efficient in maintaining long-term glycemic control. However, after pharmacotherapy is initiated, nutrition continues to be an important component of the overall treatment plan of a T2DM patient. Therefore, it is crucial that the patient is referred to a registered dietitian, or a similarly credentialed health professional, for nutrition therapy shortly after disease diagnosis and for ongoing follow-ups. Another option for many patients is referral to a comprehensive

TABLE 14.2   Goals of nutrition therapy for patients with T2DM.

Promote and support healthy eating patterns, emphasizing a variety of nutrient-dense foods in appropriate portion sizes to improve overall health and attain individualized glycemic, blood pressure, and lipid goals. Recommended goals for these markers are:[a]
- A1C <7%.
- Achieve and maintain a healthy body weight.
- Blood pressure < 130/85 mmHg.
- LDL cholesterol <100 mg/dl; triglycerides <150 mg/dl; HDL cholesterol >40 mg/dl for men and >50 mg/dl for women.
- Delay or prevent complications of diabetes.

Address individual nutritional needs based on personal and cultural preferences, health literacy and numeracy, access to healthy food choices, willingness, and ability to make behavioral changes, as well as barriers to change.

Maintain the pleasure of eating by providing positive messages about food choices while limiting food choices only when indicated by scientific evidence.

Provide the patient with practical tools for day-to-day meal planning rather than focusing on individual macronutrients, micronutrients, or single foods.

A1C, glycated hemoglobin; HDL, high-density lipoprotein; LDL, low-density lipoprotein; T2DM, type 2 diabetes mellitus.
[a] A1C, blood pressure, and cholesterol goals may need to be adjusted for the individual based on age, duration of diabetes, health history, and other health conditions.
Source: Adapted with permission from Evert et al. (2014).

diabetes self-management education program that includes counseling on dietary modification and behavioral change. Fundamental goals of nutrition therapy for T2DM are presented in Table 14.2 (Evert et al. 2014).

Although numerous studies have attempted to identify the optimal proportion of macronutrients for people with diabetes, it is well established that there is no ideal macronutrient mix that applies to all patients with T2DM. Macronutrient proportions should be individualized based on the metabolic status of the patient (e.g., lipid profile, renal function) and food preferences. For example, a slight reduction in carbohydrate content (especially sugars) might be appropriate for patients with hypertriglyceridemia, while a modest protein intake could benefit patients with an impairment in kidney function. Under this scope, a variety of dietary patterns have been shown effective in managing T2DM, including the Mediterranean-style diet, the Dietary Approaches to Stop Hypertension (DASH), and plant-based (vegan or vegetarian), low-fat, and low-carbohydrate patterns. Comorbidities, personal preferences (e.g., tradition, culture, religion, health beliefs, economics), and metabolic goals are important factors to be considered

> **Key Point**
>
> There is no ideal macronutrient mix. Macronutrient proportions should be based on the metabolic status and food preferences of each patient.

when recommending dietary patterns to patients (Evert et al. 2014; Garnett et al. 2014; Lazarou et al. 2012; Salas-Salvado et al. 2011; Gow et al. 2016.).

The type of carbohydrate is the most important factor for the dietary management of T2DM. Patients should avoid simple carbohydrates (sugars) and favor complex carbohydrates (dietary fiber) from natural, unrefined/less processed foods (Evert et al. 2014). In this context, vegetables, whole fruits, whole-grain cereal products, legumes, and dairy products should be preferred over foods that contain added sugars (such as sucrose, fructose, and high-fructose corn syrup). The use of non-nutritive sweeteners (e.g., aspartame, saccharin, sucralose, stevia, and acesulfame-potassium) is safe, when consumption is within the acceptable daily intake (ADI) established by the Food and Drug Administration (FDA). The ADI is a conservative estimate of non-nutritive sweeteners that can be safely consumed by any person in the population on a daily basis over a lifetime without significant health risks. A brief overview of widely used non-nutritive sweeteners approved by the FDA is presented in Table 14.3.

> **Key Point**
>
> The type of carbohydrate is the most important factor for the dietary management of T2DM. Patients should avoid simple carbohydrates (sugars) and emphasize complex carbohydrates (dietary fiber) from natural, unrefined/less processed foods.

In addition, substituting high-glycemic index (GI) and glycemic load (GL) foods for lower–GI and GL foods can modestly improve glycemic control and should be an additional target for patients with T2DM (Evert et al. 2014). GI is a ranking of foods on a scale from 0 to 100 according to the extent to which they raise blood glucose levels after food consumption, compared to the same quantity of a reference food (usually white bread or glucose, which have a glycemic index of 100). Table 14.4 presents the average GI of selected common foods (Atkinson et al. 2008). Foods with a high GI are rapidly digested, absorbed, and metabolized and result in marked fluctuations in blood glucose levels, while low-GI foods produce smaller fluctuations in blood glucose and insulin levels (Figure 14.2). Unprocessed foods with a high dietary fiber content, such as whole fruits, vegetables, whole grains, and legumes, have a low GI and should be preferred over processed foods rich in sugars, such as refined grains, pastries, sweets, fruit juices, and sugar-sweetened beverages. Although GI is a useful index to compare different foods with regard to their ability to raise blood glucose, the portion size and total carbohydrate amount consumed is more important. For

> **Key Point**
>
> Substituting high-glycemic index (GI) and glycemic load (GL) foods for lower GI and GL foods can modestly improve glycemic control.

TABLE 14.3 **Widely used non-nutritive sweeteners.**

	Aspartame	Acesulfame-K	Saccharin	Sucralose	Steviosides
Definition	Synthetic sweetener composed of aspartic acid and phenylalanine.	A combination of an organic acid and potassium.	Synthetic sweetener in forms of sodium or calcium saccharin.	A sugar derivative by replacing 3 hydroxyl groups with 3 chlorine atoms on the sugar molecule.	Derived from the leaves of *Stevia rebaudiana* plant in South America. Known as "sweet leaf."
Characteristics	Loses sweetness with high heat.	Highly heat stable for cooking and baking. Metallic aftertaste.	Highly heat stable for cooking and baking. Bitter metallic aftertaste.	Highly heat stable for cooking and baking.	Heat stable. Licorice aftertaste. Enhances sweet and savory flavors. Lacks bulking property.
Metabolism	Broken down into aspartic acid, phenylalanine, and methanol upon digestion. All compounds are metabolized normally, except in individuals with PKU.	Not metabolized and excreted unchanged by the kidneys.	Not metabolized and excreted unchanged by the kidneys.	Not randomized and excreted by the kidneys and in feces.	Not absorbed in small intestine. Degraded into steviol by bacteria in the colon, where it is absorbed. Excreted in the feces and urine.
Relative sweetness compared to sucrose[a]	180	200	300	600	200–300
kcal/g	4	0	0	0	0
ADI (mg/kg/d)	50	15	5	5	0–4 (as steviol)
ADI for 70 kg person/cans of soda equivalent	3500 mg/28	1050 mg/21	350 mg/4	350 mg/6	0–280 mg/5
Uses	Tabletop sweetener, ingredients in foods and diet soft drinks. Limited use in bakery products.	Tabletop sweetener, baked goods, frozen desserts, candies, beverages, cough drops, and breath mints.	Tabletop sweetener, soft drinks, baked goods, jams, chewing gum, canned fruit, candy, dessert toppings, salad dressings.	Tabletop sweetener, beverages, chewing gum, frozen desserts, fruit juices, gelatins.	Tabletop sweetener, juices, tea beverages. Used extensively in Japan for pickles, dried seafoods, and confections.
Health concerns	All should be used at levels below the ADI.				

ADI, acceptable daily intake; PKU, phenylketonuria.
[a] Relative sweetness as compared to sucrose (table sugar). 1 = reference value, which is the sweetness of sucrose.
Source: Adapted with permission from Dwyer et al. (2000).

example, although 100 g of a raw apple has a lower GI compared to 100 g of boiled potatoes (36 vs. 78), consuming three raw apples (~180 g; ~45 g of carbohydrates) will lead to a greater increase in blood glucose compared to the consumption of ½ cup of boiled potatoes (~80 g; ~15 g of carbohydrates). The glycemic load (GL) is an alternate index that takes into account the consumed portion size of a food and the GI of that food and can be used to compare the blood-glucose-raising effects of different quantities of various foods (Augustin et al. 2015). The GL can be calculated as: GL = GI × carbohydrate (g) content per portion (minus the dietary fiber) ÷ 100.

Besides carbohydrate quality, the quantity of carbohydrates for patients with T2DM has been a matter of intense debate. Although data on the ideal amount of carbohydrate intake are inconclusive, the amount of carbohydrates consumed, combined with the available insulin, may be an important factor determining the glycemic response of a diabetic patient and should be considered when developing the eating plan. For patients with T2DM on oral antidiabetic medications, daily carbohydrate intake must be relatively consistent with respect to time of consumption and amount to achieve an optimal glycemic control. Therefore, monitoring carbohydrate intake by experience-based estimation is also a

TABLE 14.4   The average glycemic index of common foods.

High-carbohydrate foods		Breakfast cereals		Fruits and fruit products		Vegetables	
White wheat bread	75±2	Cornflakes	81±6	Apple, raw	36±2	Potato, boiled	78±4
Whole-wheat/whole-meal bread	74±2	Wheat-flake biscuits	69±2	Orange, raw	43±3	Potato, instant mash	87±3
Corn tortilla	46±4	Porridge, rolled oats	55±2	Banana, raw	51±3	Potato, French fries	63±5
White rice, boiled	73±4	Instant oat porridge	79±3	Pineapple, raw	59±8	Carrots, boiled	39±4
Brown rice, boiled	68±4	Rice porridge/congee	78±9	Watermelon, raw	76±4	Sweet potato, boiled	63±6
Spaghetti, white	49±2	Millet porridge	67±5	Apple juice	41±2	Pumpkin, boiled	64±7
Spaghetti, whole meal	48±5	Muesli	57±2	Orange juice	50±2	Taro, boiled	53±2
Dairy products and alternatives		**Legumes**		**Snack products**		**Sugars**	
Milk, full fat	39±3	Chickpeas	39±3	Chocolate	40±3	Fructose	15±4
Milk, skim	37±4	Kidney beans	24±4	Popcorn	65±5	Sucrose	65±4
Ice cream	51±3	Lentils	32±5	Potato chips	56±3	Glucose	103±3
Yogurt, fruit	41±2	Soya beans	16±1	Soft drink/soda	59±3	Honey	61±3

Source: Adapted with permission from Atkinson et al. (2008).

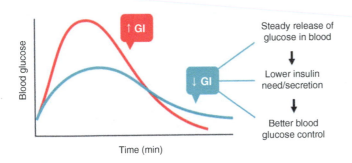

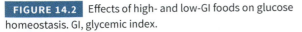

FIGURE 14.2 Effects of high- and low-GI foods on glucose homeostasis. GI, glycemic index.

useful strategy in achieving normoglycemia in T2DM (Evert et al. 2014). Table 14.5 provides an overview of the average carbohydrate content of basic food groups, which can serve as a tool for the education of the diabetic patient. In general, dairy products, fruits, vegetables, grains, and legumes are important sources of carbohydrates, while white meat, red meat, fish and seafood, and fats, oils, and nuts have negligible carbohydrate content. For packaged foods and beverages, information on their exact carbohydrate content can be obtained from food labels.

> **Key Point**
>
> The amount of carbohydrates consumed, combined with the available insulin, may be an important factor determining the glycemic response of a diabetic patient.

Evidence is inconclusive regarding the ideal amount of daily fat (dietary lipids) intake for people with T2DM; however, the type and quality of fat in the diet appear to be far more important than quantity. A Mediterranean-style dietary pattern, rich in monounsaturated fatty acids (especially from extra-virgin olive oil, olives, and nuts) and polyunsaturated fatty acids (e.g., omega-3 fatty acids from fish and green leafy vegetables) has been shown to improve glycemic control and reduce cardiovascular risk; this diet is recommended for T2DM patients compared to a lower-fat, higher-carbohydrate dietary pattern. More information on the Mediterranean diet can be found in Chapter 7. Evidence does not support recommending omega-3 fatty acid supplements for patients with T2DM. However, the recommendation for the general population to eat at least two servings of fish (particularly fatty fish) per week is also appropriate for people with T2DM. Emphasis must also be given to minimizing the intake of trans-fatty acids from refined and processed foods, such as commercial sweets, pastries, baked goods, salty snacks, and fast food, to lower cardiovascular risk (Evert et al. 2014).

> **Key Point**
>
> The type and quality of fat in the diet appear to be far more important than quantity.

> **Key Point**
>
> Emphasis must be given to minimizing the intake of trans-fatty acids from refined and processed foods.

TABLE 14.5 Carbohydrate content of major food groups.

Food group	Examples of foods and portions	Carbohydrates (g)
Dairy products	1 cup of milk, sour milk or kefir, 200 g of yogurt	12
Fruits	1 medium apple, pear, or peach, 1 small banana, 2 figs, kiwis, or mandarins, 1 cup of strawberries or cherries, 1 slice of melon or watermelon, ½ cup of fruit juice	15
Vegetables	1 cup of raw vegetables (tomato, cucumber, lettuce, pepper, carrot, cabbage, etc.) or ½ cup of boiled vegetables (zucchini, cauliflower, beetroot)	5
Starchy vegetables	½ cup of potatoes (boiled, roasted, or mashed), corn, or peas	15
Grains[a]	1 slice (30 g) of bread, 2 small rusks, ½ pita bread, ½ bagel, ½ cup of breakfast cereals or oatmeal, ½ cup of cooked rice or pasta, 1 tablespoon (15 g) of flour	15
Legumes	½ cup of beans, fava beans, chickpeas, lentils	15
Sugars	1 teaspoon of sugar, honey, or marmalade	5

[a] Although grains are rich in carbohydrates, choosing whole-grain instead of refined-grain products can produce more stable glycemic levels, avoiding blood sugar spikes.

With regard to proteins, if there is no evidence of diabetic kidney disease, daily protein intake should be individualized in accordance with current guidelines for the general population (e.g., 0.8 g/kg or 1.0–1.2 g/kg for older adults; a further increase might be required for exercising individuals and athletes). People with diabetic kidney disease (either micro- or macroalbuminuria) may decrease protein intake but not below 0.6 g/kg; no significant improvements are expected in glycemic control, cardiovascular risk, or the course of glomerular filtration rate decline when protein intake is very low. Furthermore, significant decreases in protein intake can lead to additional complications, including malnutrition (Evert et al. 2014).

> **Key Point**
>
> Daily protein intake should be individualized in accordance with current guidelines for the general population.

All things considered, there is no standard meal plan or eating pattern that works for all people with T2DM. In order to be effective, nutrition therapy for T2DM should be individualized, based on the patient's comorbidities, individual health goals, personal and cultural preferences, access to healthy choices, and readiness, ability, and self-efficacy to change. Nutrition interventions should propose a variety of minimally processed foods in appropriate portion sizes as part of a healthy eating pattern and provide the patient with practical tools for day-to-day meal planning and behavior change that can be maintained in the long term. Table 14.6 provides a summary of nutritional recommendations for patients with T2DM, based on general guidelines for diabetes management and medication-specific advice (Evert et al. 2014).

> **Key Point**
>
> There is no standard meal plan or eating pattern that works for all people with T2DM.

> **Key Point**
>
> Nutrition therapy for T2DM should be individualized for each patient based on his/her comorbidities, individual health goals, personal and cultural preferences, access to healthy choices, and readiness, ability, and self-efficacy to change.

According to Mr. AM's dietary assessment, individualized counseling toward a healthy diet for T2DM management should focus on taking these steps:

- Consume only moderate amounts of complex carbohydrates at each meal and snacks.
- Increase the consumption of plant-based, fiber-rich, low-GI/GL foods:
  a. Fruits, e.g., one fruit/day and gradual increase to two to three fruits/day with emphasis on a variety of fresh, whole, seasonal fruits.
  b. Vegetables, e.g., a seasonal salad accompanying lunch and dinner with emphasis on a variety of fresh seasonal raw vegetables.
  c. Whole grains, such as whole-grain pasta and brown rice, instead of refined ones.
  d. Legumes, e.g., one meal/week and gradual increase to two meals/week instead of pasta.
- Consume only moderate amounts of sweets and sugar-sweetened beverages. Given Mr. AM's daily consumption of sweets, a realistic goal would be to gradually decrease the frequency of consumption to two to three portions/week and emphasize smaller portion sizes (e.g., one chocolate cookie or ½ glass of soda), with a longer-term goal of eliminating them. Other less energy-dense and lower-GI choices could be considered, such as sweets based on milk and yogurt, nuts with honey, smoothies with fresh fruits and milk/yogurt, or other low-sugar beverages, such as herbal infusions and artificially sweetened beverages.

TABLE 14.6   Key topics for nutrition education in patients with T2DM.

Strategies for all people with T2DM:
- Portion control should be recommended for glycemic control and weight loss and maintenance.
- Amount and type of ingested carbohydrate-containing foods and beverages and endogenous insulin production are the most important determinants of the post-meal blood glucose level; therefore, it is important to know the carbohydrate type and content in the foods we consume, i.e., starchy vegetables, whole grains, fruit, milk and milk products, vegetables, and sugar.
- When choosing carbohydrate-containing foods, whenever possible choose nutrient-dense, high-fiber instead of processed foods with added sodium, fat, and sugars. Nutrient-dense foods and beverages provide calorie-free vitamins, minerals, and other healthy micronutrients.
- Avoid sugar-sweetened beverages.
- For most people, it is not necessary to subtract the amount of dietary fiber or sugar alcohols from total carbohydrates when carbohydrate counting.
- Substitute foods higher in unsaturated fat (liquid oils, especially olive oil) for foods higher in trans or saturated fat (such as margarine and butter).
- Select leaner protein sources and meat alternatives, such as white meat and fish.
- Vitamin and mineral supplements, herbal products, or cinnamon intake are not recommended in the management of T2DM due to lack of evidence.
- Moderate alcohol consumption (one drink/day or less for adult women and two drinks or less for adult men) has minimal acute or long-term effects on blood glucose in people with T2DM. To reduce risk of hypoglycemia for individuals using insulin or insulin secretagogues, alcohol should be consumed with food.
- Limit sodium intake to 2300 mg/day.

Strategies for individuals on insulin secretagogues:
- Consume moderate amounts of carbohydrate at each meal and snacks.
- To reduce risk of hypoglycemia:[a]
  - Eat a source of carbohydrate at meals.
  - Do not skip meals.
  - Physical activity may result in low blood glucose. Always carry a source of carbohydrates with you to reduce risk of hypoglycemia.

Strategies for individuals on biguanides (metformin):
- Consume moderate amounts of carbohydrate at each meal and snacks.
- Gradually titrate to minimize gastrointestinal side effects[b] when initiating use:
  - Take medication with food or 15 min after a meal if symptoms persist.
  - If side effects do not resolve over time (a few weeks), talk to your doctor.
  - If taking along with an insulin secretagogue or insulin, may experience hypoglycemia.

Strategies for individuals on a-glucosidase inhibitors:
- Gradually titrate to minimize gastrointestinal side effects[b] when initiating use.
- Take at start of meal to have maximal effect:
  - If taking along with an insulin secretagogue or insulin, patients may experience hypoglycemia.
  - If hypoglycemia occurs, eat something containing monosaccharides such as glucose tablets, as the drug will prevent the digestion of polysaccharides.

Strategies for individuals on incretin mimetics (GLP-1):
- Gradually titrate to minimize gastrointestinal side effects[b] when initiating use:
  - Injection of daily or twice-daily GLP-1s should be premeal.
  - If side effects do not resolve over time (a few weeks), talk to your doctor.
  - If taking along with an insulin secretagogue or insulin, patients may experience hypoglycemia.
  - Once-weekly GLP-1s can be taken at any time during the day regardless of mealtimes.

Strategies for individuals with insulin-requiring T2DM:
- Learn how to count carbohydrates or use another meal-planning approach to quantify carbohydrate intake. The objective of using such a meal-planning approach is to "match" mealtime insulin to carbohydrates consumed.
- If on a multiple-daily injection plan or on an insulin pump:
  - Take mealtime insulin before eating.
  - Meals can be consumed at different times.
  - If physical activity is performed within 1–2 h of mealtime insulin injection, this dose may need to be lowered to reduce risk of hypoglycemia.
- If on a premixed insulin plan:
  - Insulin doses need to be taken at consistent times every day.
  - Meals need to be consumed at similar times every day.
  - Do not skip meals to reduce the risk of hypoglycemia.
  - Physical activity may result in low blood glucose depending on when it is performed. Always carry a source of quick-acting carbohydrates with you to reduce risk of hypoglycemia.
- If on a fixed insulin plan:
  - Eat similar amounts of carbohydrates each day to match the set doses of insulin.

GLP-1, glucagon-like peptide 1; T2DM, type 2 diabetes mellitus.

[a] Treatment of hypoglycemia: current recommendations to treat hypoglycemia include the use of glucose tablets or carbohydrate-containing foods or beverages (such as fruit juice, sports drinks, regular soda pop, or hard candy). A commonly recommended dose of glucose is 15–20 g. When blood glucose levels are ~50–60 mg/dl, treatment with 15 g of glucose is expected to raise blood glucose levels by ~50 mg/dl. If the hypoglycemia persists after 15-20 from the glucose intake, the treatment should be repeated.

[b] Gastrointestinal symptoms are commonly reported as side effects of oral hypoglycemic drugs. Although such symptoms have been reported with the use of various categories of antidiabetic agents, the most pronounced are related to the use of metformin. Metformin is a biguanide class of drugs and has been recommended as first-line therapy for T2DM. It has a good safety profile, efficacy, low cost, and potential cardiovascular benefits; however, its gastrointestinal side effects can negatively affect patients' quality of life and treatment adherence. The most common symptoms are diarrhea and fecal incontinence, heartburn, and nausea, followed by abdominal pain, bloating, and retching. The exact mechanism(s) for the gastrointestinal intolerance when taking metformin is unclear; possible mechanisms include the stimulation of intestinal secretion of serotonin and malabsorption of bile salts.

Source: Adapted with permission from Evert et al. (2014) and McCreight et al. (2016).

Meal	Current dietary habits	Recommended alternatives
TABLE 14.7	**Recommended dietary changes for the management of T2DM.**	
Breakfast	1 cup of full-fat milk and 1 slice of white bread with 1 tablespoon of orange jam	1 cup of full-fat milk and 2 whole seasonal fruits
Morning snack	1 slice of cheese pie and 1 milk chocolate	1 whole-grain sandwich with cheese and vegetables
Lunch	3 cups of pasta carbonara with parmesan, 2 slices of white bread, 1 cup of lettuce salad with 2 tablespoons of olive oil, and 2 glasses of Coca-Cola	1 roasted fish filet with potatoes, 1 slice of whole-grain bread, 1 seasonal salad with olive oil, and water or 1 glass of sugar-free beverage (e.g., artificially sweetened soda)
Afternoon snack	1 cup of coffee with 3 teaspoons of sugar and 1 milk chocolate	1 cup of coffee with 1 teaspoon of sugar and 1–2 whole seasonal fruits
Dinner	1 medium sandwich with ham, cheese, and mayonnaise, a handful of oregano potato chips, and 2 glasses of Coca-Cola	Omelet with 2 eggs and cheese, 1 slice of whole-grain bread, and 1 seasonal salad with olive oil

- *Consume healthy fat sources, such as extra-virgin olive oil (in cooking and salads), olives, and nuts, instead of margarine and butter.*
- *Consume lean protein sources, such as fish/seafood, white meat, and eggs (in moderation) instead of red meat.*
- *Follow a balanced meal pattern with emphasis on home cooking and nutritional variety, combined with portion control to achieve a gradual modest weight loss.*

Table 14.7 summarizes beneficial dietary changes for Mr. AM toward managing T2DM based on his 24-hour dietary recall.

Physical Activity Modification

It is well established that participation in regular physical activity improves blood glucose control and can prevent or delay T2DM; this is in addition to positively affecting lipids, blood pressure, cardiovascular events, mortality, and quality of life. Structured interventions combining physical activity and modest weight loss have been shown to lower T2DM risk by up to 60% in high-risk populations, and to contribute to an efficient disease management when combined with appropriate pharmacological treatments. Most of the benefits of exercise on T2DM management can be attributed to acute and chronic improvements in insulin sensitivity; aerobic and resistance types of exercise can be used, provided they are sustained in the long term. In general, most adults with T2DM should engage in ≥150 min of moderate-to-vigorous-intensity aerobic activity weekly, spread over ≥3 days/week, with no more than 2 consecutive days without activity. Both high-intensity interval training and continuous exercise training are appropriate for most patients (Colberg et al. 2016). Resistance exercise (such as free weights, resistance bands, and/or use of body weight as resistance) should also be performed 2–3 times/week with moderate (e.g., 10–15 repetitions to near fatigue) to vigorous (e.g., 6–8 repetitions to near fatigue) intensity; at least 8–10 exercises with completion of 1–3 sets of 10–15 repetitions to near fatigue per set should be performed (Colberg et al. 2016).

Adults with T2DM are frequently treated with multiple medications. The use of oral antidiabetic drugs does not require modifications in response to exercise. On the other hand, some medications for diabetes comorbidities (e.g., CVD, hypertension) may need to be adjusted when exercise is planned. Although changes should be individualized, patients on antihypertensive medication should generally check their blood glucose before and after exercise and treat hypoglycaemia, and avoid dehydration through proper fluid replacement In addition, patients treated for dyslipidemia with fibrates should avoid exercise if muscle conditions such as myositis or rhabdomyolysis are present (Colberg et al. 2016).

Macrovascular and microvascular diabetes-related complications develop, depending on the age and comorbidities of the patient prior to diagnosis, and can worsen with inadequate blood glucose control. Vascular and neural complications of T2DM often cause physical limitations and varying levels of disability requiring precautions during exercise. In patients with cardiovascular diseases, physical activity is generally regarded as safe, especially if it is of light to moderate intensity However, patients with coronary artery disease, myocardial infarction, and stroke should preferably exercise in a supervised cardiac rehabilitation program, at least initially, starting at a low intensity and progressing , if the patient is able, to more moderate activities. Patients with exertional angina and congestive heart failure should avoid activities that cause an excessive rise in heart rate Patients with peripheral neuropathy and foot

> **Key Point**
>
> It is well established that participation in regular physical activity improves blood glucose control and can prevent or delay T2DM.

> **Key Point**
>
> Most of the benefits of exercise on T2DM management can be attributed to acute and chronic improvements in insulin sensitivity.

> **Key Point**
>
> The use of oral antidiabetic drugs does not require modifications in response to exercise.

deformities/ulcers should always exercise with proper foot care, in order to avoid infections, ulceration, and amputation. Although moderate walking is not likely to increase risk of foot ulcers or reulceration, jogging should be avoided and emphasis should be placed on non–weight-bearing activities to reduce undue plantar pressures. Feet should be examined daily to detect and treat blisters, sores, or ulcers early Moreover, in the presence of autonomic neuropathy, patients may experience a variety of complications during exercise, such as postural hypotension, chronotropic incompetence, delayed gastric emptying, altered thermoregulation, and dehydration. Therefore, they should ideally obtain medical approval and undergo symptom-limited exercise testing before commencing exercise, avoid exercising in hot environments, stay hydrated, and avoid activities with rapid postural or directional changes to avoid fainting or falling

> **Key Point**
>
> Vascular and neural complications of T2DM often cause physical limitations and varying levels of disability requiring precautions during exercise.

In the presence of severe nonproliferative and unstable proliferative retinopathy, patients should be counseled to avoid vigorous activities that significantly elevate blood pressure, jumping, jarring, and head-down activities Cataracts do not impact the ability to exercise, only the safety of doing so due to loss of visual acuity. In this case, activities that can be dangerous due to limited vision, such as outdoor cycling, should be avoided For patients with diabetic kidney disease, all activities are considered safe (exercise does not accelerate the progression of kidney disease, even though protein excretion acutely increases following exercise), but exercise should begin at a low intensity and volume if aerobic capacity and muscle function are substantially reduced. Vigorous exercise should best be avoided the day before urine protein tests are performed to prevent false positive readings. In the presence of end-stage renal disease, performing supervised, moderate aerobic physical activity during dialysis sessions may be beneficial and increase patients' compliance, but electrolytes should be closely monitored to prevent complications.

According to Mr. AM's comorbidities and physical activity assessment, key points for individualized counseling toward a physically active lifestyle include the following:

- *Mr. AM is completely sedentary at the time of evaluation; any increase in physical activity would be beneficial.*
- *Exercise training volume and intensity should progress appropriately according to his capabilities in order to minimize risks of injury.*
- *Given his unhealed foot wound, non–weight-bearing activities should be chosen. Examples include using a stationary bicycle, lifting weights or using resistance bands while seated, using a stationary hand cycling machine to work the upper body muscles, a wide range of motion exercises for joint flexibility, isometric exercises that tighten and relax muscles, and yoga exercises that do not require supporting one's weight on the feet.*
- *Given his blurry sight resulting from mild retinopathy, intense activities that result in dramatic increases in blood pressure, such as heavy weight lifting, should be avoided.*
- *When his foot wound is healed, walking is the easiest and more sustainable form of aerobic physical activity. A realistic goal would be to aim for a 20-minute walk 2–3 days/week, with a gradual increase to a 30-minute walk on most days of the week to achieve the recommended 150 minutes/week of aerobic physical activity.*
- *Other advice should focus on using stairs instead of elevators whenever possible, taking a short walk after lunch, engaging in family activities with his children and grandchildren that involve physical activity, or any kind of light exercise he enjoys.*

Sleep Modification

Abnormal sleep duration, including short (<7 hours/day) and long sleep (>9 hours/day), and the presence of sleep disorders – mainly obstructive sleep apnea – have evolved as major public health concerns, due to their high prevalence and significant links with mortality and comorbid conditions. There is an independent association of sleep disturbances with the development and progression of disorders affecting glucose metabolism, mainly T2DM (Ogilvie and Patel 2018; Ryan 2018). Experimental short-term sleep restriction in humans has been shown to lead to increased calorie intake, weight gain, insulin resistance, and possibly impaired insulin secretion. Sympathetic excitation, inflammation, and alterations of the 24-hour cortisol profile with blunting of the usual nocturnal decline have been proposed as the underlying mechanisms for these disorders. The results of the available well-designed epidemiological studies also point to a U-shaped association between sleep duration and diabetes risk, meaning that diabetes risk is higher for short- and long-sleepers compared to individuals in the intermediate category of sleep duration. A late sleep pattern (i.e., going to bed late) is also associated with higher insulin resistance in T2DM patients and healthy individuals.

> **Key Point**
>
> There is compelling evidence of an independent association of sleep disturbances with the development and progression of disorders affecting glucose metabolism, mainly T2DM.

> **Key Point**
>
> Diabetes risk is higher for both short- and long-sleepers compared to individuals in the intermediate category of sleep duration.

According to Mr. AM's assessment, counseling toward the improvement of sleep habits should focus on the following:

- T2DM often coexists with sleep disorders, mainly obstructive sleep apnea, an obesity-related chronic disease characterized by repetitive pauses of breathing during sleep due to obstructions of the upper airways. According to the assessment using the Berlin questionnaire, Mr. AM was found to be at high risk for obstructive sleep apnea and should be referred to a sleep specialist for a more comprehensive sleep assessment and treatment.
- Mr. AM usually sleeps 5–6 hours during the night. He should be encouraged to gradually increase his daily sleep duration to 7 hours as recommended for adults, and perhaps have a siesta in the middle of the day.
- Besides total sleep duration, a shift toward an earlier sleep pattern, e.g., from 23:00 to 07:00 instead of 12:30 to 08:30, could be beneficial for glycemic control.
- Education on sleep hygiene to promote sleep quality. Sleep hygiene practices include: (i) limiting daytime naps to 30–40 minutes; (ii) avoiding stimulants, such as caffeine and nicotine, 4–6 hours before bedtime; (iii) avoiding of alcohol before bedtime; (iv) a short (10-minute) interval of light aerobic exercise, such as walking, before sleep; (v) avoiding foods that can trigger indigestion and gastrointestinal symptoms before sleep; (vi) ensuring adequate exposure to sunlight during the day and darkness at night; (vii) establishing a regular relaxing bedtime routine; (viii) making sure that the sleep environment is pleasant: cool bedroom, avoidance of noises, dark and quiet environment, etc.

Stress Management

Psychological stress is common in many physical illnesses and is increasingly recognized as a risk factor for disease onset and progression. An emerging body of literature suggests that stress may play a significant role in the development of T2DM (Hackett and Steptoe 2017; Sharif et al. 2018). Stress triggers biological responses that exacerbate insulin resistance, including the release of glucose and lipids into the circulation, inflammatory cytokine expression, and increased blood pressure. Repeated or sustained stress exposure leads to chronic allostatic load, with dysregulation of glucose metabolism and neuroendocrine function and chronic low-grade inflammation. Moreover, among individuals with established T2DM, stress and depression are associated with poor glycemic control and increased risk of cardiovascular complications. Stress management interventions, including group-based stress management training, mindfulness, cognitive behavioral interventions, and collaborative care, may alleviate stress symptoms in diabetes, improve glycemic control, and have a favorable effect on the disease progression. Although more research is needed, stress relief is increasingly recognized as an important part of diabetes management and should be included in multicomponent diabetes interventions.

> **Key Point**
> Stress may play a significant role in the development of T2DM.

> **Key Point**
> Stress management interventions may alleviate stress symptoms in diabetes, improve glycemic control, and have a favorable effect on the disease progression.

Counseling for Mr. AM toward stress management should focus on the following:

- *Flexibility and balance exercises, such as yoga and tai chi, could be recommended in addition to aerobic exercise to improve mobility and contribute to stress relief.*
- *Social/convivial activities with family and friends. Being connected to others is a fundamental human need crucial to both well-being and survival; on the other hand, social isolation has been shown to significantly increase risk for morbidity and premature mortality.*
- *Referral to a mental health specialist for a more intensive stress management intervention should be considered in case depressive symptoms are evident.*

Take-Home Messages

- T2DM is the most common type of diabetes, in which insulin resistance, caused by genetic factors but also by obesity and an unhealthy lifestyle, leads to impaired glucose control.
- A comprehensive clinical and lifestyle assessment is crucial for all patients with T2DM. Emphasis should be placed on diabetes symptoms and comorbidities, as well as modifiable behaviors that are linked to overweight and impaired glucose metabolism.
- A multidisciplinary team approach is essential for the efficient management of a patient with T2DM.
- Treatment goals should include glucose, blood pressure, lipid, and weight control; lifestyle modification; and regular follow-ups and screening for the prevention of comorbidities.
- There is no standard meal plan or eating pattern that is appropriate for all patients with T2DM. Nutrition therapy should be individualized for each patient.
- A healthy dietary pattern for diabetes should focus on weight control if necessary, low-GI high-fiber plant-based foods (fruits, vegetables, whole grains, and legumes), healthy fats (olive oil and nuts), lean protein

foods (fish-seafood, white meat, and eggs), and avoiding processed, refined, and sugar-sweetened drinks and foods.

- Several healthy dietary patterns, e.g., the Mediterranean diet, can be used for the management of T2DM.
- Regular physical activity lowers the risk of developing T2DM and can contribute to its management, when combined with proper nutritional and pharmacological treatment.
- The beneficial effects of physical activity on T2DM are mediated from acute and chronic improvements in insulin action, provided that an adequate level of physical activity is sustained in the long term.
- Exercise interventions in patients with T2DM must always be individualized and take into account special considerations, such as medications and comorbidities.
- Most patients with T2DM should engage in ≥150 minutes of moderate-to-vigorous-intensity activity weekly, spread over at least 3 days/week, with no more than 2 consecutive days without activity. Resistance exercise should also be performed 2–3 times/week.

- Flexibility and balance training are additionally recommended 2–3 times/week for older patients with T2DM. Yoga and tai chi may be included based on individual preferences to improve flexibility, muscular strength, and balance, and to decrease stress levels.
- Abnormal sleep is associated with impaired glucose metabolism. Patients with T2DM should aim for an adequate sleep duration, a normal sleep schedule, and optimal sleep hygiene.
- Referral to a sleep specialist for a more comprehensive sleep assessment should be considered in case symptoms related to sleep-disordered breathing are evident.
- Stress has a role in the etiology of T2DM, both as a predictor of new-onset diabetes and as a prognostic factor in people with existing disease.
- Despite being an understudied topic, the available stress management interventions have been found modestly efficient in alleviating stress symptoms, improving glycemic control, and having a favorable effect on diabetes progression.

Self-Assessment Questions

1. Provide the definition and outline the main types of diabetes mellitus.
2. What kind of physical activity advice would you give to a patient with T2DM with unstable proliferative retinopathy?
3. Which of the following statements are true for the link between sleep and diabetes?
   a. Patients with T2DM are protected from sleep disorders due to hyperglycemia.
   b. Sleep restriction can lead to increased calorie intake, weight gain, insulin resistance, and possibly impaired insulin secretion.
   c. Going to bed early is associated with higher risk for insulin resistance.
   d. T2DM risk is higher for both short- and long-sleepers, compared to those in the intermediate category of sleep duration.
   e. Patients with T2DM require more sleep compared to the general population due to their chronic disease burden.
4. What are the current recommendations for the acute treatment of hypoglycemia?
   a. Consumption of 3 tablespoons of sugar or honey in water.
   b. Use of glucose tablets or foods/beverages containing 15–20 g of carbohydrates.
   c. Consumption of a snack rich in dietary fiber and proteins.
   d. No food consumption and reevaluation of blood glucose levels every 15 minutes until hypoglycemia is corrected by liver glucose production.

   e. Consumption of a meal with ≥ 50 g of carbohydrates, such as two cups of boiled pasta or rice.
5. Provide an overview of the basic physical activity guidelines for patients with T2DM in terms of type, frequency, duration, and intensity.
6. Which of the following statements about the glycemic index (GI) are true?
   a. It is a ranking of foods on a scale from 0 to 300.
   b. The GI of a food is a measure of the extent to which it raises blood glucose levels after consumption, compared to the same quantity of a reference food.
   c. Foods with low GI are rapidly digested, absorbed, and metabolized and result in marked fluctuations in blood glucose levels.
   d. High-GI foods lead to a steady release of glucose in blood.
   e. Unprocessed foods with a high dietary fiber content, such as whole fruits, vegetables, whole grains, and legumes, have a lower GI compared to processed foods rich in simple carbohydrates.
7. What are the main goals of nutrition therapy for patients with T2DM?
8. A female patient with T2DM who drinks ~1 L of sugar-sweetened soda on a daily basis visits your office for lifestyle modification. Outline the main points of dietary counseling that you would provide to this patient.
9. Characterize the following statements as true (T) or false (F).
   a. Carbohydrate quantity is crucial for diabetes management, and all patients should consume ≤150 g of carbohydrates daily to avoid hyperglycemia ( ).

b. Use of metformin can cause muscle weakness and cramping ( ).

c. Whole-grain products can produce a better glycemic response compared to refined-grain products ( ).

d. Omega-3 fatty acid supplements are routinely recommended for the management of diabetes mellitus along with the adoption of a balanced diet ( ).

e. Eye cataracts do not impact the ability of a diabetic patient to exercise, only the safety of doing so due to loss of visual acuity ( ).

10. Which of the following foods contain ~30 g of carbohydrates?
    a. two medium fruits
    b. 200 g of roasted chicken
    c. 1 cup of breakfast cereals
    d. 2 cups of boiled pasta
    e. 60 g of cheese
    f. one thin slice of whole-grain bread

11. Which of the following foods/beverages is expected to result in greater increases in blood glucose levels?
    a. 100 g of a raw apple
    b. 100 g of whole-grain pasta
    c. 100 g of full-fat milk
    d. 100 g of boiled potatoes
    e. 100 g of chocolate

12. Briefly outline the main complications of T2DM.

13. Which of the following statements about oral antidiabetic medications are true?
    a. They act at the pancreas and boost the production of insulin.
    b. Their use does not require major modifications in response to exercise.
    c. They aim at decreasing the production of glucose by the liver and making muscle more sensitive to insulin.
    d. They only work when carbohydrate intake is reduced to <50% of total energy intake.
    e. All of the above

14. What are the criteria for the diagnosis of T2DM?

15. Characterize the following statements as true (T) or false (F).
    a. Patients with T2DM should abstain from all kinds of physical activity to avoid episodes of hypoglycemia ( ).
    b. There is no ideal dietary macronutrient composition for the management of T2DM ( ).
    c. Ideal protein intake should be about 50% higher in patients with T2DM compared to the general population ( ).
    d. Non-nutritive sweeteners are dangerous for patients with T2DM because they are linked to detrimental metabolic changes ( ).
    e. T2DM is the result of an autoimmune pancreatic β-cell destruction, which leads to a complete insulin deficiency ( ).

16. How is stress related to T2DM?

17. Which of the following statements about patients with T2DM and foot ulcers are true:
    a. Moderate walking is likely to increase reulceration and should be avoided.
    b. Intense weight-bearing activities should be avoided in the presence of unhealed ulcers.
    c. Feet must be examined daily to detect and treat blisters, sores, or ulcers early.
    d. Jogging is the optimal exercise for skin regrowth and healing.
    e. The patient should avoid any kind of physical activity until the wound is healed.

18. What kind of advice would you give to a patient with T2DM about the GI of foods?

19. Which of the following are potential side effects of metformin?
    a. diarrhea and fecal incontinence
    b. fatigue and muscle weakness
    c. blurry vision
    d. abdominal pain, bloating, and retching
    e. tachycardia and hypertension

20. A male patient with diabetic chronic kidney disease presents at your office for lifestyle counseling. What are your recommendations on protein intake and exercise?

Bibliography

American Diabetes Association. (2010). Diagnosis and classification of diabetes mellitus. *Diabetes Care* 33 (Suppl 1): S62–S69. https://doi.org/10.2337/dc10-S062.

American Diabetes Association. (2020a). 9. Pharmacologic approaches to glycemic treatment: standards of medical care in diabetes-2020. *Diabetes Care* 43 (Suppl 1): S98–S110. https://doi.org/10.2337/dc20-S009.

American Diabetes Association. (2020b). 2. Classification and diagnosis of diabetes: standards of medical care in diabetes-2020. *Diabetes Care* 43 (Suppl 1): S14–S31. https://doi.org/10.2337/dc20-S002.

American Diabetes Association. (2020c). 8. Obesity management for the treatment of type 2 diabetes: standards of medical care in diabetes-2020. *Diabetes Care* 43 (Suppl 1): S89–S97. https://doi.org/10.2337/dc20-S008.

Atkinson, F.S., Foster-Powell, K., and Brand-Miller, J.C. (2008). International tables of glycemic index and glycemic load values: 2008. *Diabetes Care* 31 (12): 2281–2283. https://doi.org/10.2337/dc08-1239.

Augustin, L.S., Kendall, C.W., Jenkins, D.J. et al. (2015). Glycemic index, glycemic load and glycemic response: an international scientific consensus summit from the International Carbohydrate Quality Consortium (ICQC). *Nutr. Metab. Cardiovasc. Dis.* 25 (9): 795–815. https://doi.org/10.1016/j.numecd.2015.05.005.

Boulton, A.J.M. and Whitehouse, R.W. (2000). The diabetic foot. In: K.R. Feingold, B. Anawalt, A. Boyce, G. Chrousos, W.W. de Herder, K. Dhatariya, K. Dungan, A. Grossman, J.M. Hershman, J. Hofland, S. Kalra, G. Kaltsas, C. Koch, P. Kopp, M. Korbonits, C.S. Kovacs, W. Kuohung, B. Laferrere, E.A. McGee, R. McLachlan, J.E. Morley,

M. New, J. Purnell, R. Sahay, F. Singer, C.A. Stratakis, D.L. Trence & D.P. Wilson (Eds.), *Endotext*. South Dartmouth, MA: MDText.com, Inc.

Colberg, S.R., Sigal, R.J., Yardley, J.E. et al. (2016). Physical activity/ exercise and diabetes: a position statement of the American Diabetes Association. *Diabetes Care* 39 (11): 2065–2079. https://doi.org/10.2337/dc16-1728.

Dwyer, J.T., Melanson, K.J., Sriprachy-anunt, U. et al. (2000). Dietary treatment of obesity. In: K.R. Feingold, B. Anawalt, A. Boyce, G. Chrousos, W.W. de Herder, K. Dhatariya, K. Dungan, A. Grossman, J.M. Hershman, J. Hofland, S. Kalra, G. Kaltsas, C. Koch, P. Kopp, M. Korbonits, C.S. Kovacs, W. Kuohung, B. Laferrere, E.A. McGee, R. McLachlan, J.E. Morley, M. New, J. Purnell, R. Sahay, F. Singer, C.A. Stratakis, D.L. Trence & D.P. Wilson (Eds.), *Endotext*. South Dartmouth, MA: MDText.com, Inc.

Evert, A.B., Boucher, J.L., Cypress, M. et al. (2014). Nutrition therapy recommendations for the management of adults with diabetes. *Diabetes Care* 37 (Suppl 1): S120–S143. https://doi.org/10.2337/dc14-S120.

Faselis, C., Katsimardou, A., Imprialos, K. et al. (2020). Microvascular complications of type 2 diabetes mellitus. *Curr. Vasc. Pharmacol.* 18 (2): 117–124. https://doi.org/10.2174/1570161117666190502103733.

Garnett, S.P., Gow, M., Ho, M., Baur, L.A., Noakes, M., Woodhead, H.J. et al. (2014). Improved insulin sensitivity and body composition, irrespective of macronutrient intake, after a 12 month intervention in adolescents with pre-diabetes; RESIST a randomised control trial. BMC Pediatr, 14, 289. doi: 10.1186/s12887-014-0289-0.

Goisser, S., Kiesswetter, E., Schoene, D. et al. (2020). Dietary weight-loss interventions for the management of obesity in older adults. *Rev. Endocr. Metab. Disord.* 21 (3): 355–368. https://doi.org/10.1007/s11154-020-09577-2.

Gow, M.L., Garnett, S.P., Baur, L.A., and Lister, N.B. (2016). The effectiveness of different diet strategies to reduce type 2 diabetes risk in youth. *Nutrients* 8 (8): 486. doi: 10.3390/nu8080486.

Hackett, R.A. and Steptoe, A. (2017). Type 2 diabetes mellitus and psychological stress – a modifiable risk factor. *Nat. Rev. Endocrinol.* 13 (9): 547–560. https://doi.org/10.1038/nrendo.2017.64.

Lazarou, C., Panagiotakos, D., and Matalas, A.L. (2012). The role of diet in prevention and management of type 2 diabetes: implications for public health. *Crit. Rev. Food Sci. Nutr.* 52 (5): 382–389. doi: 10.1080/10408398.2010.500258.

McCreight, L.J., Bailey, C.J., and Pearson, E.R. (2016). Metformin and the gastrointestinal tract. *Diabetologia* 59 (3): 426–435. https://doi.org/10.1007/s00125-015-3844-9.

McGill, M., Blonde, L., Chan, J.C.N. et al. (2017). The interdisciplinary team in type 2 diabetes management: challenges and best practice solutions from real-world scenarios. *J. Clin. Transl. Endocrinol.* 7: 21–27. https://doi.org/10.1016/j.jcte.2016.12.001.

Ogilvie, R.P. and Patel, S.R. (2018). The epidemiology of sleep and diabetes. *Curr. Diab. Rep.* 18 (10): 82. https://doi.org/10.1007/s11892-018-1055-8.

Ryan, S. (2018). Sleep and diabetes. *Curr. Opin. Pulm. Med.* 24 (6): 555–560. https://doi.org/10.1097/MCP.0000000000000524.

Salas-Salvado, J., Martinez-Gonzalez, M.A., Bullo, M., and Ros, E. (2011). The role of diet in the prevention of type 2 diabetes. *Nutr. Metab. Cardiovasc. Dis.* 21 Suppl 2: B32–48. doi: 10.1016/j.numecd.2011.03.009.

Sharif, K., Watad, A., Coplan, L. et al. (2018). Psychological stress and type 1 diabetes mellitus: what is the link? *Expert Rev. Clin. Immunol.* 14 (12): 1081–1088. https://doi.org/10.1080/1744666X.2018.1538787.

Viigimaa, M., Sachinidis, A., Toumpourleka, M. et al. (2020). Macrovascular complications of type 2 diabetes mellitus. *Curr. Vasc. Pharmacol.* 18 (2): 110–116. https://doi.org/10.2174/1570161117666190405165151.

Zheng, Y., Ley, S.H., and Hu, F.B. (2018). Global aetiology and epidemiology of type 2 diabetes mellitus and its complications. *Nat. Rev. Endocrinol.* 14 (2): 88–98. https://doi.org/10.1038/nrendo.2017.151.

CHAPTER 15

Hypertension Case Study

Mrs. MW is an African-American 45-year-old female who was diagnosed with hypertension (average blood pressure measurements, 168/102 mmHg) 6 months ago. At that time she visited her family doctor due to a stressful event at her job that resulted in a modest headache that was later resolved. Her height was 1.60 m, her body weight was 85.5 kg, she was sedentary, and she smoked approximately 15 cigarettes/day. Her doctor initially suggested a nonpharmacological approach for the management of hypertension and advised her to lose some weight, quit smoking, avoid work-related stress, and come back for reassessment after one month. Mrs. MW did not make any changes in her dietary habits, but quit smoking and started a modest physical activity program. During several follow-ups over a period of 6 months, her blood pressure was still high, and her doctor prescribed blood pressure–lowering medication (angiotensin-converting enzyme inhibitor) and referred her to you for lifestyle assessment and modification.

Assessment

Clinical Assessment

Hypertension is a pathophysiologic process characterized by chronically elevated systolic blood pressure (SBP), diastolic blood pressure (DBP), or both. It constitutes a common and serious risk factor for the development of cardiovascular diseases, including stroke, coronary heart disease and heart failure, and chronic kidney disease. There is no evidence of a BP threshold when examining the relationship between BP and risk for the development of cardiovascular and renal disease. In other words, the risk of cardiovascular and renal disease has been shown to increase progressively throughout a wide range of BP values, including "normal" BP values. However, in clinical practice, cut-off BP values are used to simplify diagnosis and decision-making about treatment; "hypertension" is defined as the level of BP at which the benefits of treatment outweigh the risks associated with treatment, as documented by available clinical trials. Table 15.1 summarizes the current BP cut-off points for the diagnosis and classification of adult hypertension, as recommended by American and European medical societies (Whelton et al. 2018; Williams et al. 2018).

Auscultatory or oscillometric semiautomatic or automatic sphygmomanometers are the preferred method for measuring BP in clinical practice. These devices should be validated according to standardized conditions and protocols. BP should initially be measured at rest in both upper arms, using an appropriate cuff size for the arm circumference. A consistent and significant SBP difference between arms (i.e., >15 mmHg) is associated with an increased cardiovascular risk, most likely due to atheromatous vascular disease. When there is a difference in BP between arms, ideally established by a simultaneous measurement, the arm with the higher BP values should be used for all subsequent measurements. Table 15.2 summarizes fundamental points for an accurate assessment of BP in clinical practice (Whelton et al. 2018; Williams et al. 2018).

Mrs. MW initially presented at her doctor's office with BP values averaging 168/102 mmHg over several measures and classified as stage 2 (American)/grade 2 (European) hypertension. Further in-office and out-of-office BP monitoring confirmed the diagnosis of stage/grade 2 hypertension.

Accumulated epidemiological evidence suggests that the global prevalence of hypertension is currently estimated to be 1.4 billion, i.e., affecting approximately 30% of the world adult population. The prevalence of hypertension is consistent across the world, and it becomes progressively more common with advancing age, with a prevalence of >60% in people aged >60 years (Whelton et al. 2018; Williams

> **Key Point**
>
> Hypertension is a common and serious risk factor for the development of cardiovascular diseases, including stroke, coronary heart disease and heart failure, and chronic kidney disease.

Textbook of Lifestyle Medicine, First Edition. Labros S. Sidossis and Stefanos N. Kales.
© 2022 John Wiley & Sons Ltd. Published 2022 by John Wiley & Sons Ltd.

et al. 2018). Elevated BP is a leading global contributor to premature death, accounting for more than 10 million deaths and 200 million disability-adjusted life years. Despite advances in diagnosis and treatment of hypertension over the past decades, the disability-adjusted life years attributable to hypertension have increased by 40% since 1990. SBP ≥ 140 mmHg is the leading cause for the mortality and disability burden (70%). The largest number of SBP-related deaths/year are due to ischaemic heart disease (4.9 million), hemorrhagic stroke (2.0 million), and ischemic stroke (1.5 million) (Whelton et al. 2018; Williams et al. 2018). The continuous relationship between BP and risk of events has been shown at all ages and in all ethnic groups and extends from high BP levels to relatively low values. Both SBP and DBP levels can predict morbidity risk; however, SBP appears to be a better predictor of risk events than DBP after the age of 50 years High DBP levels are associated with increased cardiovascular risk and are more commonly elevated in younger (<50 years) vs. older patients. DBP tends to decline from midlife as a consequence of arterial stiffening; consequently, SBP assumes even greater importance as a risk factor after the age of 50. In middle-aged and older people, increased pulse pressure (the difference between SBP and DBP values) has additional prognostic value.

Hypertension rarely occurs in isolation; it often clusters with other cardiometabolic risk factors, such as dyslipidemia and glucose intolerance. This metabolic risk factor clustering, also known as the metabolic syndrome, has a multiplicative effect on cardiovascular risk (i.e., the likelihood of a person developing a cardiovascular event over a defined period). More information about the metabolic syndrome can be found in Chapter 12. Consequently, quantification of total cardiovascular risk is an important part of the risk stratification process

> **Key Point**
>
> The global prevalence of hypertension is currently estimated to be 1.4 billion; i.e., affecting approximately 30% of the world adult population.

> **Key Point**
>
> Elevated BP is a leading global contributor to premature death.

> **Key Point**
>
> SBP appears to be a better predictor of risk events than DBP after the age of 50 years.

TABLE 15.1 Guidelines for the classification of blood pressure levels.

American guidelines	Systolic BP (mmHg)		Diastolic BP (mmHg)
Normal	<120	and	<80
Elevated	120–129	and	<80
Hypertension stage 1	130–139	or	80–89
Hypertension stage 2	≥140	or	≥90
European guidelines			
Optimal	<120	and	<80
Normal	120–129	and/or	80–84
High normal	130–139	and/or	85–89
Grade 1 hypertension	140–159	and/or	90–99
Grade 2 hypertension	160–179	and/or	100–109
Grade 3 hypertension	≥180	and/or	≥110
Isolated systolic hypertension	≥140	and	<90

Source: Adapted from Whelton et al. (2018) and Williams et al. (2018).

TABLE 15.2 Protocol for blood pressure evaluation in clinical practice.

- Patients should be seated comfortably in a quiet environment for at least 5 min before beginning BP measurements.
- Three BP measurements should be recorded, with a 1–2 min interval, and additional measurements should be performed if the first two readings differ by >10 mmHg. BP is recorded as the average of the last two BP measurements.
- Additional measurements may have to be performed in patients with unstable BP values due to arrhythmias, such as in patients with atrial fibrillation. In these patients, manual auscultatory methods should be used, as most automated devices will overestimate BP.
- Use a standard bladder cuff (12–13 cm wide and 35 cm long) for most patients, but have larger and smaller cuffs available for larger and thinner arms, respectively.
- The cuff should be positioned at the level of the heart, with the back and arm supported to avoid muscle contraction and isometric exercise-dependent increases in BP.
- When using auscultatory methods, use phases I and V (sudden reduction/disappearance) Korotkoff sounds to identify SBP and DBP, respectively.
- Measure BP in both arms at the first visit to detect possible between-arm differences. Use the arm with the higher value as the reference.
- Record heart rate and use pulse palpation for regularity to exclude arrhythmia.

Source: Adapted from Williams et al. (2018).

for all patients with hypertension. Many cardiovascular risk assessment systems are available, and most are able to project a 10-year risk. The European Association of Preventive Cardiology (EAPC) and the European Society of Cardiology (ESC) have developed a Systematic Coronary Risk Evaluation (SCORE) system. This system estimates the 10-year risk of a first fatal atherosclerotic event for Europeans aged 40–65 years, in relation to the country of origin, age, sex, smoking habits, total cholesterol level, and SBP. Similarly, the American College of Cardiology (ACC) and the American Heart Association (AHA) have developed the risk score for atherosclerotic cardiovascular disease (ASCVD). This score provides the 10-year risk estimates for developing a first ASCVD event for black and white men and women aged 40–79 years, based on age, sex, total cholesterol, high-density lipoprotein cholesterol, SBP (including treated or untreated status), history of diabetes mellitus, and smoking habits.

Mrs. MW is African-American, 45 years old, has recently (6 months ago) quit smoking, is currently on antihypertensive medication, and her latest biochemical evaluation revealed a total cholesterol of 212 mg/dl and high-density lipoprotein cholesterol of 55 mg/dl. During the current visit at your office, her BP was 163/95 mmHg. Based on the ASCVD risk score, her 10-year risk of developing a first ASCVD event is 7.5%.

Anthropometric Assessment

Detailed instructions on how to perform anthropometric assessments have been presented in Chapter 13.

Mrs. MW's height is 1.60 m, and she initially presented at her doctor's office with a body weight of 85.5 kg. After her doctor advised her on lifestyle modification, Mrs. MW quit smoking and started exercising, aiming to lose weight and manage her high BP. During your assessment, 6 months after the initial diagnosis of hypertension, her body weight was 87.3 kg. Based on her current body weight, Mrs. MW's body mass index (BMI) is 87.3 kg ÷ (1.60 m)² = 34.10 kg/m², and according to the classification of BMI values, she is considered obese class I with increased risk of morbidity. In addition, her waist circumference is 112.5 cm, which is considered very high (indicative of abdominal adiposity). After discussing with Mrs. MW about her body weight history, you recorded the following information: Mrs. MW usually weighed ~65 kg as a young adult, and she had never experienced any problems with her body weight until the age of 30, when she got a new job as a sales manager

at a multinational corporation. She stated that her long working hours and stressful job have contributed to a gradual weight gain of approximately 25 kg over the past 10 years. A few years ago, she tried to lose weight under the supervision of a health professional, and although she managed to lose ~8 kg in 3 months, she stopped the regimen because she had to move to another city to work on a new company facility. Ever since, her usual weight is ~85 kg. During the last 6 months, she has been struggling to lose weight in order to improve her BP; however, she admits that after quitting on smoking her appetite has increased and her efforts have been unsuccessful.

Dietary Assessment

Detailed instructions on how to perform dietary assessments have been presented in Chapter 13.

After interviewing Mrs. MW about her dietary habits, you recorded the following information: Mrs. MW lives alone, and she rarely cooks due to long working hours. Her breakfast includes coffee and some kind of sandwich, and her typical lunch is a fast-food choice consumed during lunch break at the office. Her dinner is usually smaller and consists of a cup of yogurt with cereals, unless she has to attend a business dinner (~1–2 times/week). She particularly likes red meat and potatoes, she eats fish and chicken ~2 times/month, and although she likes fruits and vegetables, she admits not consuming them on a regular basis due to lack of time for grocery shopping. She drinks alcohol (2–3 drinks) on a daily basis in the evening when she tries "to relax from a long working day", and she reports consuming at least three alcoholic drinks at business meals with colleagues. During the past 6 months she has been experiencing strong urges for food, usually in the afternoon and before bedtime, which she attributes to smoking cessation.

In the context of the 24-hour dietary recall (Appendix D.1), Mrs. MW described the consumption of foods and beverages of the previous day as follows:

- _Breakfast_: 1 cup of instant coffee with 1 teaspoon of sugar and one medium chicken nugget sandwich (white bread) with cheese, tomato, and mayonnaise
- _Morning snack_: 1 cup of instant coffee with 1 teaspoon of sugar
- _Lunch_: one cheeseburger with bacon, one serving of French fries, and two glasses of regular Coca-Cola
- _Afternoon snack_: one cup of instant coffee with 1 teaspoon of sugar and 1 cup of salted peanuts
- _Dinner_: 1 cup of low-fat yogurt (2%) with 3 tablespoons of breakfast cereals
- _Late evening snack_: four salted breadsticks, 60 g of parmesan cheese, four slices of smoked turkey ham, and three glasses of red wine

Physical Activity Assessment

Detailed instructions on how to perform physical activity assessments have been presented in Chapter 13.

After interviewing Mrs. MW about her physical activity habits, you recorded the following information: Mrs. MW has never exercised systematically, and her job is highly sedentary due to extended screen time and long meetings with her colleagues. She always uses her car for transportation to and from work, shopping, and other daily activities. Since the diagnosis of hypertension 6 months ago, she has been trying to become as physically active as possible and started walking in her neighborhood for 15 minutes/day on most weekdays.

Sleep Assessment

Detailed instructions on how to perform sleep assessments have been presented in Chapter 13.

After interviewing Mrs. MW about her sleep habits, you recorded the following information: During a typical day, Mrs. MW usually wakes up around 06:00, goes for a short walk in her neighborhood around 06:30, and then drives to work and reaches her office around 08:00. Her working schedule is 08:00–18:00, with a lunch break between 12:00 and 13:00. After work, she usually returns home around 19:00, she has dinner, does house chores, relaxes in front of the TV for a couple of hours, and goes to bed around midnight. During weekends, she usually travels to visit her parents in a nearby city or meets with friends, and she sleeps for ~6 hours/night. Mrs. MW does not report any severe sleep problems; however, she usually feels sleepy during most days, a fact that she attributes to long working hours. Using the Berlin questionnaire (Appendix D.8), Mrs. MW was categorized as at high risk for the presence of obstructive sleep apnea (OSA).

Stress Assessment

Detailed instructions on how to assess stress levels have been presented in Chapter 13.

Mrs. MW has a demanding job that keeps her busy throughout the weekdays. As she stated, "My job has been my first priority for the past decade, and my work-related responsibilities usually leave me no time to rest, relax, or socialize during the week." After completing the Perceived Stress Scale (Appendix D.10), Mrs. MW's score was 30, indicative of high stress levels.

Hypertension Management

General Principles

The primary goal of hypertension management is to reduce and eventually normalize BP values. The first objective should be to bring BP to <140/90 mmHg in all patients; if successful, and the regimen is well tolerated, a new target of 130/80 mmHg is set. However, as previously mentioned, hypertension is a major risk factor for morbidity and mortality, and consequently treatment goals should go beyond normalizing BP values; they should expand to clinically meaningful reductions in hypertension-related health risks, management of comorbidities (e.g., T2DM and cardiovascular diseases), and improvements in patients' quality of life and well-being.

Meta-analyses of clinical trials have shown that a 10-mmHg reduction in SBP or a 5-mmHg reduction in DBP are associated with significant reductions in all major cardiovascular events (~20%), all-cause mortality (~10–15%), stroke (~35%), coronary events (~20%), and heart failure (~40%) (Whelton et al. 2018; Williams et al. 2018). These reductions in relative risk are consistent irrespective of baseline BP values, the level of cardiovascular risk, the presence of comorbidities, age, sex, and ethnicity Therefore, both BP values and total cardiovascular risk should be the core endpoints of treatment strategies for patients with hypertension.

Management of hypertension involves lifestyle interventions and drug treatment. Lifestyle interventions should represent the first-choice therapy for all hypertensive patients, as they have been shown to be efficient as the sole treatment for borderline/elevated and stage/grade 1 hypertension (Whelton et al. 2018; Williams et al. 2018). In higher stages/grades of hypertension, lifestyle modification alone is unlikely to yield significant improvements in BP; in these cases drug therapy is also recommended.

Heathy lifestyle choices can prevent or delay the onset of hypertension and may be sufficient to delay or prevent the need for drug therapy in patients with stage 1/grade 1 hypertension, and augment the effects of BP-lowering therapy. Healthy lifestyle changes can also improve other cardiovascular risk factors and offer protection against cardiometabolic diseases, which is important for all high-risk hypertensive patients. Recommended lifestyle measures that have been shown to reduce BP include weight loss and maintaining a healthy body weight, salt/sodium restriction, moderation of alcohol

> **Key Point**
> The primary goal of hypertension management is to reduce and eventually normalize BP values.

> **Key Point**
> BP values and total cardiovascular risk should be the core endpoints of treatment strategies for patients with hypertension.

> **Key Point**
> Heathy lifestyle choices can prevent or delay the onset of hypertension and may be sufficient to delay or prevent the need for drug therapy in patients with stage 1/grade 1 hypertension, and augment the effects of BP-lowering therapy.

TABLE 15.3   Suggested lifestyle interventions for patients with hypertension.

Healthy body weight	• Hypertensive patients should aim at a healthy BMI and waist circumference to reduce blood pressure and total cardiovascular risk. • Approximate impact on SBP: expect ~ −1 mmHg in SBP for every 1 kg reduction in body weight.
Healthy diet	• Increased consumption of vegetables, fruits, whole grains, legumes, fish, nuts, and healthy oils. • Approximate impact on SBP: −10 mmHg.
Salt	• Salt restriction to ≤5 g/day, corresponding to a sodium intake of ≤2 g/day. • Optimal sodium intake is <1500 mg/day, but aim for at least a 1000 mg/day reduction in most adults. • Approximate impact on SBP: −5 mmHg.
Alcohol	• Alcohol intake should be restricted to <14 units/week for men and < 8 units/week for women. One unit of alcohol equals to ~10 g of pure alcohol and corresponds to 12 oz of beer (5% alcohol), 5 oz of wine (12% alcohol), or 1.5 oz of distilled spirits (40% alcohol). • Approximate impact on SBP: −4 mmHg. • Binge drinking, i.e., a pattern of drinking that brings blood alcohol concentration to ≥0.08 g/dl (typically happens when men consume ≥5 drinks or women consume ≥4 drinks in about 2 hours) should be avoided.
Exercise	• Regular aerobic exercise, e.g., ≥30 min of moderate intensity (65–75% heart rate reserve) on 5–7 days/week. • Addition of dynamic resistance and isometric exercises is recommended. • Approximate impact on SBP: −5 mmHg.
Smoking	• Counseling on abstinence from active and passive smoking and referral to smoking cessation programs.

Source: Adapted from Whelton et al. (2018) and Williams et al. (2018).

> **Key Point**
>
> Healthy lifestyle changes can also improve other cardiovascular risk factors and offer protection against cardiometabolic diseases.

consumption, the adoption of a healthy diet characterized by high consumption of plant-based foods, mainly vegetables and fruits, and regular physical activity. In addition, tobacco smoking has an acute prolonged pressor effect that may raise daytime ambulatory BP; smoking cessation is therefore recommended for all hypertensive patients as a means to lower daytime BP values and the risk for cardiovascular diseases and cancer. Table 15.3 provides a summary of lifestyle-related modifications that can effectively lower BP (Whelton et al. 2018; Williams et al. 2018).

Most patients will require drug therapy in addition to lifestyle measures to achieve optimal BP control. To date (2021), five major drug classes are recommended for the treatment of hypertension: angiotensin-converting enzyme inhibitors, angiotensin receptor blockers, beta-blockers, calcium channel blockers, and diuretics (e.g., thiazides). Because there are compelling or possible contraindications for each medication, the choice of medication should be individualized. Other classes of drugs that have been less widely studied in clinical trials or are known to be associated with a higher risk of adverse effects include alpha-blockers, centrally acting agents, and mineralocorticoid receptor antagonists. These agents may be useful additions to the common antihypertensive medications in patients whose BP cannot be controlled by combinations of the aforementioned major drug classes.

Weight Control

A substantial and consistent body of evidence from observational studies and clinical trials documents that body weight is directly associated with BP. Excessive weight gain increases the risk of developing hypertension, while moderate weight loss decreases BP levels and can help manage hypertension (Hall et al. 2015). Reductions in BP occur even with a modest weight loss, irrespective of attainment of a desirable body weight, i.e., even if BMI values do not fall below 27.5 kg/m². In a representative meta-analysis that aggregated results across 25 clinical trials, weight loss of 5.1 kg reduced mean SBP and DBP by 4.4 and 3.6 mmHg, respectively; in subgroup analyses, BP reductions were similar for nonhypertensive and hypertensive subjects but were greater in those who had lost more weight (Neter et al. 2003). The BP-lowering effect of weight loss appears to present a dose–response relationship of approximately −1 mmHg/kg of weight loss. Additional trials have documented that modest weight loss, with or without sodium reduction, can prevent the onset of hypertension by ~20% among overweight, prehypertensive individuals and can facilitate medication step-down or even complete drug withdrawal in hypertensive patients (Whelton et al. 2018; Williams et al. 2018).

> **Key Point**
>
> Excessive weight gain increases the risk of developing hypertension, while moderate weight loss decreases BP levels and can help manage hypertension.

> **Key Point**
>
> The BP-lowering effect of weight loss appears to present a dose-response relationship of about −1 mmHg/kg of weight loss.

Key Point

Weight reduction is recommended in all overweight and obese hypertensive patients to lower BP levels, control metabolic complications, and lower total cardiovascular risk.

Key Point

A multidisciplinary approach to weight loss and weight-loss maintenance in hypertensive patients should include dietary advice and motivational counseling toward a modest reduction in caloric intake.

Key Point

Adherence to a prudent diet rich in plant-based foods and low in red meat products, saturated fatty acids, and cholesterol is essential for lowering BP.

Key Point

The MedD is associated with a significant reduction in ambulatory BP, blood glucose, and lipid levels, and a significant reduction in cardiovascular events and all-cause mortality.

Key Point

The DASH diet has been advocated as the first-line dietary therapy for hypertension.

Therefore, weight reduction is recommended in all overweight and obese hypertensive patients to lower BP levels, control metabolic complications, and lower total cardiovascular risk. Although the optimal BMI is unclear, maintenance of a healthy body weight (BMI of approximately 20–27.5 kg/m² in people <60 years of age; higher in older patients) and waist circumference (<94 cm for men and <80 cm for women) is recommended for nonhypertensive individuals to prevent hypertension, and for hypertensive patients to reduce BP (Piepoli et al. 2016). More importantly, in view of the well-recognized difficulty of maintaining the lost weight, efforts to prevent weight regain among those who have lost weight are critically important. As with obesity management, a multidisciplinary approach to weight loss and weight-loss maintenance in hypertensive patients should include dietary advice and motivational counseling toward a modest reduction in caloric intake. Achievement and maintenance of weight loss through behavior change are challenging but feasible over prolonged periods of follow-up. For those who do not meet their weight-loss goals with nonpharmacological lifestyle interventions, pharmacotherapy or bariatric surgery can also be considered.

Detailed instructions on weight-loss goals, how to estimate a patient's energy needs, and how to achieve energy restriction have been presented in Chapter 13.

Mrs. MW is 42 years old and weighs 87.3 kg. Based on the Schofield equations for women aged 30–60 years old, her basal metabolic rate (BMR) is estimated to be 8.126 × 87.3 + 845.6 = ~1555 kcal. Given that she is mildly active, her BMR should be multiplied with a 1.5 physical activity factor, leading to a total daily energy expenditure of ~2330 kcal. An energy deficit of 500–750 kcal would lead to a target daily energy intake of ~1600–1800 kcal, enough to achieve the desired weight loss.

Dietary Modification

Adoption of a healthy dietary pattern is fundamental for the management of hypertension (Sacks and Campos 2010). Adherence to a prudent diet, rich in plant-based foods and low in red meat products, saturated fatty acids, and cholesterol, is essential for lowering BP. A plant-based diet would emphasize the consumption of vegetables, legumes, fresh fruits, grains, nuts, and unsaturated oils, especially olive oil. Two healthy dietary patterns, the Mediterranean diet (MedD) and the Dietary Approaches to Stop Hypertension (DASH) diet, comply with most of the aforementioned recommendations. Both have been studied for the treatment of hypertension, and both can be used as nutritional tools not only for the control of BP but also for the improvement of cardiovascular and total health. The MedD can be described as the dietary pattern adopted in the olive-growing areas of the Mediterranean region in the late 1950s and early 1960s, when the region was recovering from the effects of World War II (Trichopoulou 2001). The MedD has evolved throughout time. Currently, it can be defined as a dietary pattern characterized by high consumption of olive oil (as the main edible fat), vegetables, legumes, whole grains, fruits and nuts, moderate consumption of poultry and fish (varying with proximity to the sea), low consumption of full-fat dairy products and red meat, and low-to-moderate consumption of wine as the main source of alcohol accompanying meals (Figure 15.1) (Sofi 2009). A number of studies and meta-analyses have shown that the MedD is associated with a significant reduction in ambulatory BP, blood glucose, and lipid levels, and a significant reduction in cardiovascular events and all-cause mortality (Domenech et al. 2014; Sofi et al. 2010). More information on the MedD can be found in Chapter 7.

On the other hand, the DASH diet (Figure 15.1) was developed in the 1990s as the outcome of a study funded by the National Institutes of Health to identify dietary interventions for the treatment of hypertension. The DASH diet may decrease SBP by 6–11 mmHg; this effect was evident in hypertensive and normotensive people (Challa et al. 2020). Based on these results, the DASH diet has been advocated as the first-line dietary therapy for hypertension, and several subsequent studies have confirmed its beneficial effects on BP (Filippou et al. 2020), total cardiovascular risk, morbidity, and mortality (Soltani et al. 2020). The DASH diet emphasizes the intake of plant-based products, such as fruits, vegetables, whole grains, legumes, nuts and seeds, and lean animal products, such as low-fat dairy products, poultry, and fish, and can be characterized as a low-fat (especially saturated fat) dietary pattern rich in potassium, magnesium, calcium, and dietary fiber. More information on the DASH diet can be found in Chapter 6.

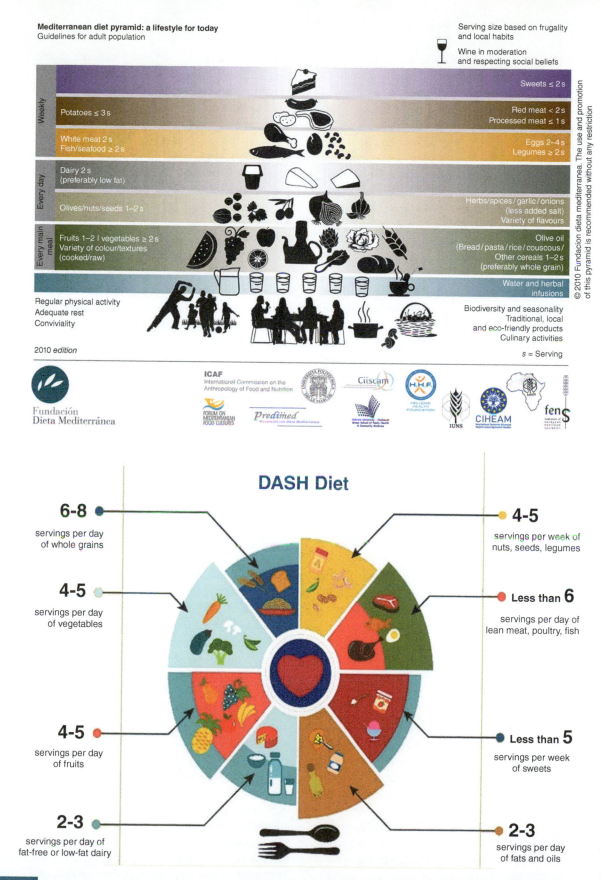

Mediterranean diet pyramid: a lifestyle for today
Guidelines for adult population

Serving size based on frugality and local habits

Wine in moderation and respecting social beliefs

Sweets ≤ 2 s

Weekly

Potatoes ≤ 3 s

Red meat < 2 s
Processed meat ≤ 1 s

White meat 2 s
Fish/seafood ≥ 2 s

Eggs 2–4 s
Legumes ≥ 2 s

Every day

Dairy 2 s
(preferably low fat)

Olives/nuts/seeds 1–2 s

Herbs/spices/garlic/onions
(less added salt)
Variety of flavours

Every main meal

Fruits 1–2 I vegetables ≥ 2 s
Variety of colour/textures
(cooked/raw)

Olive oil
(Bread/pasta/rice/couscous/
Other cereals 1–2 s
(preferably whole grain)

Water and herbal
infusions

Regular physical activity
Adequate rest
Conviviality

Biodiversity and seasonality
Traditional, local
and eco-friendly products
Culinary activities

2010 *edition*

s = Serving

© 2010 Fundacion dieta mediterranea. The use and promotion of this pyramid is recommended without any restriction

Fundación
Dieta Mediterránea

ICAF
International Commission on the
Anthropology of Food and Nutrition

FORUM ON MEDITERRANEAN FOOD CULTURES

Predimed

Ciiscam

H.H.F.
HELLENIC HEALTH FOUNDATION

IUNS

CIHEAM

fen**s**

DASH Diet

6-8
servings per day
of whole grains

4-5
servings per day
of vegetables

4-5
servings per day
of fruits

2-3
servings per day of
fat-free or low-fat dairy

4-5
servings per week of
nuts, seeds, legumes

Less than **6**
servings per day of
lean meat, poultry, fish

Less than **5**
servings per week
of sweets

2-3
servings per day
of fats and oils

FIGURE 15.1 **Schematic illustration of the Mediterranean diet (above) and the DASH diet (below).** The Mediterranean pyramid depicts the recommended daily or weekly intake of food groups based on the Mediterranean diet pattern, along with several other healthy behaviors (such as increased physical activity, culinary activities, adequate hydration, conviviality, and adequate sleep) proposed in the context of the healthy Mediterranean lifestyle pattern. Serving sizes are not strictly defined and, according to the pyramid, should be based on frugality, local habits, and individual needs to achieve and maintain a healthy body weight. The DASH eating plan depicts the recommended daily or weekly food group intake for a 2000-cal diet. Serving sizes, and recommended food group intake for other levels of energy intake, can be found at the NIH website (DASH Eating Plan).

Besides the adoption of a prudent dietary pattern, other efficient interventions for lowering BP include reduction in sodium intake, moderate alcohol consumption, and increased potassium intake. There is data to suggest that other nonpharmacological dietary interventions may be successful in lowering BP, but more studies are needed to confirm their effectiveness. Such interventions include consumption of probiotics, increased intake of protein, fiber, flaxseed, or fish oil, supplementation with calcium or magnesium, the consumption of garlic, dark chocolate, tea, and coffee, and the adoption of other dietary patterns, such as low-carbohydrate and vegetarian diet (Whelton et al. 2018; Williams et al. 2018).

With regard to sodium, there is strong evidence of its causal relationship with BP, and excessive sodium consumption has been associated with an increased prevalence of hypertension (Elliott et al. 1996). Conversely, sodium restriction has been shown to have a BP-lowering effect. A meta-analysis of 34 randomized trials showed that a reduction of ~1.75 g sodium/d (4.4 g salt/day) was associated with a 4.2/2.1 mmHg reduction in SBP/DBP, with a more pronounced effect (−5.4/−2.8 mmHg) in individuals with established hypertension (He et al. 2013). Moderate dietary sodium restriction may also reduce the number or dose of BP-lowering drugs that are necessary to control BP, although this requires maintenance of the lifestyle change and warrants careful monitoring (Graudal et al. 2012; He and MacGregor 2003). Therefore, all hypertensive patients should be encouraged to limit their sodium intake to ≤2 g/day (equivalent to approximately ≤5.0 g salt/day), with the optimal goal being set at <1.5 g/day (Whelton et al. 2018; Williams et al. 2018; Tsirimiagkou et al. 2021; Elijovich et al. 2016; Whelton et al 2012).

Maintaining the lifestyle changes necessary to reduce sodium intake is challenging, but even a small decrease in sodium intake is likely to be beneficial, especially in patients whose BP is salt sensitive; all patients should aim for at least a 1000 mg/day reduction in daily sodium intake. Extremely strict sodium restrictions have an adverse effect on cardiovascular risk and result in an unpalatable diet that is difficult to maintain in the long term. Thus, severe restrictions should be avoided. In the context of sodium restriction, it is very important to educate patients on the sodium content of the various foods. Table 15.4 provides an overview of the sodium content of

major food groups. Hypertensive patients should try to avoid using salt in their meals during cooking or serving, and avoid overconsumption of foods that are naturally rich in sodium, such as grain products, dairy products (especially cheese), and meat products (especially processed); fats/oils should also be consumed in moderation. However, ~80% of salt consumption comes from hidden salt in processed foods. For packaged foods, information on sodium content can be obtained through food labels; salty snacks, ready-to-eat meals, sauces, and canned foods should be avoided by patients with hypertension, as they contain high amounts of sodium that serves as a taste enhancer and a preservative.

Epidemiological data show a strong positive relationship between alcohol intake and BP levels, especially above an intake of three standard drinks/day. Binge drinking, i.e., drinking large amounts of alcohol in a short time interval, can also have a strong pressor effect. Meta-analyses of the available interventional studies suggest that reduction of alcohol consumption, even for light to moderate drinkers, is beneficial for BP; the most prominent benefits incur to those consuming ≥6 drinks/day. In this case, a reduction of alcohol intake by about 50% results in an average reduction in SBP/DBP of approximately 5.5/4.0 mmHg (Roerecke et al. 2017; Xin et al. 2001). In contrast to its effect on BP, alcohol seems to have a beneficial effect on several biomarkers for cardiovascular risk when consumed in moderation (Estruch et al. 2005). On balance with the aforementioned data, hypertensive individuals who do not consume alcohol should not be advised to start drinking, while hypertensive men and women who regularly drink should be advised to limit their alcohol consumption to less than 14 and 8 units/week, respectively (1 unit is equal to 125 ml of wine or 250 ml of beer) (Whelton et al. 2018; Williams et al. 2018). Alcohol-free days during the week and avoidance of binge drinking are also advised for an optimal management of hypertension.

Potassium has also emerged as a significant nutrient for BP regulation. Studies have documented a significant inverse relationship between potassium intake and BP in nonhypertensive and hypertensive individuals. Furthermore, potassium supplementation of ~1400 mg has shown to decrease BP by ~2 mmHg and 4–5 mmHg in adults with normotension and hypertension, respectively (Filippini et al. 2020). Although in most trials potassium supplementation was achieved by administration of potassium chloride pills, the preferred strategy to increase potassium intake is

> **Key Point**
> Moderate dietary sodium restriction may reduce the number or dose of BP-lowering drugs that are necessary to control BP.

> **Key Point**
> All hypertensive patients should be encouraged to limit their sodium intake to ≤2 g/day.

> **Key Point**
> Extremely strict sodium restrictions have an adverse effect on cardiovascular risk and result in an unpalatable diet that is difficult to maintain in the long term.

> **Key Point**
> Epidemiological data show a strong positive relationship between alcohol intake and BP levels, especially above an intake of three standard drinks/day.

> **Key Point**
> Hypertensive individuals who do not consume alcohol should not be advised to start drinking, while hypertensive men and women who regularly drink should be advised to limit their alcohol consumption.

TABLE 15.4   Sodium content of major food groups.

Food group	Examples of foods and portions	Sodium (mg)/per portion
Dairy products	1 cup of milk, sour milk, or kefir, 200 g of yogurt, 1 small piece (~30 g) of cheese	160
Vegetables	1 cup of raw vegetables (tomato, cucumber, lettuce, pepper, carrot, cabbage), ½ cup of boiled vegetables (zucchini, cauliflower, beetroot, potatoes, corn)	15
Grains	1 slice (30 g) of bread, 2 small rusks, ½ pita bread, ½ bagel, ½ cup of breakfast cereals or oatmeal, ½ cup of cooked rice or pasta, ½ cup of legumes (e.g., beans)	80
Meat products	30 g of cooked white meat (e.g., chicken and turkey), red meat (pork, veal, lamb, etc.), or fish and seafood, 1 medium egg, 2 slices of processed meat (e.g., ham), or 1 small (20 g) sausage	25
Fats and oils	1 teaspoon of oil (e.g., olive oil or sunflower oil), butter or margarine, a few pieces (4–6) of nuts, 5–10 olives	55
Salt	1 teaspoon of salt	~2000

to consume foods that are rich in potassium. Fruits rich in potassium include bananas, oranges, apricots, and raisins, while high-potassium vegetables include potatoes, mushrooms, peas, zucchini, spinach, and broccoli. For example, four to five servings of fruits and vegetables will usually provide 1500 to >3000 mg of potassium; the current recommendation for potassium intake for adults is 4700 mg/d. It must be noted that the effects of potassium intake on BP depend on the concurrent intake of salt, and vice versa. Specifically, increased intake of potassium is more effective in hypertensive patients with high salt intake compared to patients with lower salt intake. Conversely, the BP reduction from a reduced salt intake is greatest when potassium intake is low. Therefore, increasing dietary potassium intake can be an effective strategy in hypertensive individuals who cannot meet guidelines for optimal sodium intake. *Hyperpotassemia* (increased blood levels of potassium) is a common finding among patients with chronic kidney disease; in this case, dietary potassium intake should remain moderate, and management of hypertension should mainly focus on dietary sodium restriction.

Several other individual nutrients and food components have been studied in relation to BP. Particular importance has been given to caffeine, which has been shown to have an acute pressor effect; however, the consumption of typical sources of caffeine, such as coffee and tea, has been associated with cardiovascular benefits, and their consumption should not be discouraged in hypertensive patients (Ding et al. 2014; Greyling et al. 2014; Xu et al. 2020). Omega-3 polyunsaturated fatty acids have also been shown to exhibit a BP-lowering effect; however, the dosage required to achieve this effect is high (≥3 g/d), and fish oil

supplements cannot be routinely recommended as a means to lower BP (Appel et al. 2006). Finally, the intake of calcium, magnesium, and dietary fiber has also been shown to be inversely associated with BP levels in epidemiological studies; however, available data from clinical trials on the effect of their supplementation on BP levels remain largely inconclusive and insufficient to warrant a recommendation for increased intake as a means to lower BP (Appel et al. 2006).

> **Key Point**
>
> The preferred strategy to increase potassium intake is to consume foods that are rich in potassium.

> **Key Point**
>
> The effects of potassium intake on BP depend on the concurrent intake of salt, and vice versa.

> **Key Point**
>
> Studies have documented a significant inverse relationship between potassium intake and BP in nonhypertensive and hypertensive individuals.

According to Mrs. MW's dietary assessment, individualized counseling toward a healthy diet for hypertension management should focus on:

- Balanced meal pattern with emphasis on nutritional variety. Advise on daily breakfast consumption preferably at home (e.g., toast with cheese and vegetables, yogurt with fruits, etc.); consumption of healthy snacks, such as fruits, unsalted nuts, and dairy products, at the office; consumption of a healthier lunch at the office with incorporation of lean white meat-, fish-, and legume-based dishes instead of fast-food choices; reduction in sugar intake; and limitation of sugar-sweetened beverages.

- Portion control to achieve a 5–10% weight loss. Mrs. MW has one big main meal/day (lunch) at the office; restriction of the typical portion size would create a significant energy deficit. Ways to achieve this portion decrease include the consumption of an abundant portion of a salad with green leafy or other vegetables at the beginning of the meal; salads are usually rich in dietary fiber and contribute to satiety. Another *way to decrease the portion of the main meal is by choosing a healthier, less-energy-dense choice, such as a lean protein meal (chicken or fish). However, it is important that the meal is large enough to cause satiety. Restraint from nibbling throughout the day, especially before bedtime, is also important in achieving an energy deficit; this can be attained through education on the correct identification of hunger and satiety, and through the consumption of low-calorie snacks when the urge for food consumption cannot be avoided (such as homemade popcorn without salt, fruits, vegetable sticks with vinegar, whole grain rusks, etc.).*

- *Decrease in salt intake. Mrs. MW currently consumes foods that are rich in sodium, such as salted nuts, breadsticks, parmesan cheese, cold cuts, and fast-food choices based on red meat products and French fries for lunch. Low-sodium alternatives should be identified for every meal to substitute the high-sodium choices.*

- *Prudent alcohol consumption. Alcohol intake should be limited to ≤1 serving/day (e.g., 1 glass of wine). Consumption of alcohol with a main meal, rather than before bedtime, is also recommended. During social occasions, e.g., business meals, alcohol intake should be kept to a minimum, e.g., 1 unit of alcohol could be diluted with water to provide double volume; alcoholic beverages could be substituted with nonalcoholic choices, such as mineral water, alcohol-free beer, or artificially sweetened beverages.*

Table 15.5 summarizes beneficial dietary changes for Mrs. MW toward managing hypertension based on her 24-hour dietary recall.

Physical Activity Modification

Even though physical activity induces a transient, acute rise in SBP, followed by a short-lived decline in BP below baseline, many epidemiological studies suggest that regular aerobic physical activity is beneficial for the prevention of hypertension (Huai et al. 2013). Aerobic exercise is the most extensively studied type of exercise for the management of hypertension. The average reductions in SBP following aerobic training are approximately 2–4 and 5–8 mmHg in adult patients with normotension and hypertension, respectively (Cornelissen and Smart 2013). With respect to other types of exercise, a meta-analysis of clinical trials has shown that aerobic endurance training, dynamic resistance training, and isometric resistance training reduce resting SBP and DBP by 3.5/2.5, 1.8/3.2, and 10.9/6.2 mmHg, respectively, in the general population, with benefits being greater for hypertensive compared to healthy individuals (Cornelissen and Smart 2013). Although more research is required, available data tend to suggest that isometric resistance training has the potential for the largest reductions in SBP and should therefore be recommended. In isometric exercise there is static contraction of a muscle without any visible movement in the angle of the joint. The three main types of isometric exercise are isometric presses, pulls, and holds. Isometric presses and pulls refer to the effort to push or pull against another part of your body that pushes or pulls back with equal force, or attempts to move an immovable object.

Besides improvements in BP, it must be noted that regular physical activity, even of low intensity and duration, is associated with significant improvements in cardiovascular morbidity and mortality, with health risks decreasing as the frequency and duration of exercise increases (Kraus et al. 2019; Rossi et al. 2012). Hypertensive patients should follow the physical

> **Key Point**
>
> Regular aerobic physical activity is beneficial for the prevention of hypertension.

> **Key Point**
>
> Isometric resistance training, in which there is a static contraction of muscle without any visible movement in the joint angle, has the potential for the largest reductions in SBP.

TABLE 15.5 **Recommended dietary changes for the management of hypertension.**

Meal	Current dietary habits	Recommended alternatives
Breakfast	1 cup of instant coffee with 1 teaspoon of sugar and 1 medium chicken nugget sandwich (white bread) with cheese, tomato, and mayonnaise	1 cup of instant coffee with 1 teaspoon of sugar and 1 small sandwich with whole-grain bread, low-salt cheese, and vegetables
Morning snack	1 cup of instant coffee with 1 teaspoon of sugar	2 whole seasonal fruits
Lunch	1 cheeseburger with bacon, 1 serving of French fries, and 2 glasses of regular Coca-Cola	1 roasted chicken filet with 1 cup of potatoes, 1 seasonal salad with olive oil, and 1 glass of wine
Afternoon snack	1 cup of instant coffee with 1 teaspoon of sugar and 1 cup of salted peanuts	1 cup of instant coffee with 1 teaspoon of sugar and 1 cup of low-fat yogurt (2%) with 2 tablespoons of oatmeal
Dinner	1 cup of low-fat yogurt (2%) with 3 tablespoons of breakfast cereals	1 seasonal salad with olive oil, 2 whole-grain rusks, 60 g of low-salt cheese, and 1 boiled egg
Late evening snack	4 salted breadsticks, 60 g of parmesan cheese, 2 slices of smoked turkey ham, and 3 glasses of red wine	2 whole seasonal fruits

> **Key Point**
>
> Regular physical activity, even of low intensity and duration, is associated with significant improvements in cardiovascular morbidity and mortality.

activity guidelines for the general population and be advised to accumulate at least 30 minutes/day of moderate-intensity aerobic exercise (walking, jogging, cycling, or swimming) for 5–7 days/week. For additional health benefits, patients should be advised to perform isometric resistance exercises 2–3 days/week, gradually increase moderate-intensity aerobic physical activity to 300 minutes/week, or gradually increase vigorous-intensity exercise to 150 minutes/week (World Health Organization 2010).

According to Mrs. MW's physical activity assessment, key points for individualized counseling toward a physically active lifestyle should include:

- *Encouragement to sustain a physically active lifestyle with a gradual increase in physical activity level to achieve at least 30 minutes/day of moderate intensity exercise on 5–7 days/week. Examples of advice toward this goal include:*
  - *A gradual increase in morning walking time from 15 to 30 minutes/day.*
  - *An additional short walk after lunch break and/or before bedtime on weekdays. This will increase daily physical activity time and could alleviate work-related stress.*
  - *Using stairs instead of elevators whenever possible. For example, if the building allows it, she could take bathroom breaks one or two floors up, using the stairs.*
  - *Walking instead of driving for daily activities, such as shopping.*
  - *Bicep/tricep exercises with hand weights or sit/stand exercises while at the office.*
  - *Group outdoor activities with family and friends that involve convivial aerobic exercise or any kind of organized exercise (e.g., jogging, swimming, cycling, etc.) during weekends that can be maintained in the long term.*
  - *Engagement in isometric exercises. Isometric exercises have a strong BP-lowering effect and can be done on a daily basis before bedtime.*

Sleep Modification

The relationship between sleep and BP is less well studied; however, accumulating evidence suggests that sleep deprivation and insomnia are positively linked to increased BP levels and the presence, severity, and incidence of hypertension. In addition, a relationship between sleep disorders and hypertension is increasingly recognized, with the strongest data being available for OSA. OSA is characterized by repetitive pauses of breathing during sleep due to obstructions of the upper airways that result in intermittent hypoxia. Hypoxia, in turn, leads to an abnormal increase in sympathetic activation, which contributes to increased vascular resistance and cardiac output and, eventually, increases in BP that are also sustained during wakefulness.

Approximately 50% of patients with OSA are hypertensive. Moreover, the presence of OSA has been indicated as a significant risk factor for the development of hypertension in prospective studies. Treatment of sleep apnea with available therapies (e.g., continuous positive airway pressure) has been shown to result in a decrease in sympathetic activity and modest reductions in BP. The greatest benefits were shown in patients with the highest adherence (Calhoun and Harding 2010).

> **Key Point**
>
> OSA is characterized by repetitive pauses of breathing during sleep due to obstructions of the upper airways that result in intermittent hypoxia.

> **Key Point**
>
> Approximately 50% of patients with OSA are hypertensive.

According to Mrs. MW's assessment, counseling toward the improvement of sleep habits should focus on the following:

- *Mrs. MW is at increased risk for the presence of OSA. Referral to a sleep specialist for a sleep study is advised.*
- *Mrs. MW sleeps for about 6–7 hours on a regular basis. She should be encouraged to gradually increase her daily sleep duration to 7–8 hours as recommended for adults.*
- *Avoidance of alcohol close to bedtime. Mrs. MW frequently consumes at least two glasses of wine with her late evening snack. Alcohol is a central nervous system depressant that can induce feelings of relaxation and sleepiness, but the consumption of alcohol in excess has been linked to poor sleep quality and duration. Research has shown that people who drink large amounts of alcohol before going to bed are often prone to delayed sleep onset, sleep disruptions, snoring, breathing pauses, and overall poor sleep quality.*
- *Education on other sleep hygiene techniques to promote sleep quality, such as avoiding stimulants, e.g., caffeine and nicotine, 4–6 hours before bedtime, a short (10-minute) interval of light aerobic exercise before sleep, avoidance of overeating and consumption of foods that can trigger indigestion and gastrointestinal symptoms before sleep, establishing a regular relaxing bedtime routine, and making sure that the sleep environment is pleasant.*

Stress Management

Exposure to chronic stress is a risk factor for hypertension; occupational stress, stressful impact of the social environment, and low socioeconomic status have all been associated with increased risk for the development of hypertension. Overall, there is growing support of the hypothesis that exposure to chronic stress contributes to the development of hypertension,

> **Key Point**
>
> Exposure to chronic stress contributes to the development of hypertension, and thinking about or experiencing stressful events can delay BP recovery.

and that thinking about or experiencing stressful events can delay BP recovery (Spruill 2010). Several stress management techniques, such as biofeedback, progressive muscle relaxation, stress management training, and transcendental meditation, have been explored in the context of hypertension treatment, and evidence suggests that transcendental meditation is associated with significant BP reductions, possibly due to its strong effect in reducing rumination (Rainforth et al. 2007).

Counseling for Mrs. MW toward stress management should focus on the following:

- *Engagement in activities that contribute to relaxation and stress relief, such as yoga and tai chi. Many yoga poses, such as the chair and tree pose, fall into the category of isometric training and can contribute to significant decreases in BP and stress relief. Yoga, developed thousands of years ago, is recognized as a form of mind–body medicine. In yoga, physical postures and breathing exercises improve muscle strength, flexibility, blood circulation, oxygen uptake, and hormone function. In addition, the relaxation induced by meditation helps to stabilize the autonomic nervous system with a tendency toward parasympathetic dominance. The resulting physiological benefits help yoga practitioners become more resilient to stressful conditions and reduce a variety of important risk factors for various diseases, especially hypertension and cardiorespiratory diseases (Parshad 2004).*
- *Mrs. MW presented at her doctor 6 months ago with symptoms of a mild anxiety attack caused by a stressful event at her work. Targeting factors that influence the impact of stress on BP, such as an individual's coping responses, may be a useful intervention strategy, particularly when exposure to stress cannot be completely avoided, as is the case of work-related stress. In this context, mindfulness-based stress reduction is an efficient strategy for stress and anxiety management. It uses a combination of mindfulness meditation, body awareness, yoga, and exploration of patterns of behavior, thinking, feeling, and action. Mindfulness can be understood as the nonjudgmental acceptance and investigation of present experience, including body sensations, mental states, thoughts, emotions, impulses, and memories, in order to reduce distress and promote well-being. Referral to a mental health specialist for an in-depth stress evaluation and management intervention should be considered in case stress symptoms are evident and increasing in intensity.*

Smoking Cessation

Smoking is positively associated with increases in BP and represents a major risk factor for cardiovascular diseases. Studies have shown that both normotensive subjects and untreated hypertensive smokers have higher daily BP values than non-smokers (Groppelli et al. 1992). In addition, smoking is second only to BP as a contributing risk to the global burden of disease;

therefore, smoking cessation is probably the single most effective lifestyle measure for the prevention of cardiovascular diseases (Doll et al. 1994; Lim et al. 2012). This is of special importance for hypertensive patients, who have high cardiovascular risk, due to hypertension-related organ damage.

History of tobacco use should be established at each patient visit, and patients with hypertension who are smokers should be counseled toward smoking cessation. In this context, brief advice from a health professional can have a small but significant effect of 1–3% over and above the unassisted 12-month quit rate among smokers (Stead et al. 2013). This can be improved by the use of available pharmacological measures, such as nicotine replacement therapy, bupropion, and varenicline (Cahill et al. 2013). Combining behavioral support with pharmacotherapy can further increase the chance of success by 70–100%, compared with brief advice alone, and is the ideal approach for smoking cessation in hypertensive patients (Stead et al. 2016). Table 15.6 provides an overview of the 5-A system proposed by the World Health Organization as a smoking cessation strategy for routine practice.

> **Key Point**
>
> Smoking is positively associated with increases in BP and represents a major risk factor for cardiovascular diseases.

> **Key Point**
>
> Smoking cessation is probably the single most effective lifestyle measure to prevent cardiovascular diseases.

> **Key Point**
>
> History of tobacco use should be established at each patient visit, and patients with hypertension who are smokers should be counseled toward smoking cessation.

Mrs. MW recently quit smoking when she was first diagnosed with hypertension, and she should be motivated to maintain this beneficial lifestyle change through constant education on smoking-related risks, encouragement, and support. Since she quit smoking, Mrs. MW has been experiencing urges for food

TABLE 15.6	The "Five As" for a smoking cessation strategy for routine practice.
ASK: Systematically inquire about smoking status at every opportunity.	
ADVISE: Unequivocally urge all smokers to quit.	
ASSESS: Determine the person's degree of addiction and readiness to quit.	
ASSIST: Agree on a smoking cessation strategy, including setting a quit date, behavioral counseling, and pharmacological support.	
ARRANGE: Arrange a schedule of follow-up.	

consumption and has gained a total of 1.8 kg within 6 months. It must be noted that smoking cessation usually results in weight gain. Thus, smokers should be advised that weight gain of 5% or more of body weight is highly possible; however, the health benefits of tobacco cessation far outweigh the risks from this mild weight gain.

Take-Home Messages

- Hypertension is a pathophysiologic process characterized by chronically elevated SBP, DBP, or both.
- Hypertension is a risk factor for the development of cardiovascular diseases, including stroke, coronary heart disease and heart failure, and chronic kidney disease.
- A comprehensive clinical and lifestyle (dietary, physical activity, and sleep) assessment is crucial for all hypertensive patients. Emphasis must be placed on comorbidities and behaviors that are linked to obesity and BP and can be modified.
- Reduction of BP values and decline of total cardiovascular risk are the two major goals of treatment strategies for patients with hypertension.
- The first objective of treatment should be to lower BP to <140/90 mmHg in all patients and, provided that the treatment is well tolerated, BP values should be further decreased to 130/80 mmHg or lower in most patients.
- Lifestyle interventions represent the first-choice therapy for all hypertensive patients and are likely to be sufficient as the sole treatment in the case of DBP/SBP levels of <160/100. In higher grades/stages of hypertension, drug therapy is usually necessary.
- Hypertensive patients should try to attain a healthy BMI and waist circumference values to reduce BP and total cardiovascular risk. Reductions in BP occur even with a modest weight loss, irrespective of attainment of a desirable body weight.
- Adoption of a healthy diet is fundamental for the management of hypertension.
- Hypertensive patients should be advised to adopt a diet rich in plant-based foods, such as vegetables, legumes, fresh fruits, whole grains, nuts, and unsaturated oils (especially olive oil), and low in red meat products and highly processed foods.
- The MedD and the DASH diet comply with most of the aforementioned recommendations on single dietary components and can be used as promising nutritional tools, not only for the control of BP but also for the improvement of cardiovascular and total health.
- Sodium restriction has a strong BP-lowering effect and can reduce the number or dose of BP-lowering drugs that are necessary to control BP.
- Increased potassium intake can help toward hypertension management, especially when sodium intake is high.
- Hypertensive patients who drink alcohol should be advised to limit their consumption to less than 14 and 7 units/week, for men and women, respectively. Binge drinking should be avoided.
- Regular aerobic physical activity is beneficial for the prevention and treatment of hypertension and the decrease of cardiovascular risk.
- Hypertensive patients should aim to participate in at least 30 minutes/day of moderate-intensity aerobic exercise 5–7 days/week.
- Isometric exercises have a strong BP-lowering effect and should be advised on top of aerobic training.
- Sleep deprivation, insomnia, and the presence of sleep disorders are positively linked to increased BP levels and the presence, severity, and incidence of hypertension.
- Hypertensive patients should aim for an adequate sleep duration along with a normal sleep schedule and optimal sleep hygiene. In case of a sleep disorder, such as OSA, referral to a specialist for further evaluation and proper treatment is crucial.
- Smoking is associated with increases in BP and represents a major risk factor for cardiovascular diseases.
- The history of tobacco use should be assessed in clinical practice, and all hypertensive smokers should be counseled toward smoking cessation using available behavioral and pharmacological interventions.
- Exposure to chronic psychosocial stress contributes to the development of hypertension.
- Stress management techniques, such as meditation and yoga, are useful complementary interventions for hypertension management.

Self-Assessment Questions

1. Provide the definition and diagnostic criteria of hypertension.
2. Which of the following BP measurements are indicative of isolated systolic hypertension?
   a. SBP 165 mmHg and DBP 95 mmHg
   b. SBP 122 mmHg and DBP 82 mmHg
   c. SBP 150 mmHg and DBP 85 mmHg
   d. SBP 115 mmHg and DBP 98 mmHg
   e. SBP 134 mmHg and DBP 75 mmHg
3. Which of the following statements about potassium are true?
   a. An increased intake of potassium has a greater BP-lowering effect when our diet is high in salt.
   b. Potassium has an acute pressor effect, and its intake should ideally be limited by hypertensive patients.
   c. Potassium supplementation is a preferred strategy to increase potassium intake compared to consuming foods naturally rich in potassium.
   d. Fruits (e.g., bananas oranges, apricots, and raisins) and vegetables (potatoes, mushrooms, peas, zucchini, spinach, and broccoli) are rich in potassium.
   e. Current recommendation for potassium intake for adults is ~2000 mg/day.
4. What is the DASH diet?
5. Characterize the following statements as true (T) or false (F).
   a. All hypertensive smokers should be counseled toward smoking cessation ( ).
   b. When there is a difference in BP between arms, the arm with the lowest BP values should be used for all subsequent measurements ( ).
   c. Dynamic resistance training has the potential for the largest reductions in SBP compared to aerobic exercise and isometric resistance training ( ).
   d. Calcium has a strong BP-lowering effect, and its supplementation is routinely used for hypertension management in clinical practice ( ).
   e. The presence of OSA is a risk factor for hypertension ( ).
6. Briefly describe the protocol for an accurate assessment of BP in clinical practice.
7. Which of the following diets can have a beneficial impact on BP?
   a. a Mediterranean-style diet
   b. a diet rich in vegetables, fruits, fish, nuts, and healthy oils
   c. the DASH diet
   d. a diet rich in plant-based products and low in sodium
   e. all of the above
8. Provide a brief overview of effective lifestyle changes for the management of hypertension.
9. Characterize the following statements as true (T) or false (F).
   a. Although smoking is a major risk factor for cardiovascular diseases, it is negatively associated with BP levels and hypertension risk ( ).
   b. The MedD is associated with a significant reduction in BP, blood glucose and lipid levels, cardiovascular events, and all-cause mortality ( ).
   c. Coffee consumption should be discouraged in patients with hypertension ( ).
   d. Hypertensive patients should follow the physical activity guidelines for the general population and be advised to participate in ≥30 minutes of moderate-intensity dynamic aerobic exercise on 5–7 days/week ( ).
   e. The DASH diet is rich in calcium, magnesium, and vitamin D, but low in saturated fat, dietary fiber, and potassium ( ).
10. What are the goals of hypertension management?
11. Which of the following statements about alcohol are true?
    a. Alcohol intake should be restricted to <14 units/week for men and <8 units/week for women in patients with hypertension.
    b. A reduction of alcohol intake by about 50% results in an average reduction in SBP/DBP of approximately 20/15 mmHg.
    c. Alcohol has a detrimental effect on cardiovascular risk even when consumed in small-to-moderate amounts.
    d. One (1) unit of alcohol is equal to 300 ml of wine or beer.
    e. Binge drinking, i.e., drinking large amounts of alcohol in a short time interval, is detrimental for BP and should be avoided.
12. Which of the following is an accurate description of the contemporary version of the MedD?
    a. A dietary pattern characterized by high consumption of olive oil, vegetables, legumes, whole grains, fruits and nuts, moderate consumption of animal-based products, and low-to-moderate consumption of wine with meals.
    b. A predominantly plant-based low-fat dietary pattern rich in potassium, magnesium, calcium, and dietary fiber.
    c. The traditional high-protein low-fat diet adopted in the olive-growing areas of the Mediterranean region in the late 1950s and early 1960s.
    d. The diet originating in the 1990s study by the National Institutes of Health, aiming to identify dietary interventions that could be useful in treating hypertension.
13. Characterize the following statements as true (T) or false (F).
    a. Isometric exercise is a static contraction of a muscle without any visible movement in the angle of the joint ( ).
    b. Occupational stress, social stress, and low socioeconomic status have been associated with increased risk for hypertension ( ).
    c. Increased consumption of garlic, dark chocolate, and tea are well-established nonpharmacological dietary treatments for hypertension ( ).
    d. Combining behavioral support with pharmacotherapy is the most effective approach for smoking cessation ( ).
    e. Omega-3 polyunsaturated fatty acids have a BP-lowering effect; however, the dosage required to achieve this effect is very high (≥3 g/d) ( ).
14. How can weight loss contribute to hypertension management?
15. Which of the following foods contains approximately 300 mg of sodium?
    a. 1 cup of full-fat milk
    b. two small whole-grain rusks
    c. 2 teaspoons of olive oil
    d. 60 g of parmesan cheese
    e. one peach

16. Which of the following statements about sodium/salt are true?
    a. ~80% of salt consumption comes from dairy and meat products.
    b. Hypertensive patients should aim for a ≥1000-mg reduction in daily sodium intake.
    c. In people with treated hypertension, effective sodium restriction may reduce the number or dose of BP-lowering drugs that are necessary to control BP.
    d. Extremely strict sodium restrictions (<1000 mg/d) are recommended for hypertensive patients who cannot lose weight.
    e. 2 g of sodium equal to approximately 10 g of salt.
17. Characterize the following statements as true (T) or false (F).
    a. The DASH diet can be described as the dietary pattern adopted in the olive-growing areas of the Mediterranean region in the late 1950s and early 1960s ( ).
    b. A consistent and significant SBP difference between arms (i.e., >15 mmHg) is associated with increased cardiovascular risk ( ).

c. Exposure to chronic psychosocial stress contributes to hypertension, while thinking about or experiencing stressful events can delay BP recovery ( ).
d. One teaspoon of salt contains approximately 500 mg of sodium ( ).
e. DBP tends to decline from midlife as a consequence of arterial stiffening and SBP assumes even greater importance as a risk factor from midlife and on ( ).
18. What is the relationship between sleep and hypertension?
19. Which of the following have a well-established BP-lowering effect?
    a. increased consumption of low-fat dairy products, nuts, and healthy oils
    b. regular aerobic exercise, e.g., ≥30 minutes of moderate intensity 5–7 days/week
    c. increased magnesium intake
    d. abstinence from active and passive smoking
    e. maintenance of a healthy body weight
    f. all of the above
20. A hypertensive patient visits your office for lifestyle counseling. What would you recommend on sodium intake?

Bibliography

Appel, L.J., Brands, M.W., Daniels, S.R. et al. (2006). Dietary approaches to prevent and treat hypertension: a scientific statement from the American Heart Association. *Hypertension* 47 (2): 296–308. https://doi.org/10.1161/01.HYP.0000202568.01167.B6.

Cahill, K., Stevens, S., Perera, R., and Lancaster, T. (2013). Pharmacological interventions for smoking cessation: an overview and network meta-analysis. *Cochrane Database Syst. Rev.* (5): CD009329. https://doi.org/10.1002/14651858.CD009329.pub2.

Calhoun, D.A. and Harding, S.M. (2010). Sleep and hypertension. *Chest* 138 (2): 434–443. https://doi.org/10.1378/chest.09-2954.

Challa, H.J., Ameer, M.A., and Uppaluri, K.R. (2020). *DASH Diet (Dietary Approaches to Stop Hypertension)*. Treasure Island, FL: StatPearls.

Cornelissen, V.A. and Smart, N.A. (2013). Exercise training for blood pressure: a systematic review and meta-analysis. *J. Am. Heart Assoc.* 2 (1): e004473. https://doi.org/10.1161/JAHA.112.004473.

Ding, M., Bhupathiraju, S.N., Satija, A. et al. (2014). Long-term coffee consumption and risk of cardiovascular disease: a systematic review and a dose-response meta-analysis of prospective cohort studies. *Circulation* 129 (6): 643–659. https://doi.org/10.1161/CIRCULATIONAHA.113.005925.

Doll, R., Peto, R., Wheatley, K. et al. (1994). Mortality in relation to smoking: 40 years' observations on male British doctors. *BMJ* 309 (6959): 901–911. https://doi.org/10.1136/bmj.309.6959.901.

Domenech, M., Roman, P., Lapetra, J. et al. (2014). Mediterranean diet reduces 24-hour ambulatory blood pressure, blood glucose, and lipids: one-year randomized, clinical trial. *Hypertension* 64 (1): 69–76. https://doi.org/10.1161/HYPERTENSIONAHA.113.03353.

Elijovich, F., Weinberger, M.H., Anderson, C.A., Appel, L.J., Bursztyn, M., Cook, N.R. et al. (2016). Salt sensitivity of blood pressure: a scientific statement from the American Heart Association. *Hypertension* 68 (3): e7–e46. doi: 10.1161/HYP.0000000000000047.

Elliott, P., Stamler, J., Nichols, R. et al. (1996). Intersalt revisited: further analyses of 24 hour sodium excretion and blood pressure within and across populations. Intersalt Cooperative Research Group. *BMJ* 312 (7041): 1249–1253. https://doi.org/10.1136/bmj.312.7041.1249.

Estruch, R., Coca, A., and Rodicio, J.L. (2005). High blood pressure, alcohol and cardiovascular risk. *J. Hypertens.* 23 (1): 226–229. doi: 10.1097/00004872-200501000-00039.

Filippini, T., Naska, A., Kasdagli, M.I. et al. (2020). Potassium intake and blood pressure: a dose-response meta-analysis of randomized controlled trials. *J. Am. Heart Assoc.* 9 (12): e015719. https://doi.org/10.1161/JAHA.119.015719.

Filippou, C.D., Tsioufis, C.P., Thomopoulos, C.G. et al. (2020). Dietary Approaches to Stop Hypertension (DASH) diet and blood pressure reduction in adults with and without hypertension: a systematic review and meta-analysis of randomized controlled trials. *Adv. Nutr.* 11 (5): 1150–1160. https://doi.org/10.1093/advances/nmaa041.

Graudal, N.A., Hubeck-Graudal, T., and Jurgens, G. (2012). Effects of low-sodium diet vs. high-sodium diet on blood pressure, renin, aldosterone, catecholamines, cholesterol, and triglyceride (Cochrane review). *Am. J. Hypertens.* 25 (1): 1–15. https://doi.org/10.1038/ajh.2011.210.

Greyling, A., Ras, R.T., Zock, P.L. et al. (2014). The effect of black tea on blood pressure: a systematic review with meta-analysis of randomized controlled trials. *PLoS One* 9 (7): e103247. https://doi.org/10.1371/journal.pone.0103247.

Groppelli, A., Giorgi, D.M., Omboni, S. et al. (1992). Persistent blood pressure increase induced by heavy smoking. *J. Hypertens.* 10 (5): 495–499. https://doi.org/10.1097/00004872-199205000-00014.

Hall, J.E., do Carmo, J.M., da Silva, A.A. et al. (2015). Obesity-induced hypertension: interaction of neurohumoral and renal mechanisms. *Circ. Res.* 116 (6): 991–1006. https://doi.org/10.1161/CIRCRESAHA.116.305697.

He, F.J., Li, J., and Macgregor, G.A. (2013). Effect of longer term modest salt reduction on blood pressure: Cochrane systematic review and meta-analysis of randomised trials. *BMJ* 346: f1325. https://doi.org/10.1136/bmj.f1325.

He, F.J. and MacGregor, G.A. (2003). How far should salt intake be reduced? *Hypertension* 42 (6): 1093–1099. https://doi.org/10.1161/01.HYP.0000102864.05174.E8.

Huai, P., Xun, H., Reilly, K.H. et al. (2013). Physical activity and risk of hypertension: a meta-analysis of prospective cohort studies. *Hypertension* 62 (6): 1021–1026. https://doi.org/10.1161/HYPERTENSIONAHA.113.01965.

Kraus, W.E., Powell, K.E., Haskell, W.L. et al. (2019). Physical activity, all-cause and cardiovascular mortality, and cardiovascular disease. *Med. Sci. Sports Exerc.* 51 (6): 1270–1281. https://doi.org/10.1249/MSS.0000000000001939.

Lim, S.S., Vos, T., Flaxman, A.D. et al. (2012). A comparative risk assessment of burden of disease and injury attributable to 67 risk factors and risk factor clusters in 21 regions, 1990-2010: a systematic analysis for the Global Burden of Disease Study 2010. *Lancet* 380 (9859): 2224–2260. https://doi.org/10.1016/S0140-6736(12)61766-8.

Neter, J.E., Stam, B.E., Kok, F.J. et al. (2003). Influence of weight reduction on blood pressure: a meta-analysis of randomized controlled trials. *Hypertension* 42 (5): 878–884. https://doi.org/10.1161/01.HYP.0000094221.86888.AE.

Parshad, O. (2004). Role of yoga in stress management. *West Indian Med. J.* 53 (3): 191–194.

Piepoli, M.F., Hoes, A.W., Agewall, S. et al. (2016). 2016 European guidelines on cardiovascular disease prevention in clinical practice: The Sixth Joint Task Force of the European Society of Cardiology and Other Societies on Cardiovascular Disease Prevention in Clinical Practice (constituted by representatives of 10 societies and by invited experts) Developed with the special contribution of the European Association for Cardiovascular Prevention & Rehabilitation (EACPR). *Eur. Heart J.* 37 (29): 2315–2381. https://doi.org/10.1093/eurheartj/ehw106.

Rainforth, M.V., Schneider, R.H., Nidich, S.I. et al. (2007). Stress reduction programs in patients with elevated blood pressure: a systematic review and meta-analysis. *Curr. Hypertens. Rep.* 9 (6): 520–528. https://doi.org/10.1007/s11906-007-0094-3.

Roerecke, M., Kaczorowski, J., Tobe, S.W. et al. (2017). The effect of a reduction in alcohol consumption on blood pressure: a systematic review and meta-analysis. *Lancet Public Health* 2 (2): e108–e120. https://doi.org/10.1016/S2468-2667(17)30003-8.

Rossi, A., Dikareva, A., Bacon, S.L., and Daskalopoulou, S.S. (2012). The impact of physical activity on mortality in patients with high blood pressure: a systematic review. *J. Hypertens.* 30 (7): 1277–1288. https://doi.org/10.1097/HJH.0b013e3283544669.

Sacks, F.M. and Campos, H. (2010). Dietary therapy in hypertension. *N. Engl. J. Med.* 362 (22): 2102–2112. doi: 10.1056/NEJMct0911013.

Sofi, F. (2009). The Mediterranean diet revisited: evidence of its effectiveness grows. *Curr. Opin. Cardiol.* 24 (5): 442–446. https://doi.org/10.1097/HCO.0b013e32832f056e.

Sofi, F., Abbate, R., Gensini, G.F., and Casini, A. (2010). Accruing evidence on benefits of adherence to the Mediterranean diet on health: an updated systematic review and meta-analysis. *Am. J. Clin. Nutr.* 92 (5): 1189–1196. https://doi.org/10.3945/ajcn.2010.29673.

Soltani, S., Arablou, T., Jayedi, A., and Salehi-Abargouei, A. (2020). Adherence to the Dietary Approaches to Stop Hypertension (DASH) diet in relation to all-cause and cause-specific mortality: a systematic review and dose-response meta-analysis of prospective cohort studies. *Nutr. J.* 19 (1): 37. https://doi.org/10.1186/s12937-020-00554-8.

Spruill, T.M. (2010). Chronic psychosocial stress and hypertension. *Curr. Hypertens. Rep.* 12 (1): 10–16. https://doi.org/10.1007/s11906-009-0084-8.

Stead, L.F., Buitrago, D., Preciado, N. et al. (2013). Physician advice for smoking cessation. *Cochrane Database Syst. Rev.* (5): CD000165. https://doi.org/10.1002/14651858.CD000165.pub4.

Stead, L.F., Koilpillai, P., Fanshawe, T.R., and Lancaster, T. (2016). Combined pharmacotherapy and behavioural interventions for smoking cessation. *Cochrane Database Syst. Rev.* (3): CD008286. https://doi.org/10.1002/14651858.CD008286.pub3.

Trichopoulou, A. (2001). Mediterranean diet: the past and the present. *Nutr. Metab. Cardiovasc. Dis.* 11 (4 Suppl): 1–4.

Tsirimiagkou, C., Karatzi, K., Argyris, A., Chalkidou, F., Tzelefa, V., Sfikakis, P.P. et al. (2021). Levels of dietary sodium intake: diverging associations with arterial stiffness and atheromatosis. *Hellenic J. Cardiol.* doi: 10.1016/j.hjc.2021.02.005.

Whelton, P.K., Appel, L.J., Sacco, R.L., Anderson, C.A., Antman, E.M., Campbell, N. et al. (2012). Sodium, blood pressure, and cardiovascular disease: further evidence supporting the American Heart Association sodium reduction recommendations. *Circulation* 126 (24): 2880–2889. doi: 10.1161/CIR.0b013e318279acbf.

Whelton, P.K., Carey, R.M., Aronow, W.S. et al. (2018). 2017 ACC/AHA/AAPA/ABC/ACPM/AGS/APhA/ASH/ASPC/NMA/PCNA guideline for the prevention, detection, evaluation, and management of high blood pressure in adults: executive summary: a report of the American College of Cardiology/American Heart Association Task Force on Clinical Practice Guidelines. *Circulation* 138 (17): e426–e483. https://doi.org/10.1161/CIR.0000000000000597.

Williams, B., Mancia, G., Spiering, W. et al. (2018). 2018 ESC/ESH guidelines for the management of arterial hypertension: the Task Force for the Management of Arterial Hypertension of the European Society of Cardiology and the European Society of Hypertension. *J. Hypertens.* 36 (10): 1953–2041. https://doi.org/10.1097/HJH.0000000000001940.

World Health Organization. (2010). *Global Recommendations on Physical Activity for Health*. Geneva: WHO Guidelines Review Committee.

Xin, X., He, J., Frontini, M.G. et al. (2001). Effects of alcohol reduction on blood pressure: a meta-analysis of randomized controlled trials. *Hypertension* 38 (5): 1112–1117. https://doi.org/10.1161/hy1101.093424.

Xu, R., Yang, K., Ding, J., and Chen, G. (2020). Effect of green tea supplementation on blood pressure: a systematic review and meta-analysis of randomized controlled trials. *Medicine (Baltimore)* 99 (6): e19047. https://doi.org/10.1097/MD.0000000000019047.

CHAPTER 16

Dyslipidemia Case Study

Mr. KI is a 37-year-old police officer who lives with his wife and two kids. He has no significant previous medical history other than obesity. He recently visited his doctor for an annual checkup and fasting blood work; his blood glucose was 87 mg/dl, total cholesterol 270 mg/dl, high-density lipoprotein (HDL) cholesterol 34 mg/dl, low-density lipoprotein (LDL) cholesterol 198 mg/dl, triglycerides (TG) 180 mg/dl, and systolic/diastolic blood pressure 124/82 mmHg. Mr. KI does not smoke, lives a sedentary lifestyle, and rarely drinks small quantities of alcohol during social occasions. His height is 1.87 m and his current body weight is 145.6 kg. Based on the diagnosis of dyslipidemia, his doctor prescribed lipid-lowering medication (statins) and referred him to you for lifestyle assessment and modification.

Assessment

Clinical Assessment

Lipids are important macronutrients for the human body, performing three fundamental biological functions: they serve as (i) structural components of cell membranes, (ii) energy storehouses, and (iii) signaling molecules. The three main types of lipids are triacylglycerols (TG), phospholipids (PL), and sterols. In animals the most important sterol is cholesterol. Special types of proteins, called lipoproteins, transport lipids in plasma to all body cells for energy use, lipid deposition, and the production of important molecules, such as steroid hormones and bile acids. Lipoproteins consist of esterified and unesterified cholesterol, TG, and PL. In addition, lipoproteins contain apolipoproteins (Apo) that act as structural components, ligands for cellular receptor binding, and enzyme activators or inhibitors. There are six major types of lipoproteins: chylomicrons (CM), very low-density lipoproteins (VLDLs), intermediate-density lipoproteins (IDLs), low-density lipoproteins (LDLs), lipoprotein a

> **Key Point**
>
> Special types of proteins, called lipoproteins, transport lipids in plasma.

(Lp(a)), and high density lipoproteins (HDLs) (Table 16.1) (Mach et al. 2020).

Lipid metabolism is a complex function summarized in Figure 16.1 (Mach et al. 2020). In brief, the largest amount of cholesterol is synthesized in the liver, where it is either packaged together with TG into VLDLs or used for bile acid synthesis. The VLDLs are then secreted in the circulation and travel to the various tissues, where the TG stored in their core are hydrolyzed to free fatty acids (FFA) for energy production or storage. As more and more triacylglycerols are removed from the VLDL, the composition of the molecule changes, and it becomes IDL. In turn, IDLs can either be further hydrolyzed to become LDLs or can be taken up by the liver for further metabolism and secretion in the bile. Finally, the LDL particles are taken up by the liver (for cholesterol and bile acid synthesis) and peripheral cells (for hormone production, cell membrane synthesis, or storage).

HDL particles transport excess cholesterol from the peripheral cells back to the liver in a process referred to as *reverse cholesterol transport*. The HDL particles can either transport cholesterol directly back to the liver or interact with cholesterol ester transfer protein to exchange cholesterol for TG with VLDLs and LDLs.

> **Key Point**
>
> ApoA1-containing HDL particles transport excess cholesterol from the peripheral cells back to the liver in a process referred to as reverse cholesterol transport.

It is well established that lipoproteins can play a significant role in the pathophysiology of atherosclerosis, a condition in which plaque builds up inside the arteries, leading to their hardening and narrowing (Figure 16.2). The quantity of circulating lipoproteins, determined by genetic and dietary characteristics (e.g., excess intake of trans and saturated fatty acids [SFAs]), and the degree of lipid-oxidation/peroxidation (due to smoking and other factors), greatly influence the rate

> **Key Point**
>
> The quantity of circulating lipoproteins and the degree of lipid-oxidation/peroxidation greatly influence the rate and extent of atherosclerosis and endothelial damage.

TABLE 16.1 Physical and chemical characteristics of plasma lipoproteins.

	Density (g/ml)	Diameter (nm)	TG (%)	Cholesteryl esters (%)	PL (%)	Cholesterol (%)	Major Apo
CM	<0.95	80–100	90–95	2–4	2–6	1	ApoB-48
VLDL	0.95–1.006	30–80	50–65	8–14	12–16	4–7	ApoB-100
IDL	1.006–1.019	25–30	25–40	20–35	16–24	7–11	ApoB-100
LDL	1.019–1.063	20–25	4–6	34–35	22–26	6–15	ApoB-100
HDL	1.063–1.210	8–13	7	10–20	55	5	ApoA-1
Lp(a)	1.006–1.125	25–30	4–8	35–46	17–24	6–9	Apo(a)

Apo, apolipoprotein; CM, chylomicron; HDL, high-density lipoprotein; IDL, intermediate-density lipoprotein; LDL, low-density lipoprotein; Lp(a), lipoprotein(a); PL, phospholipid; TG, triacylglycerols; VLDL, very low-density lipoprotein.
Source: Adapted with permission from Mach et al. (2020).

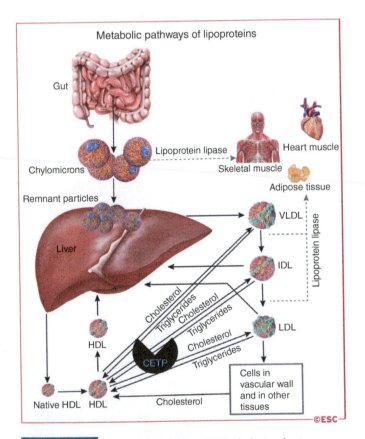

FIGURE 16.1 **Lipid metabolism.** CETP, cholesterol ester transfer protein; HDL, high-density lipoprotein; IDL, intermediate-density lipoprotein; LDL, low-density lipoprotein; VLDL, very-low-density lipoprotein. **Source:** Reprinted with permission from Mach et al. (2020).

and extent of atherosclerosis and endothelial damage. All ApoB-containing lipoproteins <70 nm in diameter, including smaller TG-rich lipoproteins and their remnant particles, can cross the endothelial barrier in the presence of endothelial dysfunction. Inside the arterial wall, the lipoproteins may be trapped after interaction with extracellular structures, such as proteoglycans. ApoB-containing lipoproteins retained in the

arterial wall provoke a complex process that leads to lipid deposition and the initiation of an atheroma. Continued exposure to ApoB-containing lipoproteins, especially oxidized, leads to additional particles being retained over time in the artery wall and to the growth and progression of atherosclerotic plaques. Eventually, the increase of the atherosclerotic plaque burden, along with changes in the composition of the plaque, reaches a critical point when the plaque ruptures, forming a thrombus that can acutely obstruct blood flow. The possible consequences are unstable angina, myocardial infarction, or even death (Figure 16.2) (Libby 2002; Brown et al. 2015; Rodriguez et al. 2019; Rosenson et al. 2018.).

Given the important role of lipoproteins in the pathophysiology of atherosclerosis, their quantification in plasma is crucial for the estimation of cardiovascular risk. In clinical practice, the concentration of plasma lipoproteins is estimated by measuring their cholesterol content. Total cholesterol (TC) in humans is distributed primarily among three major lipoprotein classes: VLDL, LDL, and HDL. A standard serum lipid profile measures the concentration of TC, HDL cholesterol (HDLC), LDL cholesterol (LDLC), and TG. LDLC should ideally be directly measured in blood, but it can also be calculated indirectly using the Friedewald formula: LDLC = TC − HDLC − (TG/5) in mg/dl or TC − HDLC − (TG/2.2) in mmol/l (Friedewald et al. 1972); this indirect calculation is used often in clinical practice, but the result can be erroneous, especially in the presence of hypertriglyceridemia.

Table 16.2 presents the range of the blood lipid profile values, used to establish the diagnosis of dyslipidemia. In general, dyslipidemias can be classified as familial, i.e.,

> **Key Point**
>
> Lipoproteins play a significant role in the pathophysiology of atherosclerosis.

> **Key Point**
>
> A standard serum lipid profile measures the concentration of total cholesterol (TC), HDL cholesterol (HDLC), LDL cholesterol (LDLC), and triglycerides (TG).

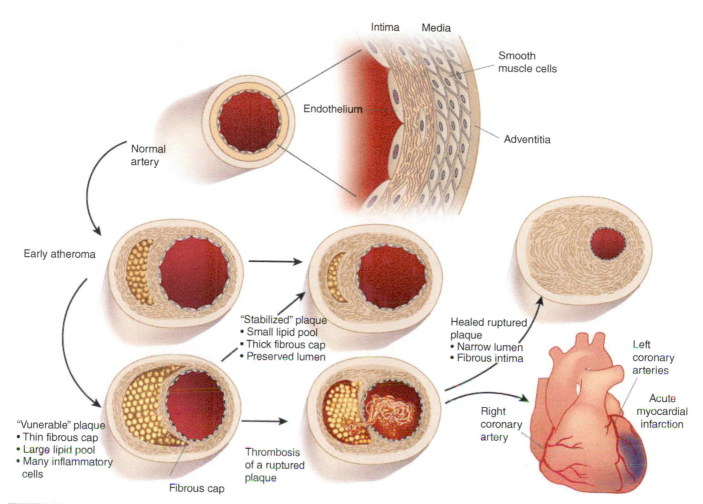

FIGURE 16.2 **Schematic of the life history of an atheroma.** The normal human coronary artery has a typical trilaminar structure. The endothelial cells in contact with the blood in the arterial lumen rest on a basement membrane. The intimal layer in adult humans generally contains a smattering of smooth muscle cells scattered within the intimal extracellular matrix. The internal elastic lamina forms the barrier between the tunica intima and the underlying tunica media. The media consists of multiple layers of smooth muscle cells, much more tightly packed than in the diffusely thickened intima, and embedded in a matrix rich in elastin as well as collagen. In early atherogenesis, recruitment of inflammatory cells and the accumulation of lipids leads to formation of a lipid-rich core, as the artery enlarges in an outward, abluminal direction to accommodate the expansion of the intima. If inflammatory conditions prevail and risk factors such as dyslipidemia persist, the lipid core can grow, and proteinases secreted by the activated leukocytes can degrade the extracellular matrix, while pro-inflammatory cytokines, such as interferon-g, can limit the synthesis of new collagen. These changes can thin the fibrous cap and render it friable and susceptible to rupture. When the plaque ruptures, blood coming in contact with the tissue factor in the plaque coagulates. Platelets activated by thrombin generated from the coagulation cascade and by contact with the intimal compartment instigate thrombus formation. If the thrombus occludes the vessel persistently, an acute myocardial infarction can result (the dusky blue area in the anterior wall of the left ventricle, lower right). The thrombus may eventually resorb as a result of endogenous or therapeutic thrombolysis. However, a wound-healing response triggered by thrombin generated during blood coagulation can stimulate smooth muscle proliferation. Platelet-derived growth factor released from activated platelets stimulates smooth muscle cell migration. Transforming growth factor-b, also released from activated platelets, stimulates interstitial collagen production. This increased migration, proliferation, and extracellular matrix synthesis by smooth muscle cells thickens the fibrous cap and causes further expansion of the intima, often in an inward direction, yielding constriction of the lumen. Stenotic lesions produced by the luminal encroachment of the fibrosed plaque may restrict flow, particularly under situations of increased cardiac demand, leading to ischemia, commonly provoking symptoms such as angina pectoris. Advanced stenotic plaques, being more fibrous, may prove less susceptible to rupture and renewed thrombosis. Lipid lowering can reduce lipid content and calm the intimal inflammatory response, yielding a more "stable" plaque with a thick fibrous cap and a preserved lumen (center). **Source:** Reprinted with permission from Libby (2002).

> **Key Point**
>
> Dyslipidemias can be classified as familial or acquired.

inherited diseases with a strong genetic background, or acquired, i.e., secondary to obesity, metabolic diseases, and an unhealthy lifestyle with a gradual increase in severity over time. The terms *hyperlipoproteinemia, hyperlipidemia,* and *dyslipidemia* are often used to express the same condition; however, hyperlipoproteinemia more accurately refers to increased levels of lipoprotein molecules (usually not assessed in clinical practice); hyperlipidemia refers to increased levels of TC, LDLC, and TG, while dyslipidemia also includes the presence of low

TABLE 16.2   Assessment of lipidemic profile.

Parameter	Ideal levels	Acceptable levels	Pathological levels	Alarming levels
TG	<150 mg/dl (<1.7 mmol/l)	150–200 mg/dl (1.7–5.2 mmol/l)	≥200 mg/dl (≥5.2 mmol/l)	>880 mg/dl (10.0 mmol/l) – suspected familial chylomicronemia syndrome
TC	<200 mg/dl (<5.2 mmol/l)	200–240 mg/dl (5.2–6.2 mmol/l)	≥240 mg/dl (≥6.2 mmol/l)	
LDLC	<130 mg/dl (<3.4 mmol/l)	130–160 mg/dl (3.4–4.2 mmol/l)	≥160 mg/dl (≥4.2 mmol/l)	>500 mg/dl (13 mmol/l) – suspected homozygous familiar hypercholesterolemia; >190 mg/dl (5.0 mmol/l) – suspected heterozygous familiar hypercholesterolemia
HDLC	females/males ≥60/55 mg/dl (≥1.6/1.4 mmol/l)	females/males 45–60/40–55 mg/dl (1.2–1.6/1.0–1.4 mmol/l)	females/males <45/40 mg/dl (<1.2/1.0 mmol/l)	

HDLC, high-density lipoprotein cholesterol; LDLC, low-density lipoprotein cholesterol; TC, total cholesterol; TG, triglycerides.

HDLC levels. Finally, isolated increased levels of TC or LDLC are referred to as hypercholesterolemia, whereas isolated increased TG values are referred to as hypertriglyceridemia.

Mr. KI presented to his doctor's office with a TC of 270 mg/dl, HDLC of 34 mg/dl, LDLC of 198 mg/dl, and TG of 180 mg/dl. Based on the established cut-off points of lipidemic profile indices, he was diagnosed with dyslipidemia.

Anthropometric Assessment

Detailed instructions on how to perform anthropometric assessments have been presented in Chapter 13.

Mr. KI's height is 1.87 m and current weight is 145.6 kg. His body mass index (BMI) is 145.6 kg ÷ (1.87 m)² = 41.64 kg/m², and according to the classification of BMI values, he is considered obese class III with extremely high risk of morbidity. After discussing with Mr. KI about his body weight history, you recorded the following information: Mr. KI has been overweight since his childhood and as he states, "I am used to it." He admits that he has never tried to lose weight; however, after you explain to him the relationship between excess body weight and dyslipidemia, atherosclerosis, and cardiovascular risk, he is ready to consider the possibility of changing his lifestyle to achieve a healthier weight.

Dietary Assessment

Detailed instructions on how to perform dietary assessments have been presented in Chapter 13.

After interviewing Mr. KI about his dietary habits, you recorded the following information: Mr. KI has a rotating shift schedule at work with alternating morning, afternoon, and night shifts throughout a typical working week. Given his difficult work schedule, he only consumes one meal (either lunch or dinner) at home, and all other meals and snacks are fast-food choices, such as baked goods, sandwiches, pizza, burger, and commercial sweets. Mr. KI loves food, and his wife always tries to cook whatever he wants to please him. He particularly likes all kinds of red meat and French fries, which he consumes almost on a daily basis, he does not eat fish and legumes, and after his meal at home he always has a sweet dessert. He rarely eats fruits and he drinks an average of 5 cups of coffee daily, each with added cream and sugar.*

In the context of the 24-hour dietary recall (Appendix D.1), Mr. KI described the consumption of foods and beverages of the previous day (night shift) as follows:

Breakfast: two cups of instant coffee with 1 tablespoon of sugar each and one doughnut

Lunch: 250 g of roasted beef, two cups of French fries, two slices of white bread with 1 tablespoon of butter each, and ~four chocolate-chip cookies

Afternoon snack: 1 cup of instant coffee with 1 tablespoon of sugar (at work)

Dinner: 1 large (10-piece) pizza with bacon and pepperoni (at work)

Late evening snack: 2 cups of instant coffee with 1 tablespoon of sugar each, and 10 medium-sized pretzels (at work throughout the night shift)

Physical Activity Assessment

Detailed instructions on how to perform physical activity assessments have been presented in Chapter 13.

After interviewing Mr. KI about his physical activity habits, you recorded the following information: Mr. KI used to do karate as a youth, from the age of 12 until the age of 18. Since then, he has never exercised systematically and his job is mainly sedentary, due to office work and driving patrol cars. Even though his work is sedentary, he usually feels exhausted after his shift and has little energy left for anything that involves physical activity. He always uses his car for transportation to/from work, shopping, and all other daily activities. His wife is very physically active, and although she has been trying to motivate him to exercise, Mr. KI does not find interest in any kind of sport activity and is afraid of potential injuries due to his increased body weight. On the weekends, he sometimes goes for a walk with his 10-year-old son at the playground near their house; however, his aerobic capacity is markedly low, and he gets easily tired even after walking for a few hundred meters.

Sleep Assessment

Detailed instructions on how to perform sleep assessments have been presented in Chapter 13.

After interviewing Mr. KI about his sleep habits, you recorded the following information: Mr. KI does not have a steady sleep schedule due to the nature of his work; he works day and night shifts, with a 3-day break in between. When on a day shift, he usually wakes up ~05:00, goes to work from 07:00 up until 18:00 and then returns home, eats dinner with his family around 21:00, watches TV for a few hours, and goes to bed around midnight. When he works the night shift, he wakes up ~17:00, eats dinner with his family ~18:00 and goes to work from 21:00 to 08:00 in the next morning. Mr. KI does not report any severe sleep problems; however, he usually wakes up dizzy and feels sleepy during most of the day. His wife sleeps in the next room due to his loud snoring and has witnessed pauses of breathing and choking-like episodes when she used to share the same bed with him. After completing the STOP-BANG questionnaire (Appendix D.9), Mr. KI was categorized as at high risk for obstructive sleep apnea (OSA).

Stress Assessment

Detailed instructions on how to assess stress levels have been presented in Chapter 13.

Mr. KI did not report any symptoms of stress or anxiety. Although his work schedule is difficult, he likes his job and has a good relationship with his colleagues and superiors. After completing the Perceived Stress Scale (Appendix D.10), Mr. KI's score was 8, indicative of low stress levels.

Dyslipidemia Management

General Principles

The risk of experiencing an acute atherosclerotic cardiovascular event rises rapidly as more ApoB-containing lipoproteins are deposited in the subendothelial region of the coronary arteries and the atherosclerotic plaque burden increases. This provides a rationale for maintaining low levels of lipoproteins throughout life to slow the progression of atherosclerosis and recommending treatment to lower lipoproteins for both the primary and secondary prevention of cardiovascular diseases. Among the various ApoB-containing lipoproteins, LDLC is probably the most important lipoprotein in terms of cardiovascular health. Epidemiological and clinical evidence have consistently demonstrated a positive relationship between the plasma LDLC and the risk of atherosclerotic cardiovascular events. Therefore, lowering LDLC levels is key to the prevention of cardiovascular disease.

On the other hand, an inverse association between plasma HDLC and the risk of atherosclerotic cardiovascular events has been consistently shown in epidemiological studies, suggesting the important role of HDLC in cardiovascular disease prevention. However, there is currently only weak evidence to suggest that raising plasma HDLC alone is likely to significantly reduce cardiovascular risk. Therefore, HDLC levels are currently used only secondary to LDLC levels as an intervention target for patients with dyslipidemia. Elevated plasma TG levels are also associated with an increasing risk of atherosclerotic cardiovascular events, but this association becomes null after adjusting for non-HDLC, calculated by subtracting the HDL from total cholesterol. Similarly, lowering TG levels reduces cardiovascular risk by the same amount as lowering LDLC levels when measured per unit change of non-HDLC, suggesting that the effect of plasma TG on atherosclerotic cardiovascular events is mediated by changes in the concentration of TG-rich lipoproteins.

Table 16.3 summarizes treatment goals for high LDLC plasma levels according to the 2017 American Association of Clinical Endocrinologists (AACE) and American College of Endocrinology (ACE) guidelines for the management of dyslipidemia and prevention of cardiovascular disease (Jellinger et al. 2017) and the 2019 European Society of Cardiology (ESC) and European Atherosclerosis Society (EAS) guidelines for the management of dyslipidemias (Mach et al. 2020). There is no universal target for LDLC levels for all patients with dyslipidemia. Optimal LDLC values depend on the patient's total cardiovascular risk. In general, the higher the cardiovascular risk

> **Key Point**
> LDLC is probably the most important lipoprotein in terms of cardiovascular health.

> **Key Point**
> Lowering LDLC levels is key to the prevention of cardiovascular disease.

TABLE 16.3 Treatment goals for increased plasma LDLC levels.

	Risk category		LDLC goals	
			mg/dl	mmol/l
Extreme risk	AACE/ACE	• Progressive ASCVD after achieving an LDLC <70 mg/dl • Established clinical CVD in patients with DM, CKD stages 3/4, or HeFH • History of premature ASCVD (males <55 years, females <65 years)	<55	<1.4
	ESC/EAS	• ASCVD with a second vascular event within 2 years while taking maximally tolerated statin-based therapy	<40	<1.0
Very high risk	AACE/ACE	• Established or recent hospitalization for ACS • Coronary, carotid, or peripheral vascular disease • ASCVD 10-year risk >20% • DM or CKD stages 3/4 with one or more risk factor(s) • HeFH	<70	<1.8
	ESC/EAS	• Documented ASCVD (ACS: MI or unstable angina, stable angina, coronary revascularization, stroke, TIA, and peripheral arterial disease), either clinical or unequivocal on imaging • DM with target organ damage, or ≥3 major risk factors, or early onset of T1DM of long duration (>20 years) • Severe CKD (eGFR <30 ml/min/1.73 m^2) • A calculated SCORE ≥ 10% for 10-year risk of fatal CVD • FH with ASCVD or with another major risk factor	< 55 or reduction of at least 50% from baselined	<1.4
High risk	AACE/ACE	• >2 risk factors and ASCVD 10-year risk 10–20% • DM or CKD stages 3/4 with no other risk factors	<100	<2.6
	ESC/EAS	• Markedly elevated single risk factors, in particular TC >310 mg/dl (8 mmol/l), LDLC >190 mg/dl (4.9 mmol/l), or BP ≥180/110 mmHg • Patients with FH without other major risk factors • Patients with DM without target organ damage, with DM duration ≥10 years or another additional risk factor • Moderate CKD (eGFR 30–59 ml/min/1.73 m^2) • Calculated SCORE ≥ 5% and < 10% for 10-year risk of fatal CVD	<70 or reduction of at least 50% from baselined	<1.8
Moderate risk	AACE/ACE	• <2 risk factors and ASCVD 10-year risk <10%	<100	<2.6
	ESC/EAS	• Young patients (T1DM <35 years; T2DM <50 years) with duration <10 years, without other risk factors • Calculated SCORE ≥ 1% and < 5% for 10-year risk of fatal CVD	<100	<2.6
Low risk	AACE/ACE	• No risk factors	<130	<3.4
	ESC/EAS	• Calculated SCORE < 1% for 10-year risk of fatal CVD	<115	<3.0

AACE, American Association of Clinical Endocrinologists; ACE, American College of Endocrinology; ACS, acute coronary syndrome; AHA, American Heart Association; ASCVD, atherosclerotic cardiovascular disease; ASCVD score, risk score for atherosclerotic cardiovascular disease; BP, blood pressure; CKD, chronic kidney disease; CVD, cardiovascular disease; (T1/2)DM, (type 1/2) diabetes mellitus; EAS, European Atherosclerosis Society; ESC, European Society of Cardiology; eGFR, estimated glomerular filtration rate; (He)FH, (heterogenous) familial hypercholesterolemia; LDLC, low-density lipoprotein cholesterol; MI, myocardial infarction; SCORE, Systematic Coronary Risk Evaluation; TC, total cholesterol; TIA, transient ischemic attack.

of an individual, the stricter the target for LDLC levels. For example, according to the European guidelines (Mach et al. 2020), an LDLC value of <116 mg/dl is recommended for people with low cardiovascular risk, whereas the recommended level of LDLC is <55 mg/dl for patients at very high cardiovascular risk. Secondary goals have also been defined for non-HDLC, which should be 30 mg/dl (0.8 mmol/l)

> **Key Point**
>
> The higher the cardiovascular risk of an individual, the stricter the target for LDLC levels.

higher than the corresponding LDLC goal. Moreover, to date, no specific goals for HDLC or TG levels have been determined; however, increases in HDLC seem to predict atherosclerosis regression, and low HDLC levels are associated with excess events and mortality in coronary artery disease patients, even at low LDLC levels.

Management of dyslipidemia involves lifestyle interventions and drug treatment. Given that blood lipid disorders are strongly linked to increased body weight and an unhealthy lifestyle, lifestyle interventions are recommended for all patients with dyslipidemia, either as the first-line treatment or in combination with available pharmacotherapies. Drug treatment should be initiated sooner and more aggressively when the patient has a history that indicates familial dyslipidemia and a family history of early onset coronary heart disease. The main goal of the management of dyslipidemia is the reduction of cardiovascular risk. Therefore, adhering to a healthy cardioprotective lifestyle pattern is recommended for all patients with dyslipidemia.

With regard to drug treatment, established lipid-lowering drugs include statins, ezetimibe, bile acid sequestrants, fibrates, nicotinic acid, and cholesteryl ester transfer protein inhibitors. Statins are the first-line drug therapy in the treatment of hypercholesterolemia. Although LDLC goals are usually attained with monotherapy, some very-high-risk patients or those with very high LDLC levels may need additional treatment. In this case, combination therapy with statins and ezetimibe is reasonable. When goals still cannot be met, other available medications can be used in combination with statins. Statins are also the first-line treatment of hypertriglyceridemia, either alone or in combination with supplementation of n-3 fatty acids and fibrates. Cholesteryl ester transfer protein inhibitors are so far the most effective drug for increasing HDLC levels.

> **Key Point**
>
> Lifestyle interventions are recommended for all patients with dyslipidemia, either as the first-line treatment or in combination with available pharmacotherapies.

> **Key Point**
>
> Adhering to a healthy cardioprotective lifestyle pattern is recommended for all patients with dyslipidemia.

Besides blood lipid control, managing comorbidities, such as hypertension or T2DM, is also crucial in the context of cardiovascular disease prevention. Table 16.4 provides an overview of lifestyle and other health-related targets and goals for cardiovascular disease prevention that apply to all patients with dyslipidemia (Mach et al. 2020).

Weight Control

Obesity is a well-established risk factor for the development of blood lipid disorders (Figure 16.3) (Klop et al. 2013). Therefore, weight loss and maintenance of a healthy weight are important for the prevention and treatment of dyslipidemia. In the case of excess weight, even a modest (5–10% of basal body weight) weight reduction improves lipid abnormalities and favorably affects all other cardiovascular risk factors (Zomer et al. 2016). Data from clinical trials suggest that for every 1 kg decrease in body weight, there is a 2.0 mg/dl (0.05 mmol/l) decrease in TC, a 0.8 mg/dl (0.02 mmol/l) decrease in LDLC, and a 1.33 mg/dl (0.015 mmol/l) decrease in TG

> **Key Point**
>
> Obesity is a well-established risk factor for the development of blood lipid disorders.

TABLE 16.4	Treatment targets and goals for cardiovascular disease prevention.
Diet	Healthy diet low in trans/saturated fat with a focus on whole-grain products, legumes, vegetables, fruits, fish, and olive oil
Physical activity	3.5–7 h of moderate-to-vigorous physical activity per week or 30–60 min of physical activity on most days
Body weight	BMI 20–27.5 kg/m^2 and WC <94 cm (men) and <80 cm (women)
Smoking	No exposure to tobacco in any form
Blood pressure	<140/90 mmHg[a]
LDLC	See Table 16.3
Non-HDLC	30 mg/dl (0.8 mmol/l) higher than the LDLC goal
TG	<150 mg/dl (<1.7 mmol/l)
Diabetes mellitus	HbA1c <7% (<53 mmol/mol)

[a] Lower treatment targets are recommended for most treated hypertensive patients, provided that the treatment is well tolerated.
BMI, body mass index; HbA1c, glycated hemoglobin; HDLC, high-density lipoprotein cholesterol; LDLC, low-density lipoprotein cholesterol; TG, triglycerides; WC, waist circumference.
Source: Adapted with permission from Mach et al. (2020).

(Dattilo and Kris-Etherton 1992). With regard to HDLC levels, active weight loss is associated with a small decline in HDLC (1 kg of active weight loss is associated with a 0.3 mg/dl (0.007 mmol/l) decrease in HDLC); however, a 0.4 mg/dl (0.01 mmol/l) increase in HDLC is observed during the weight-maintenance phase, for every 1 kg lost (Dattilo and Kris-Etherton 1992). Although the magnitude of the effect of weight loss on blood lipids is modest, weight loss can have multiple favorable effects on other cardiovascular risk factors, especially blood pressure and glycemic control, and should be a central component of the management of obese patients with dyslipidemia.

> **Key Point**
>
> In the case of excess weight, even a modest (5–10% of basal body weight) weight reduction improves lipid abnormalities and favorably affects all other cardiovascular risk factors.

> **Key Point**
>
> Weight loss can have multiple favorable effects on other cardiovascular risk factors.

Weight reduction can be achieved primarily by decreasing caloric intake, e.g., decreasing portion sizes and limiting the consumption of energy-dense foods, and secondarily by increasing energy expenditure through physical activity, with a view to induce a negative energy balance. A combination of diet and exercise leads to the greatest improvements in physical performance and quality of life and wellness for patients with dyslipidemia, and it mitigates unintended loss of muscle

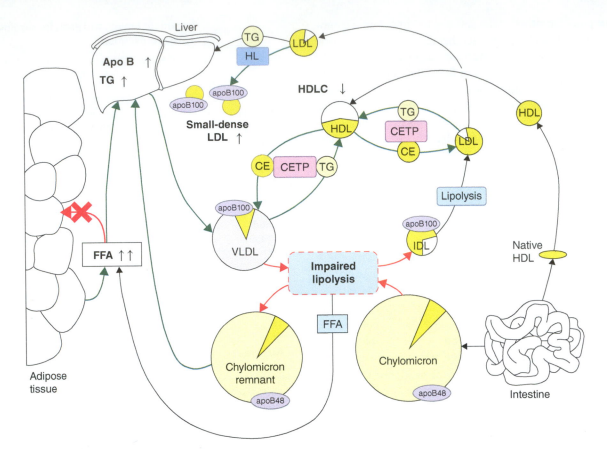

FIGURE 16.3   **Obesity and dyslipidemia.**   The hallmark of dyslipidemia in obesity is hypertriglyceridemia in part due to increased free fatty acid (FFA) fluxes to the liver, which leads to hepatic accumulation of triglycerides (TG). This leads to an increased hepatic synthesis of large, very-low-density lipoproteins (VLDL), which hampers the lipolysis of chylomicrons due to competition mainly at the level of lipoprotein lipase (LPL) with increased remnant TG being transported to the liver. Lipolysis is further impaired in obesity by reduced mRNA expression levels of LPL in adipose tissue and reduced LPL activity in skeletal muscle. Hypertriglyceridemia further induces an increased exchange of cholesterol esters (CE) and TG between VLDLs and high-density lipoproteins (HDLs) and low-density lipoproteins (LDLs) by cholesteryl ester-transfer-protein (CETP). This leads to decreased HDL cholesterol (HDLC) concentrations and a reduction in the TG content in LDLs. In addition, hepatic lipase (HL) removes TG and phospholipids from LDLs for the final formation of TG-depleted small dense LDLs. The intense yellow color represents cholesterol, whereas the light-yellow color represents the TG content within the different lipoproteins. Obesity-induced increases in metabolic processes are marked with green arrows, whereas reductions are marked with red arrows. Apo, apolipoprotein; IDL, intermediate-density lipoprotein. **Source:** Reprinted with permission from Klop et al. (2013).

and bone mass or quality (Batsis et al. 2017). Detailed instructions on weight-loss goals, how to estimate a patient's energy needs, and how to achieve energy restriction have been presented in Chapter 13.

Mr. KI is 37 years old and weighs 145.6 kg. Based on the Schofield equations for men aged 30–60 years old, his basal metabolic rate (BMR) is $11.472 \times 145.6 + 873.1 =$ *~2540 kcal. Given that he is sedentary, his BMR should be multiplied with a physical activity factor of 1.3, leading to a total*

energy expenditure of ~3300 kcal. A daily energy deficit of 1000 kcal would lead to a target daily energy intake of ~2300 kcal and achieve the desired weight loss for Mr. KI (~1 kg/week). A standard low-calorie diet providing 1500–1800 kcal/d can also be prescribed if there is a need to achieve the desired weight loss faster.

Dietary Modification

The important role of nutrition in the prevention of cardiovascular diseases has been extensively reviewed. It is well established that dietary factors influence cardiovascular risk either directly or through their action on traditional risk factors, such as plasma lipids, blood pressure, and glucose levels. Several modifications of diet macronutrient composition can have a favorable impact on blood lipid levels. These modifications, along with the magnitude of their impact on the various types of blood lipids, are summarized in Table 16.5 (Mach et al. 2020).

Most of the available data on the link between diet and dyslipidemia refer to the effects of fat quantity and quality on blood lipids. With regard to total fat quantity, a wide range of total fat intakes is acceptable for dyslipidemia and depends on individual preferences. However, fat intakes >40% of calories are generally associated with excess intakes of both saturated fat and calories, both being undesired in the case of a patient with dyslipidemia. Conversely, very low intakes of fats and oils increase the risk of inadequate intake of vitamin E and essential fatty acids and may contribute to a reduction of HDLC levels (Mensink et al. 2003; Schwingshackl et al. 2018; Sacks et al. 2017).

With regard to fat quality, trans fatty acids (TFAs) have been shown to negatively affect cardiovascular health, with every 1% energy coming from TFA resulting in a 0.8–1.6 mg/dl (0.02–0.04 mmol/l) increase in LDLC (Mensink et al. 2003; Schwingshackl et al. 2018). Natural TFA can be found in limited amounts in dairy products and in meats from ruminants; however, these types of TFA are not detrimental for health. On the other hand, TFAs are also formed during the partial hydrogenation of vegetable oils and can be found in processed foods, such as fast food, some types of margarines, baked goods, and salty snacks. Avoiding consumption of industrialized TFAs is crucial for the control of blood lipids and the prevention of cardiovascular diseases; this can be achieved through the adoption of a diet based on natural products.

As for SFA, i.e., fat present in dairy and meat products, recent data suggest that there is no robust evidence that a strict decrease in SFA intake can actually prevent cardiovascular diseases or reduce mortality (Astrup et al. 2020); therefore, a

TABLE 16.5   Impact of changes in macronutrient intake on blood lipid levels.

	Dietary interventions	Magnitude of the effect
Interventions to reduce TC and LDLC	Avoid dietary trans fats.	++
	Reduce dietary saturated fats.	+
	Increase dietary fiber.	++
	Reduce dietary cholesterol.	+
Interventions to reduce TG-rich lipoproteins	Reduce alcohol intake.	+++
	Reduce total amount of dietary carbohydrates.	+++
	Use supplements of n-3 polyunsaturated fats.	++
	Reduce intake of mono- and disaccharides.	++
	Replace saturated fats with mono- or polyunsaturated fats.	+
Interventions to increase HDLC	Avoid dietary trans fats.	++
	Reduce carbohydrates and replace with unsaturated fats.	++
	Modest consumption of alcohol in users may be continued.	+

+++ = >10%, ++ = 5–10%, + = <5%.
HDLC, high-density lipoprotein cholesterol; LDLC, low-density lipoprotein cholesterol; TC, total cholesterol; TG, triglycerides.
Source: Adapted with permission from Mach et al. (2020).

modest SFA intake in the context of a healthy diet is safe for the majority of patients with dyslipidemia. Fat intake should predominantly come from sources of unsaturated fatty acids, including monounsaturated fatty acids (MUFAs), especially from olive oil and nuts, and polyunsaturated fatty acids (PUFAs), especially omega-3 from fatty fish, although data are insufficient to make a recommendation regarding the optimal n-3:n-6 fatty acid ratio (Harris et al. 2009; Mozaffarian et al. 2013). In addition, cholesterol intake in the diet should be reduced (<300 mg/d), particularly in people with high TC/LDLC levels.

Dietary carbohydrates significantly affect blood lipids. Even though they may have a "neutral" effect on LDLC, high carbohydrate intake negatively affects plasma TG and HDLC levels. Total carbohydrate intake should range between 45% and 55% of total energy intake for patients with dyslipidemia, since both higher and lower percentages of carbohydrate diets are associated with increased mortality (Seidelmann et al. 2018). Dietary fiber (particularly the soluble type) – which is present in legumes, fruits, vegetables, and whole-grain cereals (e.g., oats and barley) – has a hypocholesterolemic effect and represents a good dietary substitute for SFA. Increased intake of fiber will maximize the effects of the diet on LDLC levels and will minimize the problematic effects of a high-carbohydrate diet on other lipoproteins. Therefore, a diet that provides 25–40 g/d of total dietary fiber, including ≥7–13 g of soluble fiber, is well tolerated, effective, and recommended for plasma lipid control.

There is no justification for recommending very-low-carbohydrate diets for the management of dyslipidemia (Dong et al, 2020). Intake of added sugars should not exceed 10% of total energy (in addition to the amount present in natural foods such as fruits); a more restrictive sugar intake may be useful for those with high plasma TG values or T2DM who want to lose weight. Excessive alcohol intake (i.e., >2 units of alcohol for men and >1 unit of alcohol for women/day) should be discouraged in all patients with

dyslipidemia as a means to lower LDLC levels. Moderate alcohol consumption (≤10 g/day [1 unit] for men and women) is acceptable for those who drink alcoholic beverages, if TG levels are not elevated, and has been associated with increases in HDLC. In the case of hypertriglyceridemia, alcohol consumption is best to be avoided.

Despite the well-established effect of macronutrient intake on blood lipids, evaluating the impact of a single dietary factor independently of any other changes in the diet is problematic. In fact, as foods are mixtures of different nutrients and other components that show strong synergistic or antagonistic effects, it is not appropriate to attribute the health effects of a food to only one of its components. Moreover, if total energy intake is kept constant, eating less of one macronutrient implies necessarily eating more of others, and the quality of the replacement can also influence the observed effect. All the aforementioned limitations warrant caution in interpreting the results of studies in relation to the effect of a single dietary change on cardiovascular risk.

In recent years, nutrition research and epidemiology has focused on the relationship between health/disease on the one hand and foods and dietary patterns – rather than single nutrients – on the other (Hodge and Bassett 2016; Hu 2002; Ocke 2013; Willett and McCullough 2008). Consistent evidence from epidemiological studies indicates that higher consumption of fruits, vegetables, nuts, legumes, fish, vegetable oils, yogurt, and whole grains, along with a lower intake of red and processed meats, foods higher in refined carbohydrates, and salt, is associated with a lower incidence of cardiovascular events (Mach et al. 2020; M. 2015.). In addition, the Prevencion con Dieta Mediterranea (PREDIMED) study, one of the few available randomized controlled clinical trials that aimed to assess the effects of diet on the primary prevention of cardiovascular disease, showed that a Mediterranean diet (with emphasis on olive oil, nuts, fresh fruits, vegetables, fish, legumes, white meat, and moderate consumption of wine with meals) supplemented with either olive oil or nuts was superior in improving the lipidemic profile and reducing cardiovascular disease risk, compared to a low-fat diet (Estruch et al. 2006). Optimal food choices for patients with dyslipidemia are presented in Table 16.6 (Mach et al. 2020).

The fact that specific nutrients have the ability to favorably affect blood lipids has also led the scientific community to investigate whether the supplementation of these nutrients or the consumption of novel types of food, enriched with these nutrients, can be part of the dietary management of dyslipidemia. So far three types of nutrients, namely, phytosterols, dietary fiber, and n-3 PUFA, have shown promising evidence for a lipid-lowering effect. In brief, daily consumption of 2 g of phytosterols can effectively lower TC and LDLC levels by 7–10% in humans (with a certain degree of heterogeneity among

TABLE 16.6   Food choices to improve the overall lipoprotein profile.

Food group	Preferred (frequent consumption)	Limited (moderate consumption)	Avoid (rare consumption)
Cereals	Whole grains	Refined bread, rice and pasta, biscuits, cornflakes	Pastries, muffins, pies, croissants
Vegetables	Raw and cooked vegetables	Potatoes	Vegetables prepared in butter or cream
Legumes	All		
Fruit	Fresh or frozen fruit	Dried fruit, jelly, jam, canned fruit, sorbets, ice popsicles, fruit juice	
Sweets and sweeteners	Non-caloric sweeteners (if caloric sweeteners cannot be reduced)	Sucrose, honey, chocolate, sweets/candies	Cakes, ice creams, fructose, soft drinks
Meat and fish	Lean and oily fish, poultry (consider removing skin), seafood, shellfish	Lean cuts of beef, lamb, pork, and veal	Sausages, salami, bacon, spare ribs, hot dogs, organ meats
Dairy food and eggs	Skimmed milk and yogurt	Low-fat milk, low-fat cheese and other milk products, eggs	Regular cheese, cream, whole milk, and yogurt
Fats and dressings	Olive oil, vinegar, mustard, fat-free dressings	Nontropical vegetable oils, soft margarines, salad dressing, mayonnaise, ketchup	Trans fats and hard margarines, palm and coconut oils, butter, lard, bacon fat
Nuts/seeds	All unsalted (except coconut)	All salted (except coconut)	Coconut
Cooking procedures	Grilling, boiling, steaming	Stir-frying, roasting	Frying

Source: Adapted with permission from Mach et al. (2020).

individuals), while it has little or no effect on HDLC and TG levels (Musa-Veloso et al. 2011). Based on their purported effect on LDLC lowering and the absence of adverse effects, functional foods with plant sterols/stanols (≥2 g/d with the main meal) may be considered: (i) in individuals with high cholesterol levels at intermediate or low global cardiovascular risk who do not qualify for pharmacotherapy; (ii) as an adjunct to pharmacological therapy in high- and very-high-risk patients who fail to achieve LDLC goals on statins or could not be treated with statins; and (iii) in adults and children (aged >6 years) with familiar hypercholesterolemia (Gylling et al. 2014). Available evidence also demonstrates that β-glucan, a viscous fiber from oat and barley, has a TC- and LDLC-lowering effect. Foods enriched with these fibers or supplements are well tolerated, effective, and are recommended for LDLC lowering (Hartley et al. 2016). However, the dosage needed to achieve a clinically relevant reduction in levels of LDLC of 3–5% varies from 3 to 10 g/day, depending on the specific type of fiber (Pirro et al. 2017). Last but not least, observational evidence indicates that consumption of fish (at least twice a week) and vegetable foods rich in n-3 PUFA (a-linoleic acid is present in walnuts, some vegetables, and some seed oils) is associated with lower risk of cardiovascular death and stroke but has no major effects on plasma lipoprotein metabolism (Mozaffarian et al. 2013; Sacks et al. 2017). Pharmacological doses of long-chain n-3 PUFA (2–3 g/day) have been shown to reduce TG levels by approximately 30% and reduce the post-prandial lipemic response, but a higher dosage may increase LDLC levels (Jacobson et al. 2012; Rivellese et al. 2003). In summary, the available evidence are not sufficient to conclusively link the intake of functional foods with clinically significant improvements in lipid metabolism and decreased cardiovascular risk.

According to Mr. KI's dietary assessment, individualized counseling toward a healthy diet for dyslipidemia management should focus on:

- *Minimize TFA intake to improve LDLC levels. Counseling toward the avoidance of processed food is crucial to minimize TFA intake. Emphasis must be given on limiting fast-food choices (e.g., pepperoni pizza with high fat cheece) and salty snacks (e.g., pretzels). Mr. KI should be motivated to eat*

> **Key Point**
>
> Daily consumption of 2 g of phytosterols can effectively lower TC and LDLC levels by 7–10%.

> **Key Point**
>
> β-glucan, a viscous fiber from oat and barley, has a TC- and LDLC-lowering effect.

> **Key Point**
>
> Pharmacological doses of long-chain n-3 PUFA (2–3 g/day) have been shown to reduce TG levels by about 30% and reduce the post-prandial lipemic response, but a higher dosage may increase LDLC levels.

home-cooked food at work (pack whatever is cooked at home to consume during his shift) or choose healthier fast-food choices, such as pizza with low fat cheece and vegetables or a whole-grain sandwich with chicken/tuna and vegetables.

- *Moderate SFA intake. Although SFA is not as detrimental as TFA for the lipidemic profile, modest consumption is recommended. Partial substitution of animal-based foods rich in SFA with other animal-based foods lower in SFA or plant-based foods can be helpful. Examples of substitutions include: (i) white meat without skin (chicken, turkey, rabbit), fish, legumes, and soy products instead of red meat (pork, veal, lamb) and cold cuts (ham, pepperoni, bacon); (ii) low-fat cheese (cottage, mozzarella, ricotta, feta) instead of high-fat cheese (parmesan, blue cheese, cheddar, Edam, Gouda, Emmental); (iii) vegetable oils (e.g., olive oil or sunflower oil) instead of butter and hard margarines; (iv) tomato sauce instead of milk cream and bechamel sauce.*

- *Decrease intake of simple carbohydrates to improve TG levels and promote weight loss. Moderation in sugar intake; this can be achieved through a reduction in the amount of sugar added in coffee (1 teaspoon instead of 1 tablespoon of sugar in each cup of coffee) or through the substitution of sugar with noncaloric sweeteners, such as aspartame, saccharin, sucralose, and stevia. Moderation in the consumption of sweets is also recommended. Given his daily consumption, a realistic goal would be to gradually reduce the frequency of desserts to 2–3 portions/week and consume smaller portions. Other less energy-dense and lower-sugar sweet choices could be considered, such as sweets based on milk and yogurt, nuts with honey, smoothies with fresh fruits, and milk/yogurt, etc.*

- *Increase dietary fiber intake. Increase in the consumption of plant-based fiber-rich foods, such as fruits (one fruit/day and gradual increase to two to three fruits/day with emphasis on a variety of fresh, whole, seasonal fruits), vegetables (a seasonal salad accompanying lunch and dinner with emphasis on a variety of fresh seasonal raw/cooked vegetables), whole grains (such as whole-grain pasta) instead of refines ones, and legumes (one meal/week and gradual increase to two meals/week instead of red-meat-based meals or fast food).*

- *Portion control to achieve a 5–10% weight loss. Mr. KI has two big meals/day (lunch and dinner), one at home and one at work. Restriction of his typical portion size could create a significant energy deficit. Ways to achieve this portion decrease include the consumption of an abundant portion of seasonal salad, which is rich in dietary fiber and contributes to satiety, or choosing a healthier, less-energy-dense choice, such as a lean protein meal (chicken or fish). The limitation of nibbling throughout the day, especially at work during night shifts, is also important to establish an energy deficit; this can be achieved through education on the correct identification of hunger and satiety, and through the consumption of low-calorie snacks when the urge for food consumption cannot be avoided (such as fruits, whole-grain rusks, low-fat dairy products, a healthy sandwich choice, etc.)*

Physical Activity Modification

Physical activity is an integral part of a healthy lifestyle, and available evidence suggests that both aerobic exercise and resistance training are effective in improving blood lipid levels (Mann et al. 2014; Tambalis et al. 2009). Aerobic training is probably the best type of exercise for the management of dyslipidemia. A meta-analysis of 51 clinical trials involving 12 weeks or more of moderate- to high-intensity aerobic training found significant positive effects in lipid profile (Leon and Sanchez 2001). On average, aerobic exercise interventions achieved a 5% increase in HDLC, a 4% decrease in TG levels, and a 5% decrease in LDLC levels. The most commonly observed change was an increase in HDLC, while reductions in TC, LDLC, and TG were less frequently observed and were evident mostly after exercise interventions of high intensity. In addition, TC remained unchanged, although the HDLC : LDLC ratio improved considerably.

Available evidence suggests that HDLC is the component of the lipidemic profile that is most likely to improve as a result of aerobic exercise (Mann et al. 2014; Tambalis et al. 2009). Although lowering LDLC is the fundamental goal for patients with dyslipidemia, an increase in HDLC can have a positive impact on atherosclerosis and total cardiovascular risk via HDLC-facilitated removal of LDLC. However, to directly reduce LDLC and TG levels, the intensity of aerobic exercise must be relatively high, something that may not be possible in individuals with a limited exercise capacity or other risk factors (Mann et al. 2014; Tambalis et al. 2009). In this context, although resistance training has been associated with smaller improvements in blood lipids compared to aerobic exercise, it may be more appropriate for less mobile groups or to provide an alternative to aerobic training when high intensity cannot be achieved. The combination of the two types of exercise has been explored only in a few studies and has been shown to be effective in lowering LDLC and increasing HDLC (Mann et al. 2014; Tambalis et al. 2009).

All things considered, available data suggest that individuals with dyslipidemia should increase physical activity to >30 minutes/day, 5 times/week. The recommended mode of exercise is a combination of moderate-intensity aerobic

>
> **Key Point**
>
> Aerobic training is probably the best type of exercise for the management of dyslipidemia.

> **Key Point**
>
> To directly reduce LDLC and TG levels, the intensity of aerobic exercise must be relatively high.

> **Key Point**
>
> Although resistance training has been associated with smaller improvements in blood lipids compared to aerobic exercise, it may be more appropriate for less mobile groups or to provide an alternative to aerobic training when high intensity cannot be achieved.

exercise at 70–80% of heart rate max (gradually increased to 85% heart rate max), combined with moderate- to high-intensity resistance training at 75–85% of one repetition maximum (Mann et al. 2014).

According to Mr. KI's physical activity assessment, key points for individualized counseling toward a physically active lifestyle include:

- *Mr. KI was sedentary at the time of evaluation. Encouragement to adopt a physically active lifestyle with a gradual increase in physical activity level to achieve at least 30 minutes of moderate-intensity aerobic exercise on 5–7 days/week is recommended to improve blood lipids. Examples of advice toward this goal include:*
  - *A 15-minute daily walking routine on any hour of the day, depending on his work schedule. Provided that Mr. KI will lose weight and improve his lifestyle, his aerobic capacity is expected to gradually increase and be sufficient to support even longer exercise durations, e.g., a 30-minute daily walking.*
  - *Using stairs instead of elevators whenever possible.*
  - *Walking instead of driving for daily activities, such as shopping.*
  - *Group outdoor activities with family and friends that involve convivial aerobic exercise during weekends.*
  - *Physical activity level should increase gradually in terms of exercise duration and intensity to avoid injuries associated with obesity.*
- *Mr. KI currently has a limited capacity for aerobic training. Resistance exercise can be recommended as an alternative to aerobic exercise until weight loss is achieved and his mobility and functionality are improved. Examples of simple resistance exercises include arm swings, seated reverse fly, seated chest press, triceps extension, toe pointing and flexion, toe raise, calf raise, leg extension, hip flexion, hip extension, and chair rise.*

Sleep Modification

Although sleep deprivation and low sleep quality have not emerged as strong predictors of blood lipid disorders, their detrimental effect on mortality and the risk of T2DM, cardiovascular disease, and obesity are well-established (Itani et al. 2017; Jike et al. 2018). Given that patients with dyslipidemia are prone to cardiovascular diseases associated with atherosclerosis, sleep of adequate duration (7–9 hours/day) and quality is an important part of the overall management

plan to lower cardiovascular risk. In addition, accumulated data suggest that a link exists between blood lipid disorders and obstructive sleep apnea (OSA), a sleep disorder mostly evident among obese individuals and characterized by pauses of breathing during sleep. Although a clear causal relationship is yet to be established, there is increasing evidence that chronic intermittent hypoxia, a major component of OSA, may be the root cause of the dyslipidemia. Potential mechanisms for this effect include the generation of reactive oxygen species, peroxidation of lipids, and sympathetic system dysfunction (Adedayo et al. 2014). In this context, management of sleep disorders is important for blood lipid control and cardiovascular health.

According to Mr. KI's assessment, counseling toward the improvement of sleep habits should focus on the following:

- *Given his high risk for OSA, Mr. KI should be referred to a sleep specialist for diagnostic sleep testing and management.*
- *Mr. KI has a rotating shift work schedule. Maintaining a steady sleep schedule is not feasible; however, he should be encouraged to gradually increase his daily sleep duration to 7–9 hours as recommended for adults.*
- *Mr. KI should be educated on sleep hygiene techniques to promote sleep quality, such as avoiding long midday naps, avoiding stimulants, e.g., caffeine, 4–6 hours before bedtime, a short (10-minute) interval of light aerobic exercise before sleep, and avoidance of foods that can trigger indigestion and gastrointestinal symptoms before sleep.*

Stress Modification

Stress has been proposed as a potential causal factor for development of dyslipidemia. Stress increases the mobiliization of lipids, glucose, and proteins and their availabilty to the various tissues and organs of the body to help maintain homeostasis and adapt to the stressor. Therefore, the increase in blood lipids induced by stress should normally return to normal levels when the stressor ends. However, when the stressor is maintained over a long period, i.e., in the case of chronic psychological stress, dyslipidemia persists and may have deleterious effects, contributing to the development of insulin resistance and atherosclerosis. Results of epidemiological studies suggest that high levels of stress, as a result of a variety of stressful events, such as loss of job and income, a period of high workload, emotional problems, or traumatizing catastrophic events, are associated with blood lipid disorders (Marcondes et al. 2012). Although the exact mechanisms are not clear, stress-induced dyslipidemia is believed to be the result of complex interactions between stress hormones, insulin, adipose tissue metabolism and cytokines, and of the impact of stress on other lifestyle habits and practices (e.g., high stress has been linked to sedentariness, sleep disorders, emotional eating, and consumption of energy-dense foods rich in TFA, SFA, and sugars) (Marcondes et al. 2012).

Mr. KI does not currently show/report any signs or symptoms of severe stress. Keeping his stress levels low is important for the management of dyslipidemia. Other goals of the intervention plan – such as increasing physical activity level, improving sleep quality, and managing sleep-disordered breathing – are also expected to offer protection against stress.

Take-Home Messages

- Lipoproteins play a significant role in atherosclerosis, a condition in which plaque builds up inside the arteries and causes their hardening and narrowing.
- ApoB-containing lipoproteins, i.e., VLDL, IDL, and LDL, are strong determinants of the initiation and progression of atherosclerosis.
- In clinical practice, the concentration of plasma lipoproteins is not usually measured directly but is estimated by measuring their cholesterol content.
- Lowering LDLC levels is the fundamental goal for a patient with dyslipidemia to lower cardiovascular risk. Secondary goals include an increase in HDLC and a decrease in TG.
- Management of dyslipidemia involves lifestyle interventions and drug treatment. Lifestyle interventions represent the first-choice therapy for all patients, since blood lipid disorders are mostly attributed to increased body weight and an unhealthy lifestyle.
- Even a modest decrease in body weight (5–10%) improves lipid abnormalities and favorably affects all other cardiovascular risk factors, often present in dyslipidemic individuals.
- For most patients with dyslipidemia, a wide range of total fat intakes is acceptable and will depend on individual preferences and characteristics.
- The quality of dietary fat is more important than the quantity. TFAs are detrimental for cardiovascular health and should be avoided. Fat intake should predominantly come from sources of unsaturated fatty acids, including n-6 and n-3 PUFA.
- Dietary fiber (particularly of the soluble type), present in high quantities in legumes, fruits, vegetables, and whole-grain cereals (e.g., oats and barley), has a hypocholesterolemic effect.
- Sugars should be avoided in all individuals with high TG levels.
- Excess alcohol intake (i.e., >2 units of alcohol for men and >1 unit of alcohol for women/day) should be discouraged in all patients with dyslipidemia as a means to lower LDLC levels. Patients with hypertriglyceridemia should limit alcohol intake to less than 2–3 drinks/week.
- Higher consumption of fruits, nonstarchy vegetables, nuts, legumes, fish, vegetable oils, yogurt, and whole grains, along with a lower intake of red and processed meats, salt, and foods higher in refined carbohydrates, is associated with a lower incidence of cardiovascular events and is the optimal diet pattern for dyslipidemic patients.
- Phytosterols, dietary fiber, and n-3 PUFA have a promising lipid-lowering effect, and their supplementation can be used as an adjunctive intervention for blood lipid control.
- Aerobic exercise and resistance training are efficient in improving blood lipid levels through various modes, frequencies, intensities, and durations of exercise.
- HDLC is most likely to improve as the result of aerobic exercise. To directly reduce LDLC and TG levels, the intensity of aerobic exercise must be high.
- Resistance training may be a more appropriate type of exercise for less mobile dyslipidemic individuals or to provide an alternative to aerobic training when high intensity cannot be achieved due to poor fitness or comorbidities.
- Given that patients with dyslipidemia are prone to atherosclerosis-related cardiovascular diseases, counseling toward an adequate sleep duration and quality is an important part of the overall management plan to lower total cardiovascular risk.

Self-Assessment Questions

1. Provide the definition and outline the main types of dyslipidemia.
2. Which of the following statements are true for the link between dietary fat and dyslipidemia?
   a. A fat intake >30% of total daily energy intake is associated with weight gain, insulin resistance, and blood lipid disorders.
   b. Pharmacological doses of long-chain n-3 PUFA (2–3 g/d) have been shown to reduce LDLC levels and increase HDLC levels.
   c. TFAs have been shown to negatively affect LDLC levels and cardiovascular health.
   d. Low-fat diets (<20% of total calories) are the best dietary approach for the management of dyslipidemia.
   e. A modest SFA intake in the context of a healthy diet is safe for the majority of patients with dyslipidemia.
3. Discuss the association between lipoproteins and atherosclerosis.
4. What is the main treatment goal for a patient with dyslipidemia?
   a. lowering HDLC
   b. lowering TG
   c. increasing HDLC
   d. lowering LDLC
   e. lowering TC
5. Provide an overview of cholesterol metabolism in the human body.
6. Hyperlipidemia refers to:
   a. increased TC or LDLC levels
   b. increased TG levels
   c. increased TG and HDLC levels
   d. increased TC and decreased HDLC levels
   e. all of the above
7. How is obstructive sleep apnea related to dyslipidemia?
8. Characterize the following statements as true (T) or false (F).
   a. HDLC is the component of the lipidemic profile that is most likely to improve as a result of aerobic exercise ( ).
   b. Lipids are important for the body because they are its sole energy substrate ( ).
   c. Resistance training has been associated with greater improvements in blood lipids compared to aerobic exercise ( ).
   d. Chronic intermittent hypoxia, a major component of OSA, is independently associated with dyslipidemia ( ).
   e. Weight loss is associated with decreases in HDLC and should be discouraged in dyslipidemic patients ( ).
9. What advice would you give to a dyslipidemic patient about the quality of dietary fat?
10. How is stress related to dyslipidemia?
11. How can weight loss contribute to the management of dyslipidemia?
12. Which of the following strategies can increase HDLC levels?
    a. decrease in dietary cholesterol
    b. supplementation of omega-3 fatty acids
    c. reduction in simple carbohydrates and replacement with unsaturated fats
    d. decrease in SFA intake
    e. modest consumption of alcohol in users
    f. aerobic exercise
    g. all of the above
13. Characterize the following statements as true (T) or false (F).
    a. Increasing dietary fiber intake can lead to increases in HDLC levels ( ).
    b. Management of sleep disorders is important for blood lipid control and cardiovascular protection ( ).
    c. β-glucan, a fiber from oat and barley, has a TC- and LDLC-lowering effect ( ).
    d. Sugars should be avoided in individuals with high TG levels ( ).
    e. Moderate alcohol consumption (≤10 g/d) has been associated with significant improvements in TG levels ( ).
14. A 42-year-old female patient with a 3-year diagnosis of T2DM and no other cardiovascular disease risk factors visits your office. What is the LDLC goal for this patient?
15. Which of the following foods should be avoided by a dyslipidemic patient?
    a. coconut oil
    b. pasta and rice
    c. olive oil
    d. boiled potatoes
    e. hard margarines
    f. all of the above
16. Functional foods with plant sterols may be considered:
    a. for patients with low HDLC levels
    b. for individuals with high cholesterol levels at intermediate or low global cardiovascular risk who do not qualify for pharmacotherapy
    c. as the sole treatment for adults and children (aged > 6 years) with familiar hypercholesterolemia
    d. as an adjunct to pharmacological therapy for high- and very-high-risk patients who fail to achieve LDLC goals on statins
    e. for patients with severe hypertriglyceridemia who cannot reduce alcohol intake
17. What are the main treatment targets and goals for cardiovascular disease prevention in patients with dyslipidemia?
18. Which of the following statements about LDLC are true?
    a. Lowering LDLC levels is the fundamental goal for a patient with dyslipidemia to lower cardiovascular risk.
    b. For every 1 kg decrease in body weight, there is an ~10 mg/dl decrease in LDLC.
    c. The higher the cardiovascular risk of a patient, the stricter the target for LDLC levels.
    d. A high-protein diet can lower LDLC levels.
    e. Isolated increases in LDLC levels are called hyperlipoproteinemia.
19. Characterize the following statements as true (T) or false (F).
    a. Dietary cholesterol intake should be reduced to <150 mg/d in patients with high TC/LDLC levels ( ).
    b. The quantity of circulating lipoproteins and the degree of lipid-oxidation greatly influence the rate

and extent of atherosclerosis and endothelial damage ( ).

c. An increase in HDLC can have a positive impact on atherosclerosis and total cardiovascular risk via HDLC-facilitated removal of LDLC ( ).

d. Boiling and steaming is preferrable to frying for dyslipidemia management ( ).

e. Very-low-carbohydrate diets (<40% of total calories) are recommended for patients with increased TG levels ( ).

20. A patient's fasting blood work revealed the following: TC 282 mg/dl, HDLC 54 mg/dl, and TG 168 mg/dl. Calculate the patient's LDLC levels.

Bibliography

Adedayo, A.M., Olafiranye, O., Smith, D. et al. (2014). Obstructive sleep apnea and dyslipidemia: evidence and underlying mechanism. *Sleep Breath.* 18 (1): 13–18. https://doi.org/10.1007/s11325-012-0760-9.

Astrup, A., Magkos, F., Bier, D.M. et al. (2020). Saturated fats and health: a reassessment and proposal for food-based recommendations: JACC state-of-the-art review. *J. Am. Coll. Cardiol.* 76 (7): 844–857. https://doi.org/10.1016/j.jacc.2020.05.077.

Batsis, J.A., Gill, L.E., Masutani, R.K. et al. (2017). Weight loss interventions in older adults with obesity: a systematic review of randomized controlled trials since 2005. *J. Am. Geriatr. Soc.* 65 (2): 257–268. https://doi.org/10.1111/jgs.14514.

Brown, L., Rosner, B., Willett, W.W., and Sacks, F.M. (1999). Cholesterol-lowering effects of dietary fiber: a meta-analysis. *Am. J. Clin. Nutr.* 69 (1): 30–42. https://doi.org/10.1093/ajcn/69.1.30.

Brown, W.V., Sacks, F.M., and Sniderman, A.D. (2015). JCL roundtable: apolipoproteins as causative elements in vascular disease. *J. Clin. Lipidol.* 9 (6): 733–740. doi: 10.1016/j.jacl.2015.10.003.

Dattilo, A.M. and Kris-Etherton, P.M. (1992). Effects of weight reduction on blood lipids and lipoproteins: a meta-analysis. *Am. J. Clin. Nutr.* 56 (2): 320–328. https://doi.org/10.1093/ajcn/56.2.320.

Estruch, R., Martinez-Gonzalez, M.A., Corella, D. et al. (2006). Effects of a Mediterranean-style diet on cardiovascular risk factors: a randomized trial. *Ann. Intern. Med.* 145 (1): 1–11. https://doi.org/10.7326/0003-4819-145-1-200607040-00004.

Friedewald, W.T., Levy, R.I., and Fredrickson, D.S. (1972). Estimation of the concentration of low-density lipoprotein cholesterol in plasma, without use of the preparative ultracentrifuge. *Clin. Chem.* 18 (6): 499–502.

Gylling, H., Plat, J., Turley, S. et al. (2014). Plant sterols and plant stanols in the management of dyslipidemia and prevention of cardiovascular disease. *Atherosclerosis* 232 (2): 346–360. https://doi.org/10.1016/j.atherosclerosis.2013.11.043.

Harris, W.S., Mozaffarian, D., Rimm, E. et al. (2009). Omega-6 fatty acids and risk for cardiovascular disease: a science advisory from the American Heart Association Nutrition Subcommittee of the Council on Nutrition, Physical Activity, and Metabolism; Council on Cardiovascular Nursing; and Council on Epidemiology and Prevention. *Circulation* 119 (6): 902–907. https://doi.org/10.1161/CIRCULATIONAHA.108.191627.

Hartley, L., May, M.D., Loveman, E. et al. (2016). Dietary fibre for the primary prevention of cardiovascular disease. *Cochrane Database Syst. Rev.* (1): CD011472. https://doi.org/10.1002/14651858.CD011472.pub2.

Hodge, A. and Bassett, J. (2016). What can we learn from dietary pattern analysis? *Public Health Nutr.* 19 (2): 191–194. https://doi.org/10.1017/S1368980015003730.

Hu, F.B. (2002). Dietary pattern analysis: a new direction in nutritional epidemiology. *Curr. Opin. Lipidol.* 13 (1): 3–9.

Itani, O., Jike, M., Watanabe, N., and Kaneita, Y. (2017). Short sleep duration and health outcomes: a systematic review, meta-analysis, and meta-regression. *Sleep Med.* 32: 246–256. https://doi.org/10.1016/j.sleep.2016.08.006.

Jacobson, T.A., Glickstein, S.B., Rowe, J.D., and Soni, P.N. (2012). Effects of eicosapentaenoic acid and docosahexaenoic acid on low-density lipoprotein cholesterol and other lipids: a review. *J. Clin. Lipidol.* 6 (1): 5–18. https://doi.org/10.1016/j.jacl.2011.10.018.

Jellinger, P.S., Handelsman, Y., Rosenblit, P.D. et al. (2017). American Association of Clinical Endocrinologists and American College of Endocrinology guidelines for management of dyslipidemia and prevention of cardiovascular disease. *Endocr. Pract.* 23 (Suppl 2): 1–87. https://doi.org/10.4158/EP171764.APPGL.

Jike, M., Itani, O., Watanabe, N. et al. (2018). Long sleep duration and health outcomes: a systematic review, meta-analysis and meta-regression. *Sleep Med. Rev.* 39: 25–36. https://doi.org/10.1016/j.smrv.2017.06.011.

Klop, B., Elte, J.W., and Cabezas, M.C. (2013). Dyslipidemia in obesity: mechanisms and potential targets. *Nutrients* 5 (4): 1218–1240. https://doi.org/10.3390/nu5041218.

Leon, A.S. and Sanchez, O.A. (2001). Response of blood lipids to exercise training alone or combined with dietary intervention. *Med. Sci. Sports Exerc.* 33 (6 Suppl): S502–S515; discussion S28-9. https://doi.org/10.1097/00005768-200106001-00021.

Libby, P. (2002). Inflammation in atherosclerosis. *Nature* 420 (6917): 868–874. https://doi.org/10.1038/nature01323.

M. (2015). Food consumption and its impact on cardiovascular disease: importance of solutions focused on the globalized food system: a report from the workshop convened by the World Heart Federation. *J. Am. Coll. Cardiol.* 66 (14): 1590–1614. doi: 10.1016/j.jacc.2015.07.050.

Mach, F., Baigent, C., Catapano, A.L. et al. (2020). 2019 ESC/EAS guidelines for the management of dyslipidemias: lipid modification to reduce cardiovascular risk. *Eur. Heart J.* 41 (1): 111–188. https://doi.org/10.1093/eurheartj/ehz455.

Mann, S., Beedie, C., and Jimenez, A. (2014). Differential effects of aerobic exercise, resistance training and combined exercise modalities on cholesterol and the lipid profile: review, synthesis and recommendations. *Sports Med.* 44 (2): 211–221. https://doi.org/10.1007/s40279-013-0110-5.

Marcondes, F., Neves, V., Costa, R., Sanches, A., Cunha, T., Moura, M. et al. (2012). Dyslipidemia induced by stress. www.intechopen.com/books/dyslipidemia-from-prevention-to-treatment/dyslipidemia-induced-by-stress.

Mensink, R.P., Zock, P.L., Kester, A.D., and Katan, M.B. (2003). Effects of dietary fatty acids and carbohydrates on the ratio of serum total to HDL cholesterol and on serum lipids and apolipoproteins: a meta-analysis of 60 controlled trials. *Am. J. Clin. Nutr.* 77 (5): 1146–1155. https://doi.org/10.1093/ajcn/77.5.1146.

Mozaffarian, D., Lemaitre, R.N., King, I.B. et al. (2013). Plasma phospholipid long-chain omega-3 fatty acids and total and cause-specific mortality in older adults: a cohort study. *Ann. Intern. Med.* 158(7):515–525.https://doi.org/10.7326/0003-4819-158-7-201304020-00003.

Musa-Veloso, K., Poon, T.H., Elliot, J.A., and Chung, C. (2011). A comparison of the LDL-cholesterol lowering efficacy of plant stanols and plant sterols over a continuous dose range: results of a meta-analysis of randomized, placebo-controlled trials. *Prostaglandins Leukot. Essent. Fatty Acids* 85 (1): 9–28. https://doi.org/10.1016/j.plefa.2011.02.001.

Ocke, M.C. (2013). Evaluation of methodologies for assessing the overall diet: dietary quality scores and dietary pattern analysis. *Proc. Nutr. Soc.* 72 (2): 191–199. https://doi.org/10.1017/S0029665113000013.

Pirro, M., Vetrani, C., Bianchi, C. et al. (2017). Joint position statement on "nutraceuticals for the treatment of hypercholesterolemia" of the Italian Society of Diabetology (SID) and of the Italian Society for the Study of Arteriosclerosis (SISA). *Nutr. Metab. Cardiovasc. Dis.* 27 (1): 2–17. https://doi.org/10.1016/j.numecd.2016.11.122.

Dong T, Guo M, Zhang P, Sun G, Chen B (2020) The effects of low-carbohydrate diets on cardiovascular risk factors: A meta-analysis. PLoS ONE 15(1): e0225348. https://doi.org/10.1371/journal.pone.0225348.

Rivellese, A.A., Maffettone, A., Vessby, B. et al. (2003). Effects of dietary saturated, monounsaturated and n-3 fatty acids on fasting lipoproteins, LDL size and post-prandial lipid metabolism in healthy subjects. *Atherosclerosis* 167 (1): 149–158. https://doi.org/10.1016/s0021-9150(02)00424-0.

Rodriguez, A., Trigatti, B.L., Mineo, C., Knaack, D., Wilkins, J.T., Sahoo, D. et al. (2019). Proceedings of the Ninth HDL (High-Density Lipoprotein) Workshop: Focus on Cardiovascular Disease. *Arterioscler. Thromb. Vasc. Biol.* 39 (12): 2457–2467. doi: 10.1161/ATVBAHA.119.313340.

Rosenson, R.S., Brewer, H.B., Jr., Barter, P.J., Bjorkegren, J.L.M., Chapman, M.J., Gaudet, D. et al. (2018). HDL and atherosclerotic cardiovascular disease: genetic insights into complex biology. *Nat. Rev. Cardiol.* 15 (1): 9–19. doi: 10.1038/nrcardio.2017.11.

Sacks, F.M., Lichtenstein, A.H., Wu, J.H.Y. et al. (2017). Dietary fats and cardiovascular disease: a presidential advisory from the American Heart Association. *Circulation* 136 (3): e1–e23. https://doi.org/10.1161/CIR.0000000000000510.

Sacks, F.M., Lichtenstein, A.H., Wu, J.H.Y., Appel, L.J., Creager, M.A., Kris-Etherton, P.M. et al. (2017). Dietary fats and cardiovascular disease: a presidential advisory from the American Heart Association. *Circulation* 136 (3): e1–e23. doi: 10.1161/CIR.0000000000000510.

Schwingshackl, L., Bogensberger, B., Bencic, A. et al. (2018). Effects of oils and solid fats on blood lipids: a systematic review and network meta-analysis. *J. Lipid Res.* 59 (9): 1771–1782. https://doi.org/10.1194/jlr.P085522.

Seidelmann, S.B., Claggett, B., Cheng, S. et al. (2018). Dietary carbohydrate intake and mortality: a prospective cohort study and meta-analysis. *Lancet Public Health* 3 (9): e419–e428. https://doi.org/10.1016/S2468-2667(18)30135-X.

Tambalis, K., Panagiotakos, D.B., Kavouras, S.A., and Sidossis, L.S. (2009). Responses of blood lipids to aerobic, resistance, and combined aerobic with resistance exercise training: a systematic review of current evidence. *Angiology* 60 (5): 614–632. https://doi.org/10.1177/0003319708324927.

Willett, W.C. and McCullough, M.L. (2008). Dietary pattern analysis for the evaluation of dietary guidelines. *Asia Pac. J. Clin. Nutr.* 17 (Suppl 1): 75–78.

Zomer, E., Gurusamy, K., Leach, R. et al. (2016). Interventions that cause weight loss and the impact on cardiovascular risk factors: a systematic review and meta-analysis. *Obes. Rev.* 17 (10): 1001–1011. https://doi.org/10.1111/obr.12433.

Appendix A

Answers to Self-Assessment Questions

Chapter 1

1. Early definitions conceptualized health primarily as the absence of disease. The World Health Organization was the first to introduce a more holistic definition of health in 1948: "Health is a state of complete physical, mental and social well-being and not merely the absence of disease or infirmity." This more holistic concept, suggesting that health has a positive component, instead of just the absence of a negative one, i.e., illness, gradually led to the use of other terms, such as wellness and well-being.
2. Wellness is an active process through which people become aware of, and make choices toward, a more successful existence.
3. Physical, occupational, social, intellectual, spiritual, and emotional wellness.
4. e
5. b
6. Many unhealthy lifestyle choices, such as poor diet, physical inactivity, tobacco use, excessive alcohol intake, and excessive stress have been associated with the development of many chronic diseases.
7. Lifestyle medicine is the use of a whole food, plant-predominant dietary lifestyle, regular physical activity, restorative sleep, stress management, avoidance of risky substances, and positive social connection as the primary therapy for chronic diseases.

Chapter 2

1. There are four types of NCDs: cardiovascular diseases (i.e., heart attack and stroke), cancers, chronic respiratory diseases (i.e., chronic obstructive pulmonary disease and asthma), and diabetes.
2. Obesity leads to adverse metabolic effects, such as increases in blood pressure, dyslipidemia (abnormal blood lipids), and insulin resistance. The risk of coronary heart disease, ischemic stroke, and T2DM increases with increasing body mass index. Obesity has also been associated with several types of cancer, namely, breast, colon, prostate, endometrium, kidney, and gall bladder cancer. Furthermore, overall mortality rates seem to be higher among obese individuals compared to those with a healthy body weight.

3. Obesity is the consequence of a long-term energy imbalance, whereby energy intake is higher than energy expenditure. A dramatic change in the way people consume food and exercise has been recorded during the past decades. Worldwide, there is an increase in the consumption of energy-dense foods and simple sugars. At the same time, physical activity has decreased, due to the sedentary character of the working environment, changes in transportation, and urbanization. Moreover, short sleep duration has been associated with an increased risk for developing obesity, possibly due to its impact on hormones that can increase hunger and food intake. Chronic stress and associated increases in the glucocorticoid stress hormone cortisol may also play a role in the development of obesity by increasing the appetite with a preference for energy-dense foods ("comfort food").
4. b
5. a, e, and f
6. c
7. T2DM is a chronic metabolic disease characterized by inefficient use of insulin from the body. T2DM development and progression is affected by both genetic and environmental factors; exposure to an obesogenic environment characterized by sedentary behavior, high levels of stress, excessive energy consumption, and unhealthy dietary habits can trigger the onset of T2DM in genetically susceptible individuals.
8. f
9. a, c, and e
10. CVDs can be attributed to a number of modifiable risk factors such as poor eating habits, physical inactivity, tobacco smoking, obesity, hypertension, dyslipidemia, diabetes, and alcohol consumption.
11. The major risk factors for cancer onset include tobacco use, increased alcohol intake, unhealthy body weight, physical inactivity, and infections.
12. b, d, and e

Chapter 3

1. b
2. a) PUFA and MUFA
   b) with whole grains
   c) no increase or even a benefit
   d) trans fatty acids
   e) little or no positive
   f) Quitting
   g) 50–55%
3. According to the 2015–2020 dietary guidelines for Americans, the adequate daily intake of fiber is 14 g per 1000 kcals, or approximately 25 g/d for women and 38 g/d for men.

Textbook of Lifestyle Medicine, First Edition. Labros S. Sidossis and Stefanos N. Kales.
© 2022 John Wiley & Sons Ltd. Published 2022 by John Wiley & Sons Ltd.

4. The World Cancer Research Fund recommends no more than three portions of red meat per week, which is equivalent to no more that 350–500 g cooked weight (or 525–750 g raw weight), and reduce consumption of processed meats to the minimum.

5. b

6. Adults should perform at least 150 minutes of moderate-intensity aerobic physical activity per week, or at least 75 minutes of vigorous-intensity aerobic physical activity throughout the week, or an equivalent combination of moderate- and vigorous-intensity activity.

7. f

8. Binge drinking is defined as ≥4 drinks for women and ≥5 drinks for men within 2 hours. Heavy drinking is defined as ≥8 drinks a week for women and ≥15 drinks a week for men, with an alcoholic drink-equivalent defined as 14 g (0.6 fl oz) of pure alcohol.

9. Stress can trigger an inflammatory response in the circulatory system, mainly in the coronary arteries, which is thought to be one of the mechanisms underlying the development of CVD.

10. The term *epigenetic mechanisms* refers to the parameters involved in the modifications of gene regulation, including DNA methylation, histone modifications, and RNA-based mechanisms.

11. Decreasing SFA intake to improve blood lipids and reduce cardiovascular risk has long been recommended by health organizations. However, accumulated research over the years has failed to support a definite detrimental effect of SFA on human health. Therefore, consuming a moderate amount of SFA in the context of a balanced diet is safe for most people. For those who overconsume SFAs, their partial substitution with omega-3 PUFAs, MUFAs, or dietary fiber can reduce CVD risk and should be encouraged.

12. The underlying mechanism by which TFAs increase CVD risk is probably related to changes in lipoprotein profile. Even moderate levels of TFA intake may lead to increased LDL concentrations, while HDL concentration usually decreases. Moreover, consumption of TFAs can increase CVD risk by increasing inflammation and endothelial dysfunction.

13. e

14. a) 20–30%
    b) Smoking
    c) Overweight
    d) Industrially produced, naturally occurring
    e) Animal, plant

15. a, c, and e

Chapter 4

1. e

2. The main characteristics of a healthy lifestyle include following a healthy diet, being physically active, maintaining a healthy weight, not smoking, not drinking excess amounts of alcohol, controlling stress, and resting adequately.

3. The quality of the diet may vary greatly, depending on dietary preferences, cultural habits, food preferences, food availability, and accessibility.

4. Physical activity is defined as any bodily movement produced by skeletal muscles that requires energy expenditure. Physical activity refers to all movement including sports or planned exercise, transportation, leisure time physical activity (like dancing), occupational (i.e., manual labor), household chores, play, games, in the context of daily, family, and community activities.

5. Alcohol causes cancer through four ways: (i) damages cells; (ii) augments the damage caused from tobacco use; (iii) affects hormones linked to breast cancer; and (iv) breaks down into cancer-causing chemicals.

6. When examining the effect of alcohol consumption with ischemic heart disease risk, the relationship follows a J-curve. This means that people who regularly consume low-to-moderate amounts of alcohol exhibit a lower risk of ischemic heart attack compared to those who do not drink. However, above this low-to-moderate alcohol consumption, the risk of ischemic heart disease rises, and excess alcohol consumption should be avoided.

7. Sleep is not just a simple absence of wakefulness. It is considered a physiologically active state in which specific processes and metabolic pathways occur that are essential for the regulation of daytime functioning and well-being. The amount and quality of sleep may significantly affect health. For example, inadequate sleep is detrimental to the process of learning and memory stabilization. Both insufficient and prolonged sleep is associated with increased risk for developing metabolic syndrome and other chronic diseases.

8. b and c

Chapter 5

1. c

2. a

3. There are two types of beriberi: wet beriberi, which affects the cardiovascular system, and dry beriberi, which affects the nervous system. Lack of thiamin (vitamin B$_1$) is considered the cause of beriberi.

4. a

5. Food components interact into the food matrix in which they are found, developing either additive or antagonistic effects on human metabolism and, by extension, on human health. This combined effect is defined as "food synergy" and "food antagonism," respectively. Therefore, assessing the impact of whole foods and food groups on health and disease is a preferable approach, compared to evaluating the effects of single nutrients.

6. Eggs were considered a risk factor for the development of CVD in the past due to their high cholesterol content. Today, it is well established that dietary cholesterol intake can only slightly affect cardiovascular risk, since most cholesterol in the human body is produced by the liver. Indeed, the effect of egg consumption, up to seven/week, on blood cholesterol is minimal when compared with the effect of trans fatty acids.

7. b and d

8. A dietary pattern can be categorized as "healthy" by the following two approaches: (i) an a priori-defined healthy diet quality score/index based on the existing dietary guidelines; or (ii) an a posteriori-derived healthy dietary pattern based on variations in food intake, extracted using principal component analysis (PCA).

9. The Healthy Eating Index (HEI) was designed to measure the extent to which Americans were following dietary recommendations. Since then, the HEI index has been revised several times. The index has several questions, each of which receives a specific score as a reflection of an important aspect of diet quality. Higher scores indicate higher consumption and better adherence to a healthy dietary pattern.

10. PCA is a statistical method that is used to identify potential patterns from weighted food frequency questionnaires or 24-hour dietary recalls within a specific population. In other words, the method clusters variables that "behave in a similar way," forming new components, instead of analyzing these variables independently. For example, someone eats a lot of vegetables but at the same time eats a lot of fruits and whole grains. Every new component can thereafter be associated with several characteristics of a study's sample.

11. d

12. b

13. The consumption of a variety of vegetables, fruits, whole grains, a variety of protein foods based on lean meats, poultry, eggs, low-fat dairy products, legumes, nuts, seafood, and soy products, and avoidance of saturated and trans fats, added sugars, and sodium.

14. The healthy Nordic dietary pattern, the healthy Asian dietary pattern, the healthy vegetarian pattern, and the healthy Mediterranean-style dietary pattern.

15. Yes, I agree, because even though most dietary patterns share common features, they differ significantly in the types of basic ingredients they use and the cooking methods. Hence, there is no healthy dietary pattern for all, but everyone can adopt the one they prefer that satisfies not only their taste but also their sociocultural identity in an attempt to achieve long-term adherence to it and, eventually, better health.

Chapter 6

The Therapeutic Lifestyle Changes (TLC) diet

1. The strategy is to replace saturated and trans fatty acids with unsaturated and monosaturated fatty acids and replace simple carbohydrates (e.g., sugars) with complex carbohydrates (e.g., whole grains, fruits, and vegetables).

2. a) 25–35%
   b) the intake of saturated fats and cholesterol
   c) LDL cholesterol goal
   d) physically active, maintain a healthy body weight

3. c

4. prevent the absorption of cholesterol

The Dietary Approaches to Stop Hypertension (DASH) diet

1. DASH is a dietary pattern originated in the 1990s to normalize BP in patients with hypertension.

2. a) four to five servings/day
   b) four to five servings/day
   c) seven to eight servings/day
   d) two to three servings/day
   e) two or fewer servings/day
   f) four to five times/week
   g) two to three servings/day

3. The current recommendation is below 2000 mg/d (i.e., 5 g/d salt) in order to reduce BP and the risk of cardiovascular diseases, stroke, and coronary heart disease.

4. In addition to the positive effects on hypertension, the DASH diet has beneficial effects on lipid profile, insulin sensitivity, inflammation, and oxidative stress, and has been inversely associated with the risk of CVD, chronic kidney disease, and several types of cancer. Moreover, even modest adherence to the DASH diet has been associated with a lower risk of all-cause mortality. An even higher adherence strengthens this risk-reducing effect.

Vegetarian diets

1. The most common types of vegetarian diets are: (i) vegan diets, devoid of all flesh foods (such as meat, poultry, seafood, and all animal products); (ii) ovovegetarian, vegan plus eggs; (iii) pesce-vegetarian, vegan plus fish and seafood; (iv) lacto-vegetarian, vegan plus dairy products; and (v) various combinations of the above (lacto-ovo-vegetarian, ovo-pescevegetarian, etc.).

2. Vegans must regularly consume foods or receive supplements high in vitamins B_{12} and D, omega-3 fatty acids, calcium, iodine, iron, and zinc, to prevent deficiencies in these vitamins and minerals. As far as the B_{12} is concerned, recent data support that not only vegans but also lacto-ovo-vegetarians are at risk of developing B_{12} deficiency, and thus all vegetarians should include a B_{12} supplement in their daily diet.

3. The mechanism(s) mediating the effect of vegetarian diets on cancer risk is not known. It has been suggested that vegetarians have lower levels of hs-CRP compared to people who eat meat; the high antioxidant and anti-inflammatory effects of the food groups included in the pattern may also result in lower inflammation, in the long term.

4. Vegetarian diets have a lower carbon footprint, meaning that they produce less greenhouse gas emissions compared to diets including meat, making this dietary choice a more environmentally friendly type of a diet.

Religious/fasting diets

1. Buddhists practice meditation and yoga, activities that have been shown to have favorable health effects; meditation has positive effects on reducing stress and increasing mindfulness, as well as improving BP and vascular endothelial function.

2. During fasting, Hindus usually avoid solid foods and follow a liquid diet with vegetable or fruit juices. A stricter fasting ritual also exists, avoiding any solids and any form of liquid but water.

3. *Kashrut,* which means "proper" or "correct," is a set of dietary laws determining the foods that Jews are permitted to eat and how they should be prepared.

4. b

5. A restriction in total energy and fat intake and an increase in the consumption of carbohydrate and fiber.

Healthy Nordic diet

1. The healthy Nordic diet is a plant-based diet adopted in the Nordic regions, namely, northern European countries, such as Denmark, Finland, Norway, Sweden, and Iceland. It is characterized by high consumption of fruits (e.g., berries, apples, and pears), vegetables (e.g., root vegetables, cabbage, potatoes, carrots), wild mushrooms, pulses (e.g., beans, peas), nuts, whole-grain foods (e.g., rye, barley, oats), rapeseed oil, oily fish (e.g., mackerel, salmon, herring), shellfish, and seaweed, while emphasis is given to low-fat choices of meat (such as poultry and game), low-fat dairy, salt restriction, and avoidance of sugar-sweetened products.

2. Compared to the MedD and the DASH diet, the Nordic diet differs on the type of the recommended oil and the vegetable and fruit choices. In the Nordic diet the added culinary fat is canola oil, a variety of rapeseed, instead of olive oil, which is used in the MedD.

3. A food is characterized as a "typical" of the Nordic diet if it fulfills a list of criteria, such as being produced within the Nordic countries, being related to Nordic dietary tradition, is superior in terms of health effects, compared to other foods of the same food group, and is consumed as food and not as dietary supplement.

Healthy Asian diet

1. The Asian diet is primarily characterized by high consumption of rice, foods of plant origin (e.g., soy products), fish and seafood, fruits and vegetables, and tea. The majority of foods are boiled, steamed, or grilled without the addition of culinary fat, or fried with minimum quantities of seed oils, or they are consumed raw.

2. The Japanese and the Chinese dietary guidelines represent two well-documented examples of the healthy Asian diets.

3. The base of the pagoda is filled with cereals, such as rice, corn, bread, noodles, and crackers, as well as tubers.

Chapter 7

1. The MedD is primarily a plant-based dietary pattern including a high consumption of whole grains, bread, fruits, vegetables, legumes, nuts, and seeds. It is characterized by a low consumption of red meat and meat products, whole-fat dairy products (mainly in the form of cheese and yogurt), processed foods, and refined cereals. Fish and seafood (that traditionally varied based on the population's proximity to the sea) is consumed in moderation. Olive oil is the main source of dietary fat, while a moderate amount of red wine is consumed with meals.

2. The MedD is considered the outcome of the interactions between the natural Mediterranean environment and major civilizations, different cultures and religions of people living in the Mediterranean basin. Consequently, there is more than one version of the MedD.

3. a – T; b – F; c – F; d – F; e – T

4. The MedD belongs to what one would call "ancient diets" but underwent significant changes over time. During the Middle Ages, eating habits of the Mediterranean populations, such as Romans, fused with those of other populations, such as German nomads who were more into hunting, farming, and gathering food resources. Although the Roman culture kept most of the "Mediterranean" style of nutrition, another food culture, the Arabic, developed on the southern shores of the Mediterranean, was slowly incorporated into the Roman culture. Muslims facilitated the introduction of yet unknown agricultural products, such as various spices and fruits, contributing greatly to the formation of several new cooking habits. The discovery of the Americas also affected the European food culture. The newly discovered land provided new kinds of foods, such as potatoes and tomatoes. Interestingly, tomatoes, thought for many years to be poisonous, later became one of the flagships of the MedD. Consequently, the MedD reflects a collection of dietary habits and food-handling practices adopted over many centuries in the countries bordering the Mediterranean Sea.

5. d

6. The Seven Countries Study is an observational cohort study initiated in 1958 by Ancel Keys. It includes data from the USA, Finland, former Yugoslavia, Japan, the Netherlands, Italy, and Greece. The primary finding of the study was that men from the USA and northern Europe experienced a much higher incidence of CHD and mortality rate from CHD compared to men of the same age in southern and central Europe. It was also found that for a cholesterol concentration of ~210 mg/dl, the risk of CHD mortality was 4–5% in the Mediterranean cohorts of southern Europe and Japan, but it reached 15% for northern Europeans.

7. a

8. An important change in the new MedD pyramid is the food group in the vertex of the pyramid. Sugary foods (such as candies, pastries, and sweetened beverages) have replaced red meat. Besides food frequency recommendations, healthy lifestyle and cultural elements were also added. Socialization, cooking with friends and family, and sharing foods, as well as seasonality, biodiversity, and the eco-friendliness characteristics of the MedD pattern, were presented at the bottom of the pyramid to highlight aspects such as relaxation, community togetherness, and sustainability. Regular physical activity is also included for balancing energy intake, weight maintenance, and other health benefits.

Food should be consumed with moderation and frugality, both key elements of the MedD following the famous Greek proverb "Μέτρον άριστον", which stands for "all in good measure," "all in moderation." There is not "a one size fits all" approach in the MedD; portion sizes are meant to adopt to the population needs related to various geographical, socioeconomic, and cultural contexts. The foods in the base of the Mediterranean pyramid should be consumed in greater frequency and quantity, while moving upward serving size shrinks and consumption frequency declines. The notion is that the foods suggested to be consumed frequently enhance satiety and provide moderate energy, along with important nutrients for a given volume, whereas foods suggested to be rarely consumed are more energy-dense.

9. b, c, and e

10. A high adherence to the MedD is inversely associated with the risk of developing cancer, cardiometabolic, neurodegenerative, mental, autoimmune, and allergic diseases. This protection is largely attributed to the synergistic effect of its components, such as fruits, vegetables, whole grains, olive oil, and wine, which are rich in numerous bioactive nutrients.

11. c, d, e

12. d

13. a – T; b – F; c – T; d – F; e – T

Chapter 8

1. The MedL can be defined as the lifestyle paradigm encompassing the various components of the daily life of the people living in the Mediterranean basin; a plant-based diet characterized by moderation, seasonality, participation in culinary activities, conviviality, daily engagement in physical activity as an inherent feature of everyday life, healthy sleeping practices, stress management practices, adequate rest, engagement in spiritual activities, active social life, and the rich cultural heritage transmitted from one generation to the next.

2. a) conviviality
   b) less
   c) decrease
   d) availability of food sources, other aspects of life

3. The four sustainable benefits of the Mediterranean diet are (i) major health and nutrition benefits; (ii) low environmental impact and richness in biodiversity; (iii) high sociocultural food values; and (iv) positive local economic returns.

4. Contrary to the popular belief that cooking is just clean, chop, and put the raw ingredients into a casserole, literature suggests that there is much more to these procedures. Culinary practices are a matter of organization, concept, perception, and technique and seem to determine individuals' food-related behavior and

dietary habits. The frequency of home-cooked meals has been associated with increased consumption of fruits, vegetables, and whole grains. Improving cooking skills have been related to reduced fast-food consumption, higher frequency of shared meals, and cooking using low-cost basic ingredients. Homemade meals are considered less energy-dense and contain lower concentrations of total fat and SFAs, dietary cholesterol, and sodium but have greater fiber, calcium, and iron content.

5. Fresh and locally grown foods are less expensive compared to imported ones, as no travel and storage expenses are added to the production cost. Nonseasonal products, usually coming from far away, require long-term storage in order to distribute them in markets all year round. As a consequence of the extended transportation and storage time, the concentration of vitamins, minerals, and other bioactive compounds may decrease. Moreover, based on the fact that plant-derived products, such as fruits and vegetables, are very vulnerable to rotting, long storage presupposes that those products may be subjected to various chemical processes to preserve them for long periods. Domestic produce is usually delivered in markets and sold within 24–48 hours after its harvest, maintaining its optimum freshness, flavor, and ripeness.

Chapter 9

1. Total energy expenditure is the arithmetic sum of resting energy expenditure, physical activity expenditure, and thermic effect of food.

2. d

3. a) four times the energy
   b) duration
   c) intensity/duration
   d) level of cardiorespiratory fitness

4. Nonexercise activity thermogenesis is defined as the energy expended for walking to work, standing, performing yard work, undertaking agricultural tasks, fidgeting, and other daily PA; i.e., everything that is not sleeping, eating, or sports-like exercise.

5. Several tools have been developed for PA evaluation, including subjective and objective methods. Subjective methods rely on the individual's recollection of activities previously or usually performed, or their willingness to record activities as they occur in PA diaries and logs. Objective methods include wearable monitors that directly measure one or more biosignals indicative of an individual's PA level, such as acceleration (accelerometers), steps (pedometers), or heart rate (heart rate monitors), as well as techniques for the estimation of physical activity expenditure (double labeled water and indirect calorimetry) as PA occurs. Feasibility and practicality, the availability of resources, and administration considerations, as well as the desired outcome of the assessment, guide the choice of an appropriate PA assessment tool, given that there is no single best instrument appropriate for every situation.

6. At least 150 minutes a week of moderate-intensity activity and at least 2 days a week of activities that strengthen muscles and activities to improve balance, such as standing on one foot.

7. Exposure to natural environments has been proposed to be associated with an increased level of vitality, defined as a positive state of physical and mental energy, characterized by a sense of enthusiasm, aliveness, and vigor.

8. a

9. The 2011 version of the Mediterranean diet pyramid recommends PA as a significant component of a healthy lifestyle. Specifically, regular practice of moderate lifestyle PA, i.e., ≥30 minutes throughout the day, is suggested as a fundamental complement to healthy dietary habits as a means to balance energy intake, maintain a healthy body weight, and attain the numerous health benefits of PA. What distinguishes the Mediterranean lifestyle PA recommendations from other formal guidelines is the promotion of the social character of PA, achieved through practicing leisure activities outdoors, preferably with company, thus making them more enjoyable and strengthening the sense of community. This is in accordance with the overall concept of conviviality and socialization of the Mediterranean lifestyle.

10. Among the determinants of PA, convenience, comfort, attractiveness, and accessibility are considered important. This notion is supported by data suggesting that barriers for PA include limited time to exercise, limited access to sports or recreation facilities, as well as displeasure against vigorous exercise and the imposed conformity or adherence to gymnasium-based exercise. On the other hand, enjoyment of the activity performed and perceived competence, as well as social environment characteristics, such as the parallel participation of and the support from friends and family, have been identified as significant positive correlates of PA. The MedL actively promotes a physically active way of life over prescribed and structured exercise programs.

11. Early recommendations on PA focused on fitness and were quite specific and strict, leading to the conclusion that a PA level not meeting these specific criteria (i.e., high-intensity PA) would be of limited or no value. As time passed, a shift of guidelines away from an exclusively "performance-related fitness" paradigm to one that also includes recommendations for health-related outcomes became evident. This change in the perception of PA recommendations further evolved and is in line with the increasing number of studies published, revealing that even moderate-intensity PA produces significant improvements in work capacity. These findings are very important; now it is clear that even people who cannot perform high-intensity or prolonged exercise can benefit from doing any kind of physical activity.

12. Adequate levels of PA among adults have been associated with reduced total and disease-specific mortality (mostly malignancy- and cardiovascular-related), a beneficial cardiometabolic profile (i.e., improved blood lipid profile, BP levels, glucose homeostasis, and inflammatory markers), lower risk for metabolic syndrome, cardiovascular disease (coronary heart disease, heart failure, and cerebrovascular disease), insulin resistance, T2DM and gestational diabetes mellitus, cancer (esophageal, gastric, colorectal, pancreatic, renal, lung, bladder, endometrial, ovarian, prostate, breast, and thyroid), and liver disease. Adequate levels of PA are also considered a key determinant of energy expenditure, and thus fundamental to energy balance and body weight regulation. The same applies to the elderly, in whom adequate PA has been additionally associated with better psychological health and quality of life (autonomy and vitality), reduced disability and fall-related injuries, as well as improved cognitive function in terms of both reduced age-related cognitive decline and reduced risk for neurological disorders, such as Alzheimer's disease. Although available scientific data for children and adolescents are more limited, the beneficial effects of PA on their physical, psychological and mental health are also evident, in terms of body weight regulation, cardiometabolic health, bone density and strength, as well as cognitive outcomes, self-esteem, self-concept, and depression.

Chapter 10

1. Specific processes and metabolic pathways are activated that are essential for the regulation of daytime functioning and overall well-being.
2. (i) The inactivity theory; (ii) the energy conservation theory; (iii) the restorative theory; and (iv) the brain plasticity theory.
3. c
4. Body temperature declines slightly before sleep and decreases even further (1–2°F) during sleep; the most significant decrease in body temperature occurs during REM sleep. Breathing rate also decreases during sleep.
5. As highlighted in the latest version of the Mediterranean diet pyramid, adequate sleep is essential for a well-functioning body. Sleep doesn't occur only at night but also during the day in the form of short naps or siestas, a typical Mediterranean practice.
6. *Siesta* is a Spanish word, derived from the Latin word *sexta* (hora), which means sixth (hour). That is midday, because counting from dawn, midday is approximately the sixth hour. The word *siesta* has been used to express the midday or afternoon rest or nap, which is taken usually after the midday meal.
7. Siestas should last between 20 and 40 minutes, before passing to the stage of deep sleep from which it is more difficult to awake. Short (below 40 minutes) daytime napping is associated with lower risk for cardiovascular disease, whereas long daytime napping (above 60 minutes) with higher risk, compared to non-nappers.
8. Adults (18–64 years old) are advised to sleep 7–9 hours/day.
9. Reduced sleep duration and/or low sleep quality is connected to increased energy intake, irregular eating habits, consumption of energy-dense snacks, especially between late evening and early morning, as well as the adoption of an unhealthy dietary pattern. The reasons for this detrimental effect of sleep deprivation on dietary habits have not been fully elucidated. It has been suggested that when the body is sleep-deprived, the level of ghrelin spikes, while the level of leptin falls, leading to an increase in hunger and the urge for energy-dense foods, such as sweets. However, increased food consumption in low-sleepers is also evident in the absence of changes in appetite-related hormones. For this reason, it has been hypothesized that the increase in food intake under conditions of sleep deprivation is also due to a physiological need to stay alert and maintain vigilance during the day.
10. Long-term shift work or frequent changes in day vs. night employment have been associated with an increased risk of diseases, including heart disease, gastrointestinal problems, depression, certain cancers, T2DM, and obesity. Studies have shown that shift workers usually have irregular eating habits and unhealthy diets and present with high triglyceride levels and insulin resistance. The mechanisms responsible for the detrimental effects of shift work on health might be related to decreased amount of sleep and the disruption of the body's circadian rhythms. Apart from the risk of developing chronic diseases, shift work may also decrease productivity and increase the risk for accidents and on-the-job injuries. The risk for accidents increases when workers start their jobs in the evenings and when their shifts last for more than 8 hours.

Chapter 11

1. a
2. There are seven proposed mechanisms: social influence and/or comparison, social control, meaning of life based on social roles, self-esteem, sense of control, belonging and companionship, and perceived support availability.
3. a) psychological and physical functioning
   b) the obligation of the other part
   c) decreased anxiety, distress, and depressive symptoms
   d) favorable physical and psychological health outcomes
4. A positive attitude can help people attain and maintain health practices and cope better with high-stress situations, including medical problems.
5. Meditation is an ancient form of stress relief that has recently been accepted as a complementary practice in modern medical science. It results in alterations in human physiology associated with a decrease in stress and anxiety and has been associated with improvements in mental health in healthy and chronically ill individuals.
6. Irrespective of what people believe in, their beliefs can comprise a lifelong guiding principle, capable of affecting health. Firmly held values and principles, religious or not, have the potential to bestow incentives, abilities, power, and hope, and in this way, they can help people to confront disease states. Among chronically ill individuals, spirituality has been shown to amplify adaptation in difficult circumstances. Moreover, finding meaning and having a purpose in life may create a positive attitude toward it, which in turn can predispose toward more sound health practices, resulting in better health.
7. The Mediterranean populations are renowned for their openness and extroversion, character traits that are believed to have an advantageous impact on their health. Even though there is limited data on the prevalence of stress and the effects of relaxation in the Mediterranean people, it has long been hypothesized that their social character influences these factors and therefore their health. It is noteworthy that this predisposition of associating with other people and being in the company of others is an inherent behavioral trait of the populations bordering the Mediterranean basin. This disposition and attitude toward sociability is not taught but constitutes a natural consequence of the way of living in the Mediterranean countries.
8. a – F; b – T; c – T; d – F; e – T

Chapter 12

1. The MetS represents the clustering of several interconnected physiological, biochemical, clinical, and metabolic disorders that directly increase the risk of adverse health outcomes related to NCDs. These disorders include impaired glucose metabolism, hypertension, dyslipidemia, central obesity, inflammation, and oxidative stress and are involved in the pathogenesis of most, if not all, major modern chronic diseases, including cardiovascular diseases and T2DM. The MetS has a rising prevalence worldwide, related to obesity, unhealthy diet, and sedentary lifestyle, and its management through lifestyle interventions should be one of the main goals of health policy in every country in the world.

2. The MetS is defined as the coexistence of three or more of the five following components: (i) increased sex-specific WC values, indicative of central obesity; (ii) increased fasting glucose levels or intake of antidiabetic medication or presence of T2DM; (iii) decreased sex-specific HDLC levels or intake of relevant medication; (iv) increased TG levels or intake of lipid-lowering medication; (v) increased systolic and/or diastolic BP levels or intake of antihypertensive medication.

3. Lifestyle medicine is the use of a whole food, plant-predominant dietary pattern, regular physical activity, restorative sleep, stress management, avoidance of risky substances, and positive social connection as a primary therapeutic modality for the prevention and treatment of chronic diseases. It is provided by a multidisciplinary team of health professionals from many fields, including medicine, nutrition, exercise, psychology, and sleep. In this setting, the patient is no longer a passive recipient of care but an active partner who makes decisions and assumes responsibility for the changes that need to take place to improve his/her health and wellness. This can be achieved through a patient/client-centered counseling style, focused on increasing motivation, health efficacy, and health literacy.

4. Conventional medicine uses medications as the core treatment for diseases. It is usually provided by health-care professionals who operate independently and treat patients as passive recipients of care, with little consideration of their environment and lifestyle. On the other hand, lifestyle medicine focuses on beneficial lifestyle changes as a means to prevent and treat diseases. It aims at promoting patients' motivation, compliance, and self-efficacy to change and is provided by a multidisciplinary team of health professionals at a user-friendly practice environment, with the patient being an active partner in care.

Chapter 13

1. Obesity is defined as the excessive accumulation of fat in the body, which poses health risks and leads to a reduced life expectancy.

2. a, c, and d

3. Sleep deprivation, even short term, has been shown to cause a variety of physiological, metabolic, and hormonal abnormalities. These abnormalities can lead to increased appetite and increased sensitivity to stimuli for food intake. Furthermore, the feeling of fatigue and exhaustion, caused by insufficient sleep, may lead to low functionality and reduced physical activity during the day. Increased energy intake and reduced levels of physical activity may result in positive energy balance and eventually weight gain in the long term.

4. b and c

5. a

6. There is no ideal weight loss target for all obese patients. The weight-loss goal must be set for each patient, based on his/her health status, desires, and motivation, and must be realistic, specific, and measurable. In general, a 5–10% weight loss over a period of 6 months is a realistic goal and of proven health benefit for most obese patients. An even greater (≥10%) weight loss may be considered for patients with higher degrees of obesity

(BMI ≥ 35 kg/m²); however, even a mild weight loss of 3–5% is beneficial for health, especially for obese patients with high cardiovascular risk or established obesity-related disorders.

7. a and c

8. a – T; b – F; c – F; d – F; e – T

9. There are no single nutrients, foods, or food groups that can promote or hinder weight loss. A balanced diet that encompasses foods from all major food groups in moderation, poses no strict restrictions, and ensures an adequate intake of all the important nutrients on a weekly basis is the cornerstone of a healthy lifestyle. Healthy eating counseling for an obese patient must emphasize the need to increase consumption of fruits, vegetables, legumes, whole grains, and fish, and the need to keep the consumption of processed meat products, ultraprocessed foods that contain added sugars, solid fats, and salt, sugar-sweetened beverages, and alcohol-containing beverages within a reasonable frequency. Other beneficial practices toward weight loss include frequent and nutritionally complete meals, correct identification of hunger and satiety, portion control, and proper meal conditions.

10. Cognitive behavioral therapy is a blend of cognitive therapy and behavioral therapy that aims to help a patient modify his/her insight and understanding of thoughts and beliefs concerning health issues, including weight regulation, obesity, and its consequences. It also directly addresses behaviors that require change for health promotion, including successful weight loss and weight-loss maintenance. It includes several components, such as goal-setting, self-monitoring, problem solving, and stimulus control, all aiming at facilitating behavior change. These elements should form the basis of specialized intervention for the management of obesity and other lifestyle-related diseases.

11. a and c

12. Energy restriction can be achieved by three major approaches. The first requires the estimation of the patient's energy requirements, usually through population-specific equations that predict BMR, and the prescription of a daily diet with an energy deficit of 500–750 kcal/d. In the second approach, we set a target energy intake that is less than the population average, i.e., <1500 kcal/d for women and <1800 kcal/d for men. The third approach is the ad libitum approach, in which a formal energy deficit target is not prescribed to the patient, but lower calorie intake is achieved through healthier food choices and the substitution of energy-dense foods with nutrient-dense food of lower caloric content.

13. c

14. All balanced hypocaloric diets result in similar, clinically significant weight loss and health benefits, regardless of which macronutrients they emphasize. Therefore, caloric restriction, achieved through reduced intake of either fat or carbohydrate or a combination of the two, leads to similar weight loss. Several dietary approaches can produce weight loss in obese adults, including a high-protein diet, a low-carbohydrate diet, a low-fat diet, a low-glycemic-load diet, a Mediterranean-style diet, and a vegetarian diet, as long as they achieve an energy deficit. Hypocaloric diets should be tailored to the individual patient on the basis of his/her personal and cultural preferences in order to have the best chance for long-term success.

15. a – F; b – F; c – T; d – F; e – T

16. The patient's BMI is 82.5 kg ÷ (1.58 m)² = 33.05 kg/m². According to the classification of BMI values, she is considered obese class I. Based on the Schofield equations for women aged 30–60 years

old, the patient's estimated BMR is 8.126×82.5+845.6 = ~1500 kcal. Given that she is mildly active, her BMR should be multiplied with a 1.5 physical activity factor, leading to a total daily energy expenditure of ~2250 kcal. An energy deficit of 500–750 kcal would lead to daily energy intake of ~1500–1750 kcal to achieve the desired weight loss. Alternatively, a standard LCD of 1500 kcal could be prescribed.

17. b, d, and e

18. Motivational interviewing is a technique in which the health-care professional becomes a helper in the change process, where the patient is the driver for change. It is a way to interact with patients that can help resolve the ambivalence that prevents patients from realizing, achieving, and maintaining personal goals. The role of a health-care professional in motivational interviewing is directive, with a goal of eliciting self-motivational statements and behavioral change from the patient. Essentially, motivational interviewing is a counseling style that activates the capacity for beneficial change that everyone possesses.

19. The patient's BMI is 102.8 kg ÷ (1.87 m)^2 = 29.40 kg/m^2. According to the classification of BMI values, he is considered overweight. His WC is very high (>102 cm). According to the combined evaluation of his BMI and WC values, he is at a high morbidity risk.

20. Stress evokes patterned, compensatory mechanisms and reactions in the human body, which are essential for survival but can also have negative effects in the case of chronic exposure to stressful stimuli. Chronic activation of the sympathetic nervous system and the hypothalamic–pituitary–adrenal axis contribute to chronically elevated cortisol levels and an anabolic state that promotes fat storage within visceral depots; this leads to increased risk of central obesity and associated comorbidities, such as hypertension, dyslipidemia, impaired glucose metabolism, MetS, and cardiovascular disease. Stress can also enhance weight gain and fat deposition through changes in eating behavior, including alterations in the pattern of food intake, emotional eating, and increased susceptibility to the rewarding properties of foods. Therefore, chronic stress is strongly linked to obesity, and its evaluation and management is crucial in the context of an efficient obesity treatment.

Chapter 14

1. Diabetes is a group of metabolic diseases characterized by hyperglycemia, resulting from defects in insulin production, insulin action, or both. It can be classified into the following general categories: (i) type 1 diabetes mellitus, also known as juvenile diabetes or insulin-dependent diabetes, which results from autoimmune pancreatic β-cell destruction, usually leading to absolute insulin deficiency; (ii) type 2 diabetes mellitus, in which insulin resistance is the fundamental feature while the pancreas partly maintains its insulin production capacity; (iii) gestational diabetes mellitus, diagnosed in the second or third trimesters of pregnancy, in the absence of diabetes mellitus prior to gestation; and (iv) other types of diabetes due to various causes, e.g., monogenic diabetes syndromes and diseases of the exocrine pancreas.

2. Individuals with unstable diabetic retinopathy are at risk for vitreous hemorrhage and retinal detachment. In general,

mild-to-moderate-intensity physical activity is considered safe; however, activities that significantly elevate BP, such as vigorous activity of any type, including weightlifting, jumping, jarring, and head-down activities should be avoided. During a vitreous hemorrhage, exercise should be completely avoided.

3. b and d

4. b

5. Participation in regular physical activity improves blood glucose control and can positively affect lipids, BP, cardiovascular events, mortality, and quality of life. Most benefits of exercise on T2DM management derive from acute and chronic improvements in insulin action; both aerobic and resistance types of exercise are beneficial, provided they are sustained in the long term. In general, most adults with T2DM should engage in ≥150 minutes of moderate-to-vigorous-intensity aerobic activity weekly, spread over ≥3 days/week, with no more than 2 consecutive days without activity. Resistance exercise should also be performed 2–3 times/week; ≥8–10 exercises with completion of 1–3 sets of 10–15 repetitions to near fatigue per set are recommended. Flexibility and balance exercises can additionally be performed ≥2–3 days/week with increasing frequency, duration, and intensity over time.

6. b and e

7. The main goal of nutrition therapy for patients with T2DM is to promote the adoption of healthy eating patterns, emphasizing a variety of nutrient-dense foods in appropriate portion sizes to improve overall health and attain individualized glycemic, BP, and lipid goals and delay or prevent diabetes complications. Individual nutritional needs should be addressed based on the patient's personal and cultural preferences, health literacy and numeracy, access to healthy food choices, willingness and ability to make behavioral changes, and barriers to change. The pleasure of eating must be maintained by providing positive messages about food choices while limiting food choices only when indicated by scientific evidence. Last but not least, the patient should be provided with practical tools for day-to-day meal planning rather than focusing on individual nutrients or foods.

8. Sugar-sweetened beverages are any liquids that are sweetened with various forms of added sugars, such as sucrose, fructose, glucose, high-fructose corn syrup, and molasses. They are a rich source of sugars and calories but have a low content of other beneficial nutrients. Frequent consumption of sugar-sweetened beverages is associated with adverse health outcomes, including weight gain/obesity and associated comorbidities. Limiting the number of sugar-sweetened beverages consumed is essential for the adoption of a balanced diet and can lead to improvements in glycemic control in patients with T2DM. Given the patient's daily consumption, a realistic initial goal would be to gradually reduce the frequency of consumption to two to three portions/week and emphasize smaller portion sizes (e.g., ½ glass of soda), with a longer-term goal of eliminating the consumption of sugar-sweetened beverages. Other less energy-dense and lower-GI choices could be considered, such as smoothies with fresh fruits and milk/yogurt, fresh fruit juices, or other low-sugar beverages, such as herbal infusions and low-sugar artificially sweetened beverages.

9. a – F; b – F; c – T; d – F; e – T

10. a and c

11. d

12. Patients with T2DM are at risk of developing complications that occur rapidly (acute) or over time (chronic) and may affect many organ systems. Acute complications include hyperglycemia, hyperosmolar state, hypoglycemia, and diabetic coma, all related to impaired glucose metabolism. Chronic complications include cardiovascular diseases (coronary heart disease, cerebrovascular disease, and peripheral vascular disease), diabetic retinopathy, diabetic nephropathy, and diabetic neuropathy. All of the above-mentioned complications result from the devastating effects of increased blood glucose to the body's vessels and nerves. Infectious diseases are also a serious complication of T2DM, caused by the hyperglycemic environment that favors immune dysfunction, micro- and macro-angiopathies, and neuropathy. The most common form of infection is foot infection, which can lead to the "diabetic foot" and, if left untreated, amputation.

13. b and c

14. Diabetes mellitus may be diagnosed based on: (i) a fasting plasma glucose of ≥126 mg/dl; (ii) a 2-hour plasma glucose of ≥200 mg/dl during a 75-g oral glucose tolerance test; (iii) a gly-cosylated hemoglobin of ≥6.5%; or (iv) a random plasma glucose of ≥200 mg/dl along with classic symptoms of hyperglycemia or hyperglycemic crisis.

15. a – F; b – T; c – F; d – F; e – F

16. Stress triggers biological responses that exacerbate insulin resistance, including the release of glucose and lipids into the circulation, inflammatory cytokine expression, and increased BP. Repeated or sustained stress exposure leads to chronic allostatic load, with dysregulation of glucose metabolism and neuroendocrine function and chronic low-grade inflammation. Moreover, among individuals with established T2DM, stress and depression are associated with poor glycemic control and increased risk of cardiovascular complications. Stress relief is increasingly recognized as an important part of diabetes management and should be included in multicomponent diabetes interventions.

17. b and c

18. The GI is a ranking of foods on a scale from 0 to 100 according to the extent to which they raise blood glucose levels after food consumption, compared to the same quantity of a reference food. Foods with a high GI are rapidly digested, absorbed, and metabolized and result in marked fluctuations in blood glucose levels, while low-GI foods produce smaller fluctuations in blood glucose and insulin levels. Substituting low-GI foods for higher–GI foods can improve glycemic control and should be a target for all patients with T2DM. Unprocessed foods with a high dietary fiber content, such as fruits, vegetables, whole grains, and legumes, have a low GI and should be preferred over processed foods rich in sugars, such as refined grains, pastries, sweets, fruit juices, and sugar-sweetened beverages.

19. a and d

20. People with diabetic kidney disease may benefit from a slight decrease in protein intake compared to that recommended for the general population. A protein intake of 0.6–0.8 g/kg is suitable for most patients. Lower protein intakes (<0.6 g/kg) are not recommended, given that they are not expected to further improve glycemic control, cardiovascular risk, or the course of glomerular filtration rate and may lead to additional complications, including malnutrition. With regard to exercise, all activities are safe and should be encouraged, depending on the patient's aerobic capacity and muscle function, but vigorous exercise should be avoided the day before urine protein tests are performed to prevent false positive readings. In end-stage renal disease, moderate-intensity aerobic physical activity undertaken during dialysis sessions may be beneficial and increase compliance.

Chapter 15

1. Hypertension can be described as a disease characterized by chronically elevated SBP, DBP, or both. Although the risk of hypertension-related diseases increases progressively throughout a wide range of BP values, in clinical practice, cut-off BP values are used to simplify the diagnosis of hypertension and decision-making about treatment. For adults, the SBP/DBP cut-off values for defining hypertension are ≥130/80 mmHg according to the latest American guidelines and ≥140/90 mmHg according to the latest European guidelines. BP centiles should be used for the diagnosis of hypertension in children and teenagers.

2. c

3. a and d

4. The DASH diet originated in the 1990s in a study funded by the National Institutes of Health in the USA, aiming to identify dietary interventions that could be useful in treating hypertension. The DASH diet showed a strong BP-lowering effect and has ever since been advocated as the first-line dietary therapy for hypertension. Subsequent studies have also highlighted its beneficial effects on cardiovascular morbidity and mortality. The DASH diet emphasizes the intake of plant-based products, such as fruits, vegetables, whole grains and nuts, low-fat dairy products, poultry, and fish and can be characterized as a low-fat (especially saturated fat) dietary pattern rich in potassium, magnesium, calcium, and dietary fiber.

5. a – T; b – F; c – F; d – F; e – T

6. Patients should be seated comfortably in a quiet environment for 5 minutes before measurements. BP should be measured in both arms at the first visit to detect possible between-arm differences, and the arm with the higher value should be used thereafter. The cuff should be positioned at the level of the heart, with the back and arm supported to avoid muscle contraction. Three BP measurements should be recorded, with a 1–2 minute interval, and additional measurements should be performed if the first two readings differ by >10 mmHg. BP should be recorded as the average of the last two BP readings.

7. e

8. Heathy lifestyle choices can prevent or delay the onset of hypertension and can reduce cardiovascular risk. Effective lifestyle changes may also be sufficient to delay or prevent the need for drug therapy in patients with stage/grade 1 hypertension, as well as augment the effects of BP-lowering therapy. Recommended lifestyle measures that have been shown to reduce BP include weight loss and maintaining a healthy body weight, salt restriction, moderation of alcohol consumption, the adoption of a healthy diet characterized by high consumption of plant-based foods, mainly vegetables and fruits, and regular physical activity. In addition, smoking cessation is recommended for all hypertensive patients as a means to lower daytime BP values and the risk for cardiovascular diseases and cancer.

9. a – F; b – T; c – F; d – T; e – F

10. The primary goal of hypertension management is to normalize BP values. The first objective should be to bring BP to <140/90 mmHg in all patients; if succeeded, and the regimen is well tolerated, a new target of 130/80 mmHg is set. Given that hypertension is a major risk factor for morbidity and mortality,

treatment goals should go beyond the normalization of BP values and expand to reductions in hypertension-related health risks, the management of comorbidities, and improvements in quality of life and well-being.

11. a and e
12. a
13. a – T; b – T; c – F; d – T; e – T
14. Body weight is directly associated with BP. Excessive weight gain is associated with increased risk of developing hypertension, while reducing body weight toward a healthy body weight range decreases BP and can help the management of hypertension. Reductions in BP occur even with a modest weight loss, irrespective of attainment of a desirable body weight, i.e., even if BMI values do not fall below $27.5 \, kg/m^2$. The BP-lowering effect of weight loss appears to present a dose–response relationship of about 1 mmHg per kg of weight loss. In addition, weight loss can facilitate medication step-down and drug withdrawal in hypertensive patients. Therefore, modest weight reduction is recommended in all overweight and obese hypertensive patients to lower BP levels but also to control other cardiometabolic complications and lower total cardiovascular risk.
15. d
16. b and c
17. a – F; b – T; c – T; d – F; e – T
18. Accumulating evidence suggests that sleep deprivation and insomnia are positively linked to increased BP levels and the presence, severity, and incidence of hypertension. In addition, a strong relationship between sleep disorders and hypertension is increasingly recognized, with the strongest data being evident for obstructive sleep apnea. Sleep apnea is characterized by repetitive pauses of breathing during sleep due to obstructions of the upper airways that result in intermittent hypoxia. Hypoxia, in turn, leads to an abnormal increase in sympathetic activation, which contributes to increased vascular resistance and cardiac output and, eventually, increases in BP, which are also sustained during wakefulness.
19. b, d, and e
20. Sodium restriction has a well-established BP-lowering effect. All hypertensive patients should be encouraged to limit their sodium intake to ≤2 g/d, with the optimal goal being set at <1.5 g/d. However, extremely strict sodium restrictions should be avoided, given that they can have an adverse effect on cardiovascular risk and result in an unpalatable diet that is difficult to maintain in the long term. In the context of sodium restriction, patients should try to avoid using salt in their meals during cooking or serving and consume foods that are naturally rich in sodium, such as grain products, dairy products, meat products (especially processed), and fats/oils. In addition, packaged foods, such as salty snacks, ready-to-eat meals, sauces, and canned foods should be avoided, as they contain high amounts of sodium that serves as a taste enhancer and a preservative.

Chapter 16

1. Dyslipidemia refers to an abnormal amount of lipids in the blood. Dyslipidemias can be classified as familiar, i.e., inherited diseases with a strong genetic background, or acquired, i.e., secondary to obesity, metabolic diseases, and an unhealthy lifestyle with a gradual increase in severity over time. Hyperlipoproteinemia refers to increased levels of lipoprotein molecules, hyperlipidemia refers to increased values of TC, LDLC, and TG (isolated increased levels of TC or LDLC are also referred to as hypercholesterolemia and isolated increased TG values are also referred to as hypertriglyceridemia), while dyslipidemia also includes the presence of low HDLC levels.
2. c and e
3. Lipoproteins play a significant role in the pathophysiology of atherosclerosis. The quantity of circulating lipoproteins and the degree of lipid-oxidation/peroxidation greatly influence the rate and extent of atherosclerosis and endothelial damage. All small ApoB-containing lipoproteins can cross the endothelial barrier in the presence of endothelial dysfunction. Inside the arterial wall the lipoproteins may be trapped and provoke a complex process that leads to lipid deposition and the initiation of an atheroma. Continued exposure to ApoB-containing lipoproteins, especially oxidized small and dense LDLs, leads to additional particles being retained over time in the artery wall and to the growth and progression of atherosclerotic plaques.
4. d
5. The majority of cholesterol present in the body is synthesized in the liver, where it is either packaged together with TG into VLDLs or is used for bile acid synthesis. The VLDLs are secreted in the circulation and travel to the various tissues, where they are hydrolyzed to liberate TG for energy production or storage; during this process VLDLs become smaller, denser, TG-rich lipoprotein remnants. These remnants can either be further hydrolyzed to become LDLs or can be taken up by the liver for further metabolism and secretion in the bile. The LDL particles are also taken up by the liver but also by peripheral cells as a source of cholesterol. The HDL particles can either transport cholesterol from peripheral cells directly back to the liver, in a process called reverse cholesterol transport, or interact with cholesteryl ester transfer protein to exchange cholesterol for TG with TG-rich ApoB-containing lipoproteins.
6. a and b
7. Obstructive sleep apnea is a sleep disorder mostly evident among obese individuals and characterized by short pauses of breathing during sleep. There is increasing evidence that chronic intermittent hypoxia, a major component of obstructive sleep apnea, is independently associated with and possibly a root cause of dyslipidemia. Intermittent hypoxia can lead to dyslipidemia via the generation of reactive oxygen species, peroxidation of lipids, and sympathetic system dysfunction. In this context, management of sleep disorders is considered important for blood lipid control and cardiovascular health in general.

8. a – T; b – F; c – F; d – T; e – F

9. The quality of dietary fat is very important for the management of dyslipidemia. Avoiding consumption of industrialized TFAs is crucial for the control of blood lipids and the prevention of cardiovascular diseases; this can be achieved through the adoption of a diet based on natural products and the minimization of processed foods, such as fast food, some types of hard margarines, baked goods, and salty or sweet snacks. SFA, i.e., fat present in animal products (dairy and meat products), can be consumed in moderation. Fat intake should predominantly come from sources of unsaturated fatty acids, including MUFA, especially from olive oil and nuts, and PUFA, especially omega-3 fatty acids from fatty fish and green leafy vegetables.

10. Stress has been proposed as a potential causal factor for dyslipidemia. Dyslipidemia induced by stress can be considered as part of the body's response to cope with stressors. The mobilization of lipids, glucose, and proteins allows the organs and tissues to maintain homeostasis and adapt to the stressor. Therefore, the increase in blood lipids induced by stress is adaptive and should return to normal levels when the stressor ends. However, when the stressor is maintained over a long period, i.e., in the case of chronic psychological stress, dyslipidemia persists and may have deleterious effects, contributing to the development of insulin resistance and atherosclerosis. Although the exact mechanisms are not clear, stress-induced dyslipidemia is believed to be the result of complex interactions between stress hormones, insulin, adipose tissue metabolism, and cytokines, and of the detrimental impact of stress on dietary, physical activity, and sleep habits.

11. Obesity is a well-established risk factor for the development of blood lipid disorders. Therefore, weight loss and maintenance of a healthy weight are important for the prevention and treatment of dyslipidemia. Data from clinical trials suggest that for every 1 kg decrease in body weight, there is a 2.0 mg/dl decrease in TC, a 0.8 mg/dl decrease in LDLC, and a 1.33 mg/dl decrease in TG. With regard to HDLC levels, active weight loss is associated with a small decline in HDLC; however, a beneficial effect is observed in the weight-maintenance phase, i.e., when weight loss has stabilized. Although the magnitude of the effect of weight loss on blood lipids is modest, weight loss can have multiple favorable effects on other cardiovascular risk factors, especially BP and glycemic control, and should be a central component of the management of obese patients with dyslipidemia.

12. c, e, and f

13. a – F; b – T; c – T; d – T; e – F

14. According to the 2017 American Association of Clinical Endocrinologists and the American College of Endocrinology guidelines, the patient is considered to have high cardiovascular risk (presence of DM with no other risk factors) and her LDLC target should be <100 mg/dl (<2.6 mmol/l). According to the 2019 European Society of Cardiology and European Atherosclerosis Society guidelines, the patient is considered of moderate cardiovascular risk (young patients with T2DM <50 years old with disease duration <10 years and without other risk factors), and her LDLC target should be <100 mg/dl (<2.6 mmol/l).

15. a and e

16. b and d

17. Dyslipidemia management mainly aims at reducing cardiovascular risk. Adhering to a healthy cardioprotective lifestyle pattern is recommended for all patients with dyslipidemia. This includes the adoption of a healthy dietary pattern low in trans/saturated fat with a focus on whole grain products, legumes, vegetables, fruits, fish, and olive oil, an adequate physical activity level (30–60 minutes of physical activity on most days), the avoidance of exposure to tobacco in any form, and the maintenance of a healthy body weight. Keeping LDLC levels within cardiovascular risk-specific goals through lifestyle modification and/or pharmacotherapy, and managing comorbidities, such as hypertension and T2DM, is also crucial in the context of cardiovascular disease prevention.

18. a and c

19. a – F; b – T; c – T; d – T; e – F

20. Using the Friedewald formula, the patient's LDLC can be calculated as TC – HDLC – (TG/5) = 282–54 – (168/5) = 194 mg/dl.

Dietary Models and One-Day Sample Meal Plans

kcal: kilocalories

oz: ounce, by weight (equivalent to 30 grams, g)

This appendix provides the dietary characteristics of 11 dietary models and samples of one-day meal plans for each model. Please note the following abbreviations:

tsp: teaspoon

Tbsp: tablespoon

B.1. The Therapeutic Lifestyle Changes (TLC) Dietary Model

Food group	Servings per day			Serving size	Examples and notes	Significance of each food group to the TLC dietary model
	1600 kcal	2000 kcal	2600 kcal			
Grains	8	11	13	½ cup of cereal, grain, or pasta, 1 oz of a bread product	Whole-grain breads and cereals, pasta, rice, potatoes, low-fat crackers, and low-fat cookies, barley, oat.	High in complex carbohydrates and fiber. Low in saturated fat, cholesterol, and total fat.
Vegetables	3	4	4	½ cup of cooked vegetables or vegetable juice, 1 cup of raw vegetables	Green leafy vegetables broccoli, Brussels sprouts, carrots, kale, eggplant, pumpkin, soy products, radishes.	Important sources of vitamins, fiber, and other nutrients. Vegetables have a higher water and fiber content, they are low in energy density (calories per gram of food) and thus, they will fill you up while providing fewer calories.
Fruits	3	4	5	1 medium fruit, ½ cup of fresh fruit, or fruit juice, ¼ cup dried fruit	Blueberries, strawberries, grapes, apples, citrus fruits, bananas, berries, nectarines, peaches, pears, plums, prunes.	Rich in fiber, vitamins (such as the antioxidants C, E, and beta-carotene), and minerals. Low in sodium. Eat raw fruit as between-meal snacks.
Fat-free or low-fat milk and milk products	2	2	3	1 cup milk or yogurt	Fat-free or low-fat milk, buttermilk, yogurt, cream cheese, low-fat cheese (with no more than 3 g of fat per ounce), such as low-fat cottage cheese, soy milk.	Sources of calcium and protein with little or no saturated fat.

(Continued)

Food group	Servings per day			Serving size	Examples and notes	Significance of each food group to the TLC dietary model
	1600 kcal	2000 kcal	2600 kcal			
Lean meats, poultry, and fish	5	7	9	1 oz (30 g) cooked poultry or fish, 1 oz of cheese, 1 egg	Poultry without skin; Lean cuts of beef: sirloin tip, round steak, and rump roast; extra lean hamburger; cold cuts made with lean meat or soy protein; lean cuts of pork are center-cut ham, loin chops, and pork tenderloin. Strictly limit organ meats, such as brain, liver, and kidneys. Oily fish: as salmon, tuna, and mackerel. Leaner fish such as cod, haddock, and catfish.	Eicosapentaenoic acid (EPA) and docosahexaenoic acid (DHA) are omega-3 fats found in oily fish. Lean cuts of meat have less fat and are rich sources of protein and iron. *Tip: Trim any fat from meat and remove skin from poultry before cooking.*
Nuts, seeds, and legumes	20–30 g unsalted nuts per day 2–3 legumes per week			½ cup beans – cooked, 2 Tbsp seeds, 6 almonds, 2 pecans, 20 peanuts (small), 2 walnuts	Black beans, kidney, chickpeas, or lentils, flaxseed, almond, walnut, peanuts, tofu.	Fiber-rich and good sources of plant protein. Nuts are important sources of polyunsaturated fat. Soy is rich in flavones/isoflavones.
Fats and oils	7	8	11	1 tsp soft margarine, 1 tsp vegetable oil	Oils including olive, canola, and peanut oil, safflower, sunflower, corn, and soybean oils, trans fat-free margarines, avocado, peanut butter without sugar. Avoid: Butter, bacon, chitterlings, coconut (shredded) Coffee whitener, (liquid/powder), cream (light, coffee, table), sour, cream (heavy, whipping), cream cheese.	When you consume fat, make it unsaturated fat – either monounsaturated or polyunsaturated. Dietary trans fats can be reduced by limiting your intake of fried restaurant foods (e.g., French fries, breaded chicken nuggets, and breaded fish).
	Saturated fat<7% of total calories Monounsaturated up to 20% of total calories Polyunsaturated up to 10% of total calories					
Sweets and added sugars	Once or twice per week			1 Tbsp sugar, jelly, or jam, ½ cup sorbet, 1 cup lemonade	Low-fat ice cream, baked goods (cookies, cakes, and pies made with unsaturated oil or soft margarines, egg whites, or egg substitutes, and fat-free milk), candies with little or no fat, such as hard candy, gumdrops, jellybeans, and candy corn.	Sweets must be low in fats.

– Less than 200 mg a day of cholesterol.
– 2 g/d of plant stanols or sterols.
– 10–25 g/d of soluble fiber.
– consume egg yolks in moderation, – including yolks in baked goods and in cooked or processed foods. Egg whites or egg substitutes have no cholesterol and fewer calories than whole eggs.

Sample Menu Plan (~ 1600 kcal)

Breakfast
Porridge with ½ cup oats and 1 cup semi-skimmed milk,
½ cup strawberries,
1 tsp sugar-free peanut butter topped with 1 Tbsp flaxseed and cinnamon

Lunch
1 cup Brussels sprouts or greens with 1 Tbsp olive oil,
5 oz grilled chicken fillet, 1 and 2/3 cup brown rice with carrots and green beans

Dinner
2 cups leafy vegetables (lettuce – spinach) salad with 2 tsp olive oil,
topped with oregano, ¼ avocado,
½ cup low-fat cheese (i.e., cottage, ricotta), and
2 oz whole-grain barley rusk

Snack
1 cup fresh fruit with 30 g almonds and walnuts

B.2. The Dietary Approaches to Stop Hypertension (DASH) Dietary Model

Food group	Servings per day			Serving size	Examples and notes	Significance of each food group to the DASH dietary model
	1600 kcal	2000 kcal	2600 kcal			
Grains	6	6–8	10–11	½ cup of cereal, grain, or pasta, 1 oz of a bread product	Whole-wheat or whole-grain breads, whole-grain breakfast cereals, brown rice, bulgur, quinoa, and oatmeal, cut back on instant or flavored rice, pasta, and cereals.	High in complex carbohydrates and fiber. Naturally low in fat. Look for products labeled "100% whole grain" or "100% whole wheat."
Vegetables	3–4	4–5	5–6	½ cup of cooked vegetables or vegetable juice, 1 cup of raw vegetables	Broccoli, carrots, collards, green beans, green peas, kale, lima beans, potatoes, spinach, squash, sweet potatoes, tomatoes.	Important sources of vitamins, fiber, and other nutrients. High in potassium. Low in sodium.
Fruits	4	4–5	5–6	1 medium fruit, ½ cup of fresh fruit or fruit juice, ¼ cup dried fruit	Apples, apricots, bananas, dates, grapes, oranges, grapefruit, mangoes, melons, peaches, pineapples, raisins, strawberries, tangerines.	Fruits are an excellent source of essential vitamins and minerals, antioxidants, and fiber.
Fat-free or low-fat milk and milk products	2–3	2–3	3	1 cup milk or yogurt	Fat-free milk or buttermilk; fat-free, low-fat, or reduced-fat cheese; fat-free/low-fat regular or frozen yogurt.	Sources of calcium, vitamin D, and protein.
Lean meats, poultry, and fish	3–4	6 or less	6 or less	1 oz (30 g) cooked poultry or fish, 1 egg	Select only lean; trim away visible fats; broil, roast, or poach; remove skin from poultry. Avoid canned or processed type.	Meat can be a rich source of protein, B vitamins, iron, and zinc.
Nuts, seeds, and legumes	3–4 per week	4–5 per week	1	½ cup beans – cooked, ⅓ cup or 1½ ounce nuts, 2 Tbsp peanut butter, 2 Tbsp or ½ ounce seeds	Almonds, hazelnuts, mixed nuts, peanuts, walnuts, sunflower seeds, peanut butter, kidney beans, peas, lentils, black peas, chickpeas, soybean-based products, such as tofu and tempeh.	Sources of magnesium, protein, fiber, and phytochemicals.
Fats and oils	2	2–3	3	1 tsp soft margarine, 1 tsp vegetable oil	Soft margarine, vegetable oil (canola, corn, olive, safflower), low-fat mayonnaise, light salad dressing.	27% of calories as fat, including fat in or added to foods.
Sweets and added sugars	3 or less	5 or less	Once or twice per week	1 Tbsp sugar, jelly, or jam, ½ cup sorbet, 1 cup lemonade	Fruit-flavored gelatin, fruit punch, hard candy, jelly, maple syrup, sorbet and ices, sugar.	Sweets must be low in fats.

- 1500 – 2300 mg sodium daily.
- 1 tsp (5 g) of table salt = 2300 mg sodium.
- About ⅔ tsp of table salt = 1500 mg sodium.
- 1 tsp of sea salt (5 g) =1960 mg of sodium.
- Use herbs, spices, and salt-free seasonings blends (basil, cinnamon, chili, dill, ginger, oregano, parsley, thyme). Rinse canned food to remove some sodium.
- Use alcohol with moderation.
- Be aware of sodium hidden sources (The AHA salty 6: Breads and rolls, pizza, poultry – chicken nuggets, cold cuts, and cured meats, canned, sandwiches).
- Add a serving of vegetables at lunch and at dinner.
- Add a serving of fruit to your meals or as a snack.
- Citrus fruits and juice, such as grapefruit, can interact with certain medications such as calcium channel blockers.

Sample Menu Plan (~ 1600 kcal)

Breakfast
Smoothie with 1 cup fresh, mixed-fruit juice and 200 g low-fat Greek yogurt,
1 Tbsp flaxseed, ½ cup raisin or redberries,
ginger or cinnamon

Lunch
1 cup steamed broccoli with 1 tsp olive oil,
1 cup whole-wheat pasta with ½ cup fresh tomato-basil sauce topped with oregano,
2 oz goat cheese or mozzarella

Dinner
1 cup lettuce – spinach salad with 1 tsp olive oil-oregano-garlic dressing,
mushrooms omelet with 2 yolks, ½ cup mushrooms, ½ cup oat,
1 oz whole-grain barley rusk

Snack
One slice whole-wheat bread with 1 tsp tahini, ½ piece sliced banana topped with grated dark chocolate

B.3. The Vegetarian Dietary Model

Food group	Servings per day			Serving size	Examples and notes	Significance of each food group to the vegetarian dietary model
	1600 kcal	2000 kcal	2600 kcal			
Grains	8	11	13	½ cup of cereal, grain, or pasta, 1 oz of a bread product	Whole-grain breads and cereals, pasta, rice, potatoes, low-fat crackers, and low-fat cookies, fortified cereals.	A good source of energy, fiber, calcium, iron and B vitamins. Fortified cereals are a good source of nonhemic iron.
Vegetables	3	4	4	½ cup of cooked vegetables or vegetable juice, 1 cup of raw vegetables	Seasonal vegetables, dark green vegetables, red and orange vegetables.	Important sources of vitamins, fiber. Dark green vegetables such as watercress, broccoli, and spring greens are a good source of non-heme iron.
Fruits	3	4	5	1 medium fruit, ½ cup of fresh fruit or fruit juice, ¼ cup dried fruit	Seasonal fruits.	Dried fruits are a good source of non-heme iron.
Dairy	2	2	3	1 cup milk or yogurt, ½ cup very low-fat cheese (e.g., cottage) - animal/plant based	Milk and dairy alternatives, such as fortified unsweetened soy, rice, and oat drinks.	Good sources of protein, calcium, vitamins A and B_{12}.
Protein: Plant-based proteins Cheese Egg	5	7	9	½ cup beans – cooked/ ½ cup plant protein (e.g., quinoa, soy products, mushrooms, etc.), 1 oz (30 g) cheese, 1 egg	Legumes: beans, peas, lentils, fortified yeast extracts, soy products, quinoa, seitan, mushrooms.	Legumes are a low-fat source of protein, fiber, vitamins (especially B_{12}), and minerals. Cheese and egg are good sources of B_{12}. Other non-dairy sources of protein include eggs and meat alternatives, such as tofu, textured vegetable protein, and tempeh.

Food group	Servings per day			Serving size	Examples and notes	Significance of each food group to the vegetarian dietary model
	1600 kcal	2000 kcal	2600 kcal			
Nuts and seeds	Once or twice daily			30 g of nuts or 2 Tbsp seeds	Almonds, walnuts, cashews, peanuts, flaxseed, pumpkin seeds, chia seeds.	Sources of protein and polyunsaturated fat.
Fats and oils	7	8	11	1 tsp soft margarine, 1 tsp vegetable oil /paste	Olive oil, flaxseed (linseed) oil, rapeseed oil, soya oil, tahini, peanut butter, avocado	Important sources of omega-3 fatty acids.
Sweets and added sugars	Once or twice per week			1 Tbsp sugar, jelly, or jam, ½ cup sorbet, 1 cup lemonade	Low-fat ice cream, baked goods, fruit compote	Sweets must be low in fats and added sugars. Fruits can satisfy craving for sweets.

- Replace the protein provided by meat by a variety of protein-rich plant foods like nuts, seeds, legumes, tempeh, tofu, and seitan.
- Combine plant proteins. Grains and legumes are called complementary protein sources because when you combine them, you get all of the essential amino acids. Nuts and seeds are also complementary to legumes because they contain tryptophan, methionine, and cystine.
- Amaranth, quinoa, hemp seed, and chia are complete proteins.

Sample Menu Plan (~ 1600 kcal)

Breakfast
200 g rice milk with 1 tsp honey, 1 Tbsp chia seeds, ½ cup oatmeal, and cinnamon

Lunch
1 cup quinoa salad with ½ cup lentils,
1 cup tomato and green – red peppers, with chopped fresh parsley,
1 Tbsp olive oil and vinegar,
½ cup cottage cheese

Dinner
1 oz whole-wheat wraps with 2 Tbsp guacamole and 1 cup grilled mushrooms and peppers

Snack
1½ cup mixed fresh fruit salad with 1 tsp sugar-free peanut butter/30 g almonds

B.4. Dietary Considerations and Requirements for Christians

(Disclaimer: the following dietary information and sample menu plan are given as generic guides and are not intended to replace specific religious dietary requirements)

Food group	Servings per day			Serving size	Examples and notes	Significance of each food group to fasting in Christianity
	1600 kcal	2000 kcal	2600 kcal			
Grains	8	11	13	½ cup of cereal, grain, or pasta, 1 oz of a bread product	Whole-grain breads and cereals, whole-grain pasta, and rice products, barley, buckwheat, bulgur, farro, millet, oats, polenta, rice, wheatberries, breads, couscous, and pastas.	Grains constitute the main source of energy, rich in fiber, and B vitamins.

(Continued)

Food group	Servings per day			Serving size	Examples and notes	Significance of each food group to fasting in Christianity
	1600 kcal	2000 kcal	2600 kcal			
Vegetables	4	5	6	½ cup of cooked vegetables or vegetable juice, 1 cup of raw vegetables	Seasonal vegetables: xorta (greens – radishes), artichokes, beets, broccoli, cabbage, carrots, celery, celeriac, chicory, collard cucumbers, dandelion eggplant, fennel, kale, leeks, lemons, lettuce, onions, peppers, pumpkin, purslane.	Important sources of vitamins, fiber, and antioxidants; variety of colors and textures provide a diversity of antioxidants and protective compounds.
Fruits	4	5	6	1 medium fruit, ½ cup of fresh fruit or fruit juice, ¼ cup dried fruit	Seasonal fruits: apples, apricots, avocados, cherries, clementines, dates, figs, grapefruits, oranges, pears, pomegranates, strawberries, tangerines.	Important sources of vitamins, fiber, and antioxidants.
Legumes, dairy products, and animal protein	4	5	7	1 oz seafood, ½ cup legumes, 1 cup milk or yogurt 1/2 cup cheese	Seafood (fish, clams, shells, octopus, etc.). Legumes: beans, lentils, chickpeas, fava beans, green beans, kidney beans. Milk, sour milk, cheese, yogurt.	Legumes are a low-fat source of protein, fiber, vitamins, and minerals. The combination of legumes and cereals is a healthy protein and lipid source.
	Fasting is personal and can vary in length and foods avoided. Meat and meat products are usually forbidden. Fish is not allowed during Easter's fasting, but it is allowed during Christmas fasting. Roman Catholics allow only fish on Fridays during the Lent season but not other meats. Shellfish, shrimps, clams, and seafood (fish roe "taramas") are allowed.					
Nuts, seeds	Nuts: once or twice daily			30 g of nuts, 2 Tbsp seeds	Almonds, walnuts, cashews, peanuts, flaxseed, pumpkin seeds, pistachios, sesame seeds.	Good sources of healthy fats, protein, and fiber. They add flavor and texture to Mediterranean dishes.
Fats and oils	11	12	13	1 tsp vegetable paste, 1 tsp vegetable oil	Olive oil, olives, peanut butter without added hydrogenated fat, tahini (sesame seed paste).	Extra-virgin olive oil is highest in health-promoting fats, phytonutrients, and other important micronutrients. High resistance to cooking temperatures.
Herbs and spices	In every meal				Anise, basil, bay leaf, chiles, cloves, cumin, fennel, garlic, lavender, marjoram, mint, oregano, parsley, pepper, pul biber, rosemary, sage, savory, sumac, tarragon, thyme.	They add flavors and aromas, reducing the need to add salt or fat. Rich in antioxidants. They contribute to the national identities of the various Mediterranean cuisines.
Sweets and added sugars	Limited sweets: once or twice per week. Sweets with animal protein (e.g., egg, butter) are not allowed.			1 Tbsp sweet spoons, 3–4 oz syrup desserts	Halva, fruit sweet spoons.	Fresh fruits are the typical daily dessert, with sweets based on nuts and made with olive oil.

- Orthodox Christian fasting incorporates voluntary abstention from specific foods for 180–200 days per year.
- Meat as well as dairy products and eggs are forbidden during fasting.
- Periodic vegetarian diet (including vegetables, legumes, nuts, fruits, olives, bread, snails, and seafood), constitutes one type of the Mediterranean diet.

Sample Menu Plan (~ 1600 kcal)

Breakfast
Herbal tea, 2 Tbsp halvah, with 2 oz whole-wheat rusk

Lunch
2 cups lettuce – tomato with 1 Tbsp olive oil, and fresh dill,
2 cups bean soup with olive oil, 30 g pickled vegetables, 1 oz whole-wheat bread and 8–10 olives

Dinner
1 cup xorta with 1 Tbsp olive oil,
2 Tbsp fish roe dip and 2 oz whole-wheat rusk

Snack
Two fresh fruits and 30 g almonds/2 oz brittle

B.5. Dietary Considerations and Requirements for Buddhists

(Disclaimer: the following dietary information and sample menu plan are given as generic guides and are not intended to replace specific religious dietary requirements)

Food group	Servings per day			Serving size	Examples and notes	Significance of each food group
	1600 kcal	2000 kcal	2600 kcal			
Grains	8	12	14	½ cup of cereal or grains, 1 oz of a bread product	Thai rice vermicelli, rice, jasmine rice, glutinous rice or sticky rice, black glutinous rice, rice noodles, rice flour, tapioca flour, narrow rice noodle, rice vermicelli (thin), wide rice noodle, cellophane noodles, or glass noodles.	Rich in fiber, vitamin B complex, and phytochemicals.
Vegetables	4	5	6	½ cup of cooked vegetables or vegetable juice, 1 cup of raw vegetables	Sweet potato, lotus root, taro, cassava, jicama, noni leaves, *luffa aegyptiaca*, luffa acutangular, piper sarmentosum, kabocha, shallot, white cabbage, cabbage sprouts, *senna siamea*, okra, pea, eggplant, tomato, bitter melon drumstick, bamboo shoot, green asparagus, water spinach, *oenanthe javanica*, bok choy, Chinese cabbage, mustard greens, Chinese broccoli or Kai-lan, *limnophila aromatica*, amaranthus spp, water mimosa, *leucaena leucocephala*, choy sum, spider plant, *marsilea crenata*, melientha suavis, tree bean, stink bean. cucumber, *limnocharis flava*, yardlong beans, bean sprouts, winged bean, soybean.	Wholesome plant foods are the base for each food. Important sources of vitamins, fiber, and antioxidants.
Fruits	5	5	6	1 medium fruit, ½ cup of fresh fruit or fruit juice, ¼ cup dried fruit	Guava, dragonfruit, Thai chestnut, jackfruit, banana, water caltrop, roselle, santol, sapodilla, longan, duku, caimito, burmese grape, tamarind, madras thorn, papaya, lotus seed, mango, lime, mangosteen, coconut, rambutan, sugar-apple, jujube, snake fruit, passionfruit, pineapple, pomelo, bilimbi, durian.	Important sources of vitamins, fiber, and antioxidants.

(Continued)

Food group	Servings per day			Serving size	Examples and notes	Significance of each food group
	1600 kcal	2000 kcal	2600 kcal			
Dairy	1	1	2	1 cup milk	Coconut milk, almond milk, rice milk, soy milk.	Sources of protein, calcium, vitamins A and D.
	Dairy are allowed, but plant-based milk is commonly used.					
Meat Poultry Egg Legumes Fish	2	3	4	1 oz (30 g) of cheese, ½ cup legumes	Beans (adzuki, edamame, mung, soy), lentils, miso, tempeh, tofu.	Legumes are a low-fat source of protein, fiber, vitamins, and minerals. Usually combined with whole-wheat grain and vegetables.
	Meat/fish/egg/poultry are usually forbidden. Buddhists who are not strict vegetarians will eat fish and/or will add it to many of their meals.					
Nuts, seeds	Daily			30 g of nuts, 2 Tbsp seeds	Almonds, cashews, hazelnuts, peanuts, sesame seeds.	Good sources of healthy fats, protein, and fiber.
Fats and oils	7	9	12	1 tsp vegetable paste, 1 tsp vegetable oil	Peanut, sesame, palm, coconut, soybean oil.	These types of oil are low-smoke, as is desirable for frying or grilling, and they do not break down quickly. Peanut oil is often used for stir-frying and deep-frying. Coconut and palm oils have the characteristic of being mostly solid at room temperature.
Herbs and spices	Onions, scallions, chives, garlic are forbidden.				Pandan or screwpine leaves, tiliacora triandra, chives, Thai sweet basil, galangal, turmeric, ginger, fingerroot, Holy basil, lemon basil, coriander/cilantro leaves, cilantro, dill, Vietnamese coriander, chili spur pepper, fresh peppercorns, wax pepper, sweet pepper, bell pepper, coriander/cilantro root. Spearmint, lemon grass, makrut lime, kaffir lime, lime.	Aroma and flavor; spices are rich in antioxidants.
Sweets and added sugars	Limited sweets			3–4 oz piece, 1 tsp maple syrup	Coconut-rice pancakes, sweet, sticky rice topped with fruits and nuts.	Meals finish with fresh fruit, sometimes sweet snacks, often eaten between meals, will also be served as a dessert.

- Alcohol is forbidden.
- Buddhists are usually vegetarian or lacto-vegetarian. In general, Buddhists abstain from meat consumption, and all of them exclude beef products from their diet. Buddhism prohibits the eating of any and all meat, because (i) the killing of animals violates the First Moral Precept, and (ii) meat is considered an intoxicant to the body.
- Herbal tea is a popular and healing drink that originates from various types of tea plants.

Sample Menu Plan (~ 1600 kcal)

Breakfast
½ cup oatmeal with 1 cup almond milk, 30 g nuts topped with 1 tsp maple syrup, 1 Tbsp sesame seeds, ½ cup shoyu, and pieces of nori

Lunch
1 cup quinoa salad with 1 cup seasonal veggies, ½ piece avocado diced, and 1 oz tempeh, topped with fresh parsley and lemon juice

Dinner
1 cup whole-wheat rice with 2 oz tofu and 1 cup carrots, asparagus, bamboo shoots, cabbage, mushrooms

Snack
Two fresh fruits and 30 g nuts

B.6. Dietary Considerations and Requirements for Hindus

(Disclaimer: the following dietary information and sample menu plan are given as generic guides and are not intended to replace specific religious dietary requirements)

Food group	Servings per day			Serving size	Examples and notes	Significance of each food group
	1600 kcal	2000 kcal	2600 kcal			
Grains	8	11	13	½ cup of cereal, grains, 1 oz of a bread product	Amaranth, pearl millet, sorghum, ragi, rice, wheat, maize, coarse cereals, roti, dosas.	Protein, fiber, minerals, calcium, iron, and B-complex vitamins.
Vegetables	3	4	4	½ cup of cooked vegetables or vegetable juice, 1 cup of raw vegetables	Okra, cauliflower, bitter-gourd, bean, cabbage, ridge gourd, spinach, fenugreek, eggplant, pumpkin, amaranth, colocasia leaves. coriander leaves, curry leaves, dill, drumstick leaves, fenugreek leaves, lettuce leaves, mint, mustard seeds, leaves, sorrel leaves, spinach.	A normal diet, to be wholesome and tasty, should include fresh vegetables and fruits, which are storehouses of micronutrients. Vegetables/fruits are rich sources of micronutrients.
Fruits	3	4	5	1 medium fruit, ½ cup of fresh fruit or fruit juice, ¼ cup dried fruit	Orange, guava, banana, pineapple, tezpur litchi, mangoes, strawberries, grapes, pomegranates, custard apple, dahanu gholvad chikoo, kachai lemon, ganganagar, mosambi (*citrus limetta*), apples, apricots, figs, pears, jungli jalebi or camachile, Japani Phal, or persimmon.	Fruits and vegetables also provide phytonutrients and fiber, which are of vital health significance.
Dairy	2	2	3	1 cup milk or yogurt	Butter, yogurt, creamy Dahi, shrikhand, mishti doi, lassi, and chaas.	Sources of protein, calcium, vitamins A and D.
	Milk and milk products are permitted.					
Meat Poultry Egg Legumes Fish	5	7	9	1 oz (30 g) cheese ½ cup legumes	Paneer chhena, pulses, green gram beans (mung beans), split green gram and skinned green gram, black-eyed beans, red lentils and split red lentils, yellow pigeon peas, adzuki beans.	Pulses are a low-fat source of protein, fiber, vitamins, and minerals. Cottage cheese is rich in protein and leucine.
	Meat is forbidden, along with all meat products. Eggs are forbidden. Cheese must not be coagulated with rennet (an animal product). Mushrooms are forbidden along with all other fungi. Fish is allowed.					
Nuts, seeds	Often			30 g of nuts, 2 Tbsp seeds	Almonds, cashews, hazelnuts, peanuts, sesame seeds, flaxseed (alsi), perilla seeds (Bhanjira), fenugreek seed (methi), mustard (sarson).	Good sources of healthy fats, protein, and fiber.
Fats and oils	7	8	11	1 tsp vegetable paste/chutney, 1 tsp vegetable oil	Chutney: Coconut/groundnuts/until ghee, mustard oil, sunflower oil, rice bran oil, flaxseed oil, groundnut oil, palm oil.	Like any clarified butter, ghee is composed almost entirely of fat, 62% of which consists of saturated fats. Mustard oil has about 60% monounsaturated fatty acids and about 21% polyunsaturated fats. Ensure moderate use of edible oils and animal foods and less use of ghee/ butter/ vanaspati.

(Continued)

Food group	Servings per day			Serving size	Examples and notes	Significance of each food group
	1600 kcal	2000 kcal	2600 kcal			
Herbs and spices	Onions – forbidden along with all other members of the *allium* genus, including garlic, scallions, chives, shallots, etc.				Black pepper, cardamom, chili peppers, cinnamon, coriander seeds, cumin seeds, turmeric.	Aroma and flavor. Recommended spices are rich in antioxidants without calories, fat, or sugar. They provide healthful phytonutrient rich antioxidants.
Sweets and added sugars	Once or twice per week			3–4 oz piece (1/2 cup)	Besan barfi, chikki fruit cake, rice puttu, sandesh double ka meetha, halwa (kesari), jelly/jam, custard (caramel) srikhand, milk chocolate, ice cream.	Many Indian desserts are fried foods made with sugar, milk, or condensed milk.

- Tamasic (heavy) foods, such as meat and fermented foods (including alcohol), promote dullness and inertia.
- Rajasic (expanding) foods, including onions, garlic, hot spices, stimulants, fish, eggs, and salt, are thought to excite intellect and passion, which interfere with meditation.
- Sattvic (ascending) foods, including fruits, vegetables, and grains, are thought to promote transcendence, sublimity, and orderliness.
- Stimulants – coffee, tea, etc.– are rajastic and to be avoided, as they interfere with meditation.
- Alcohol is not allowed.

Sample Menu Plan (~ 1600 kcal)

Breakfast
2 oz steamed rice-dough pancakes (idli), 2 Tbsp chutney, and 1 cup sambar

Lunch
1 oz roti (Indian flatbread) and 1 cup red lentil dal with 2 oz cottage cheese, 1 Tbsp chutney, and 1 oz pickles

Dinner
Two dosas (thin crepes made of rice and lentils) and 1 cup korma (curry made of yogurt, seed paste, nuts, and seasonal vegetables)

Snack
½ cup carrot halwa: carrots, milk, sugar, cashews, and raisins

B.7. Dietary Considerations and Requirements for Jews

(Disclaimer: the following dietary information and sample menu plan are given as generic guides and are not intended to replace specific religious dietary requirements)

Food group	Servings per day			Serving size	Examples and notes	Significance of each food group
	1600 kcal	2000 kcal	2600 kcal			
Grains	8	11	13	½ cup of cereal or other grains, 1 oz of a bread product	Barley, kamut, millet, teff, oats, freekeh, bulgur, sorghum, buckwheat, amaranth, quinoa, chia, farro, couscous.	Vitamins, minerals, protein, energy.
Vegetables	3	4	4	½ cup of cooked vegetables or vegetable juice, 1 cup of raw vegetables	Seasonal vegetables: tomato, cucumber, onion, pepper, celery, sweet potato, pumpkin, zucchini.	All foods that grow in the soil or on plants, bushes, or trees are viewed as kosher, with the exception of hybrid fruits and vegetables. Insects are not kosher, so foods prone to insect infestation, such as cauliflower, must be carefully examined.
Fruits	3	4	5	1 medium fruit, ½ cup of fresh fruit or fruit juice, ¼ cup dried fruit	Seasonal fruits: orange, guava, banana, pineapple, strawberries, grapes, pomegranates, apples, apricots, figs, pears.	

Food group	Servings per day			Serving size	Examples and notes	Significance of each food group
	1600 kcal	2000 kcal	2600 kcal			
Dairy	2	2	3	1 cup milk or yogurt	Low-fat soya drink, tahini from whole sesame.	Sources of protein, calcium, vitamins A and D.
	Milk and milk products are permitted.					
Meat Poultry Egg Legumes Fish	5	7	9	1 oz (30 g) meat, cheese, ½ cup legumes	Beans, soya, lupins, lentils, and chickpeas, pollock and halibut, hake, sole, salmon, tuna.	Chicken makes up the main part of the consumption of animal food products in Israel. The most consumed legume in Israel is the chickpea, mainly in salads and spreads. Cooked chickpeas are eaten less.
	Pork is forbidden. Beef, goat, lamb, poultry are allowed. Fish (but not all) are permitted. Meat must not be combined with dairy. Fish, eggs, turkey/chicken: on a weekly basis. Red meat: no more than 300 g per week.					
Nuts, seeds	Every day			30 g of nuts, 2 Tbsp seeds	Nuts, almonds, peanuts, sunflower seeds, pumpkin seeds, whole sesame seeds.	Good sources of healthy fats, protein, vitamins, minerals, and dietary fiber.
Fats and oils	7	8	11	1 tsp vegetable paste, 1 tsp vegetable oil	Olive oil, canola oil or other vegetable oils. Tahini and almonds, avocado, oil canola, oil olive.	Olive oil should be the main source of fat in the diet due to its high nutritional quality. Olive oil substitutes can be avocado, canola oil (rapeseed), and tahini from whole sesame seeds.
Herbs and spices	In every meal				Anise, cassia, cinnamon, cumin, marjoram, and myrrh. Basil, chervil, cumin, coriander, dill, marjoram, mint, oregano, poppy seed, savory, and tarragon.	It is recommended to use spices, since they contribute many flavors and assist in reducing salt consumption.
Sweets and added sugars	Once or twice per week			3–4 oz piece (1/2 cup)	Sufganiyot, babka, hamantaschen, bagel, apple cake.	Sweet snacks, sweet beverages: reduce consumption significantly.

- Menu is rich in varied foods from a vegetable source.
- Most foods are unprocessed or have undergone minimal processing.
- Infrequent use of fats, salt, and sugar for seasoning and food preparation.

Sample Menu Plan (~ 1600 kcal)

Breakfast
2 oz bagel with cinnamon, cream cheese, and apple

Lunch
1 cup couscous steamed, served with 1 cup seasonal vegetables and 1 cup beef soup

Dinner
Hummuschipsalat: 1 cup tomatoes and cucumbers dressed in olive oil, lemon juice, salt and pepper, hummus, and 10–15 French fries ("chips") served in a pita – 1 oz

Snack
Two fruits, 30 g nuts

B.8. Dietary Considerations and Requirements for Muslims during Ramadan

(Disclaimer: the following dietary information and sample menu plan are given as generic guides and are not intended to replace specific religious dietary requirements)

Food group	Servings per day			Serving size	Examples and notes	Significance of each food group during Ramadan
	1600 kcal	2000 kcal	2600 kcal			
Grains	8	11	13	½ cup of cereal or grains, 1 oz of a bread product	Barley, kamut, millet, teff, oats, freekeh, bulgur, sorghum, buckwheat, amaranth, quinoa, chia, farro.	Avoid various types of ready-made bread products rich in salt. Meals should include carbohydrates such as rice, pasta, bread, etc.
Vegetables	3	4	4	½ cup of cooked vegetables or vegetable juice, 1 cup of raw vegetables	Seasonal vegetables: olive, onion, cucumber, gourd, mustard seed.	Vegetables and fruits will keep you hydrated. It is recommended to choose appetizers that are rich in vegetables such as fatoush, green salad, and tabouleh without any added salt. Include a salad to ensure that the body's requirements for fiber, vitamins, and minerals are met.
Fruits	3	4	5	1 medium fruit, ½ cup of fresh fruit or fruit juice, ¼ cup dried fruit	Seasonal fruits: orange, banana, pineapple, strawberries, grapes, pomegranates, apples, apricots, figs, pears, dates.	Fruits are rich in fiber and are also digested slowly (raw and unpeeled). They provide fluids as they maintain water and salt levels in the body. Fruit (for breaking the fast) provides natural sugars for energy, fluid, and some vitamins and minerals.
Dairy	2	2	3	1 cup milk or yogurt	Milk, yogurt, labneh, cheese, and kefir.	Dairy products facilitate digestion and help to remain dry for longer.
	Milk and milk products are permitted.					
Meat Poultry Egg Legumes Fish	5	7	9	1 oz (30 g) cheese, 1 oz (30 g) meat, ½ cup legumes	Pork is forbidden. Beef, goat, lamb, poultry are allowed, fish.	Grilled or baked lean meat, skinless chicken, and fish, to get a good portion of healthy protein. In general, avoid fried and processed foods high in fat.
Nuts, seeds	Every day			30 g of nuts, 2 Tbsp seeds	Nuts, almonds, peanuts, sunflower seeds.	Good source of healthy fats, protein, vitamins, minerals, and dietary fiber.
Fats and oils	7	8	11	1 tsp vegetable paste, 1 tsp vegetable oil	Sunflower oil, corn oil, hazelnut oil, or olive oil.	Fatty meals must be avoided. Instead of frying and roasting, cooking methods such as grilling and baking are preferred.
Herbs and spices	In every meal				Anise, cassia, cinnamon, cumin, marjoram and myrrh, basil, chervil, cumin, coriander, dill, mint, oregano, poppy seed, savory and tarragon.	It is recommended to use spices since they contribute many flavors and assist in reducing salt consumption.
Sweets and added sugars	Avoid					Stay away from sweets that can increase your feeling of hunger a few hours after you start your fast.

- Avoid consumption of foods rich in fat, especially fatty meats, foods made with puff pastry, or pastry with added fat/margarine or butter.
- Avoid foods containing large amounts of salt, e.g., sausages, processed and salted meat and fish products, olives and pickles, snack foods, salty cheeses, various types of ready-made crackers, salads, spreads, and sauces (such as mayonnaise, mustard, ketchup).
- Eat slowly and in amounts appropriate to the needs of each individual.
- Stay hydrated.

Sample Menu Plan (~ 1600 kcal)

Suhoor (the meal eaten before sunrise)
1 cup tomato and cucumber salad with 1 egg, 1 cup bean soup (foul), ½ cup yogurt, 6–8 small olives, 1 oz whole-grain bread, and water or unsweetened drinks

Iftar (the meal eaten after sunset)
¼ cup dates, 1 cup salad with tomatoes, cucumber, and greens with lemon/vinegar dressing or olive oil dressing, 1 cup soup with 4 oz grilled or broiled chicken, 1 cup mixed vegetables and 1 cup whole-grain rice, water or unsweetened drinks

Snack
¼ cup dates/30 g walnuts, milk and water or unsweetened drinks

B.9. The Nordic Dietary Model

Food group	Servings per day			Serving size	Examples and notes	Significance of each food group to the Nordic dietary model
	1600 kcal	2000 kcal	2600 kcal			
Grains	8	11	13	½ cup of cereal or grains, 1 oz of a bread product	Oat, oat drink, pasta, rice, breakfast cereals barley, rye, wheat emmer, and spelt.	Choose cereal products that are high in fiber and whole grains and low in fat, sugar, and salt.
Vegetables	3	4	4	½ cup of cooked vegetables or vegetable juice, 1 cup of raw vegetables	Carrots, corn, cucumbers, garlic, lettuce, onions, peppers, potatoes, pumpkin, beans, tomatoes, cabbage, cauliflower, Brussels sprouts, broccoli, spinach, kohlrabi, and kale.	Make vegetables a part of all meals of the day. Potatoes contain fiber, vitamins, and minerals.
Fruits	3	4	5	1 medium fruit, ½ cup of fresh fruit or fruit juice, ¼ cup dried fruit	Lemons, apples, oranges, peaches, figs, pears, pineapples, grapes, strawberries, bananas, watermelon, plums avocados, bilberries, black currants.	Important sources of vitamins, minerals, and antioxidants.
Dairy	2	2	3	1 cup milk or yogurt	Milk, yogurt, soya milk.	Rich in protein, vitamin D, calcium.
	Choose dairy products that are low in fat, salt, and added sugar.					
Meat Poultry Egg Legumes Fish	5	7	9	1 oz (30 g) cheese, 1 oz meat/fish, ½ cup legumes	Fatty fish (salmon, rainbow trout, Baltic herring), low-fat fish (tuna, pike, perch), lean cuts of meat, white meat, chicken, game meats, free-range eggs, lentils, beans, and yellow and green peas; tofu is one vegetarian alternative to meat.	Grilled or baked lean meat, skinless chicken and fish, to get a good portion of healthy protein. In general, avoid fried and processed foods high in fat.
	Eat fish for dinner 2–3 times a week. Fish is also a great filling in sandwiches. Choose lean meat and lean meat products. Limit the amount of processed meat and red meat you consume.					
Nuts, seeds		Every day		30 g of nuts, 2 Tbsp seeds	Nuts, almonds, peanuts, sunflower seeds.	Good source of healthy fats, protein, vitamins, minerals, and dietary fiber.

(Continued)

Food group	Servings per day			Serving size	Examples and notes	Significance of each food group to the Nordic dietary model
	1600 kcal	2000 kcal	2600 kcal			
Fats and oils	7	8	11	1 tsp vegetable paste, 1 tsp vegetable oil	Canola oil, rapeseed oil, liquid margarine, and soft margarine over hard margarine and butter.	Replace foods that are high in saturated fat with foods with more unsaturated fat. The softer the margarine and butter are at fridge temperature, the higher the content of unsaturated fat.
Herbs and spices	In every meal				Parsley, mustard, horseradish, chive, thyme, cardamom, juniper, berries, and fennel, dill.	Aroma and flavor.
Sweets and added sugars	Once or twice a week				Pie with rye, pancakes, waffles.	Avoid foods and drinks that are high in sugar.

– Less saturated fat, less sugar, less salt.
– More fiber and whole grains.
– The Nordic diet is very similar to the Mediterranean diet. The biggest difference is that it emphasizes canola oil instead of extra-virgin olive oil.
– The Nordic diet wasn't designed to reflect the diet of Nordic people hundreds of years ago. Instead, it emphasizes healthy foods that are sourced locally in modern-day Scandinavia.
– Reduced food wastage and a more plant-based diet will contribute to reducing the impact on the environment.

Sample Menu Plan (~ 1600 kcal)

Breakfast
Tea and 1 slice rye bread with ½ cup cottage cheese and ½ cup berries

Lunch
1 cup cabbage with 1 tsp rapeseed oil, 3 oz grilled salmon with 1 cup boiled potatoes and carrots

Dinner
1 whole-wheat wrap with ½ cup avocado, spinach, cucumber, 2 oz tuna

Snack
1 apple sliced with 1 cup low-fat yogurt and 1 Tbsp sunflower seeds/oatmeal with egg

B.10. The Healthy Asian Dietary Model

Food group	Servings per day			Serving size	Examples and notes	Significance of each food group to the Asian dietary model
	1600 kcal	2000 kcal	2600 kcal			
Grains	8	12	14	½ cup of cereal, grains, or pasta, 1 oz of a bread product	Barley, breads (dumplings, chapatis, mantou, naan, roti), buckwheat, millet, noodles (rice, soba, somen, udon), rice.	Most important staple dishes across Asia. Rich in fiber, vitamin B complex, and phytochemicals.
Vegetables	4	5	6	½ cup of cooked vegetables or vegetable juice, 1 cup of raw vegetables	Bamboo shoots, bean sprouts, bitter melon, bok choy, broccoli, cabbage, carrots, daikon, eggplant, leeks, lettuce, lotus root, kale, kombu, mushrooms, mustard greens, peppers, seaweed, snow peas, spinach, sweet potatoes, taro root, turnips, water chestnuts, yams.	Wholesome plant foods are the base for each food. Important sources of vitamins, fiber, and antioxidants.

Food group	Servings per day			Serving size	Examples and notes	Significance of each food group to the Asian dietary model
	1600 kcal	2000 kcal	2600 kcal			
Fruits	5	5	6	1 medium fruit, ½ cup of fresh fruit or fruit juice, ¼ cup dried fruit	Apricots, bananas, cherries, coconut, dates, dragon fruit, grapes, kiwifruit, kumquat, lemons, limes, longan, lychee, mandarins, mangoes, mangosteen, melons, milk fruit, oranges, papaya, pears, pineapple, plums, pumpkin, rambutan, tangerines, yuzu.	Important sources of vitamins, fiber, and antioxidants. Basil for every meal.
Dairy	1	1	2	1 cup non-lactose milk or yogurt	Paneer yogurt (chaas, lassi), non-lactose: almond milk, rice milk, soy milk.	Good sources of protein, calcium, vitamins A and D.
	Dairy foods often but in small portions.					
Meat Poultry Egg Legumes Fish	2	3	4	1 oz of all kind of meats, 1 oz (30 g) cheese, 1 egg, ½ cup legumes	Beans (adzuki, edamame, mung, soy), lentils, miso, tempeh, tofu abalone, bonito, clams, cockles, crab, eel, king fish, mussels, octopus, oysters, roe, salmon, scallops, sea bass, shrimp, squid, tuna, whelk, yellowtail chicken, duck, quail chicken eggs, duck eggs, quail eggs, ghee, beef, pork.	Legumes are a low-fat source of protein, fiber, vitamins, and minerals. Usually combined with whole-wheat grain and vegetables. Fish are good sources of animal protein and healthy fats.
	Eggs, poultry, and some dairy foods often, but in small amounts. Red meats sparingly for special occasions, and only in small portions. Fish and shellfish at least twice a week.					
Nuts, seeds	Daily			30 g of nuts, 2 Tbsp seeds	Almonds, cashews, hazelnuts, peanuts, sesame seeds.	Good sources of healthy fats, protein, and fiber.
Fats and oils	7	9	12	1 tsp vegetable paste, 1 tsp vegetable oil	Peanut, sesame, palm, coconut, soybean oil.	Peanut and soybean oil have high smoke point and are suitable for wok cooking and deep frying. Dark sesame oil tends to have a stronger aroma, flavor, and is typically enjoyed as a condiment.
Herbs and spices	In every meal				Amchoor, asafetida, basil (Thai), cardamom, chiles, clove, coriander, curry leaves, fennel, fenugreek, galangal, garlic, ginger, ginseng, lemongrass, makrut lime leaves, masala, mint, parsley, pepper, scallion, star anise, turmeric, wasabi.	Aroma and flavor, rich in antioxidants. Used in Asian traditional medicine.
Sweets and added sugars	Limited sweets			3–4 oz piece	Chinese mooncakes, rice pudding, Japanese sugared sweet potatoes, Thai mango-coconut pudding balls.	Eaten sparingly.

- Hydrate with tea and water.
- Moderate alcohol (like sake, beer, or wine).
- Share meals with others.
- Be physically active (traditional Asian exercises, such as Tai Chi or yoga).

Sample Menu Plan (~ 1600 kcal)

Breakfast
1 cup steamed rice, ½ cup natto, and ½ cup seaweed salad

Lunch
1½ cup shiitake-mushroom soup, 2 oz rice cakes, 1 oz seared scallops, and 1 cup steamed vegetables

Dinner
1 cup miso soup, 1 cup brown rice, 1 oz vegetable tempura and 2 oz salmon or tuna sashimi

Snack
2 oz rice crackers, ½ cup wasabi peas

B.11. The Mediterranean Dietary Model

Food group	Servings per day			Serving size	Examples and notes	Significance of each food group to the Mediterranean dietary model
	1600 kcal	2000 kcal	2600 kcal			
Grains	8	9	13	½ cup of cereal, grain, or pasta, 1 oz of a bread product	Whole-grain breads and cereals, whole-grain pasta and rice products: barley, buckwheat, bulgur, farro, millet, oats, polenta, rice, wheatberries, breads, couscous, and pastas.	A good source of energy, fiber, and B vitamins; some valuable nutrients (magnesium, phosphorus, etc.) and fiber can be lost during processing.
Vegetables	4	4	5	½ cup of cooked vegetables or vegetable juice, 1 cup of raw vegetables	Seasonal vegetables: xorta (greens – radishes), artichokes, beets, broccoli, cabbage, carrots, celery, celeriac, chicory, collard cucumbers, dandelion, eggplant, fennel, kale, leeks, lemons, lettuce, onions, peppers, pumpkin, purslane.	Important sources of vitamins, fiber, and antioxidants. Variety of colors and textures provide a diversity of antioxidants and protective compounds.
Fruits	3	4	5	1 medium fruit, ½ cup of fresh fruit or fruit juice, ¼ cup dried fruit	Seasonal fruits: apples, apricots, cherries, clementines, dates, figs, grapefruits, grapes, melons, nectarines, oranges, peaches, pears, pomegranates, strawberries, tangerines.	Important sources of vitamins, fiber, and antioxidants. Should be chosen as the most frequent dessert.
Dairy	1	2	2	1 cup milk or yogurt	Milk and dairy, goat's milk and yogurt, brie, chevre, corvo, feta, haloumi, manchego, parmigiano-reggiano, pecorino, ricotta, yogurt.	Good sources of protein, calcium, vitamins A and D.
	Moderate portions of dairy foods.					
Lean cuts of meat Poultry Egg Legumes	3	4	7	1 oz meat, 1 oz (30 g) cheese, 1 egg, ½ cup legumes	Red meats, free-range goat, sheep, lamb, and poultry. Seafood (fish, clams, shells, octopus, etc.). Goat and sheep cheese (feta, halloumi, mizithra). Legumes: beans, lentils, chickpeas, fava beans, green beans, kidney beans.	Legumes are a low-fat source of protein, fiber, vitamins, and minerals. The combination of legumes and cereals is a healthy protein and lipid source. Fish and eggs are good sources of animal protein. Fish and shellfish are also good sources of healthy fats.
	Fish at least once or twice each week. Red meat (less than two servings, preferably lean cuts). Processed meat once or less per week. Moderate portions of cheese eggs (2–4 servings), and occasional poultry. Legumes: at least twice per week					

Food group	Servings per day			Serving size	Examples and notes	Significance of each food group to the Mediterranean dietary model
	1600 kcal	2000 kcal	2600 kcal			
Nuts, seeds	Nuts: once or twice daily			30 g	Almonds, walnuts, cashews, peanuts, flaxseed, pumpkin seeds, pistachios, sesame seeds.	Good sources of healthy fats, protein, and fiber. They add flavor and texture to Mediterranean dishes.
Fats and oils	11	12	13	1 tsp vegetable paste, 1 tsp vegetable oil	Olive oil, olives, peanut butter without added hydrogenated fat. Tahini (sesame seed paste).	Extra-virgin olive oil is highest in health-promoting fats, phytonutrients, and other important micronutrients. High resistance to cooking temperatures.
Herbs and spices	In every meal				Anise, basil, bay leaf, chiles, cloves, cumin, fennel, garlic, lavender, marjoram, mint, oregano, parsley, pepper, rosemary, sage, savory, sumac, tarragon, thyme.	They add flavors and aromas, reducing the need to add salt or fat. Rich in antioxidants. They contribute to the national identities of the various Mediterranean cuisines.
Sweets and added sugars	Limited sweets: once or twice per week			1 Tbsp sweet spoons, 3–4 oz syrup desserts, 1 tsp honey	Halva, fruit sweet spoons, baklava, deep-fried doughnut balls.	Fresh fruits are the typical daily dessert, with sweets based on nuts and made with olive oil.

- Biodiversity and seasonality.
- Traditional local and eco-friendly products (minimally processed).
- Culinary activities.
- Conviviality.
- Season meals with herbs and spices rather than salt.
- Snack on nuts or seeds instead of snack foods.
- Alcohol – limit it to moderate consumption with a meal (no more than one glass for women or two glasses for men).

Sample Menu Plan (~ 1600 kcal)

Breakfast
1 large orange,
2 oz whole-wheat rusk with 1 tsp honey, 1 oz feta cheese

Lunch
1 cup xorta with 2 Tbsp extra-virgin olive oil and lemon,
200 g gemista (stuffed tomatoes with rice),
1 slice of whole-wheat bread

Dinner
1 cup sliced tomatoes, cucumbers, and peppery radish, 2 Tbsp olive oil, vinegar,
2 oz barley rusks, 1 & ½ oz feta, 6–8 olives

Snack
200 g Greek yogurt with sliced apple, ½ cup oats, and 2 Tbsp raisins/30 g almonds

Bibliography

American Heart Association. (2020). The salty six infographic. https://www.heart.org/en/healthy-living/healthy-eating/eat-smart/sodium/salty-six-infographic.

Boucher, J.L. (2017). Mediterranean eating pattern. *Diabetes Spectrum* 30 (2): 72–76.

British Nutrition Foundation. (2019). A healthy Ramadan. www.nutrition.org.uk/healthyliving/seasons/ramadan.html.

CDC. (2012). Can lifestyle modifications using therapeutic lifestyle changes (TLC) reduce weight and the risk for chronic disease? https://www.cdc.gov/nutrition/downloads/r2p_life_change.pdf.

China Internet Information Center. (n.d.). Buddhist philosophy on health building. http://www.china.org.cn/english/imperial/26121.htm.

Daralliance.org. (2016). The Ramadan Nutrition Plan (RNP) for patients with diabetes. https://www.daralliance.org/daralliance/wp-content/uploads/2018/01/IDF-DAR-Practical-Guidelines_15-April-2016_low_7.pdf.

Diabetes UK. (2021). Ramadan and diabetes. www.diabetes.org.uk/guide-to-diabetes/managing-your-diabetes/ramadan.

Farrey, E. and O'Hara, N. (2000). *3 Bowls: Vegetarian Recipes from an American Zen Buddhist Monastery*. New York: Houghton Mifflin Co.

Foodandnutrition.org. (2013). Ayurveda: India's 5,000-year-old diet and wellness plan. https://foodandnutrition.org/may-2013/ayurvedaindias-5000-year-old-diet-wellness-plan.

Hewamanage, W. (2016). A critical review of dietary laws in Judaism. *Int. Res. J. Engineering, IT Scientific Res.* 2 (3): 58–65.

Hill, A. (2019). Kosher food: Everything you need to know. *Healthline* (January 25). https://www.healthline.com/nutrition/what-is-kosher.

Hindu American Foundation. (2017). 4 Things About Hinduism and Vegetarianism. https://www.hinduamerican.org/blog/4-things-about-hinduism-and-vegetarianism.

Holy Protection Orthodox Christian Church. (n.d.). Fasting throughout the year. https://www.holyorthodox.org/fastingguidelines.

Israeli Ministry of Health. (2019). Nutritional recommendations. https://health.gov.il/PublicationsFiles/dietary%20guidelines%20EN.pdf.

Jewish Visiting. (n.d.). Jewish dietary laws. www.jvisit.org.uk/jewish-dietary-laws.

Leech, J. (2019). The Nordic diet: an evidence-based review. *Healthline* (February 27). https://www.healthline.com/nutrition/thenordic-diet-review.

Matalas, A.-L., Tourlouki, E., and Lazarou, C. (2011). Fasting and food habits in the Eastern Orthodox Church. In: *Food and Faith in Christian Culture* (eds. K. Albala and T. Eden), 189–204. New York: Columbia University Press.

Mazokopakis, E. and Karagiannis, C. (2018). Investigating of the effects of Orthodox Christian fasting on human health. *Archives of Hellenic Medicine* 35 (6): 807–808.

National Health Service. (2017). What is a Mediterranean Diet? Eat well. https://www.nhs.uk/live-well/eat-well/what-is-a-mediterranean-diet.

National Health Service. (2018). The vegetarian diet. Eat well. https://www.nhs.uk/live-well/eat-well/the-vegetarian-diet.

National Heart, Lung, and Blood Institute. (2015). *DASH Eating Plan*. NIH Publication No. 06–5834. https://www.nhlbi.nih.gov/files/docs/public/heart/dash_brief.pdf.

National Institutes of Health. (2018). Does grapefruit affect my medicine? https://www.nhs.uk/common-health-questions/medicines/does-grapefruit-affect-my-medicine.

National Institutes of Health and National Heart, Lung, and Blood Institute. (2005). *Your Guide to Lowering Your Cholesterol with TLC*. NIH Publication No. 06–5235. US Department of Health and Human Services. https://www.nhlbi.nih.gov/files/docs/public/heart/chol_tlc.pdf.

Nordic Council of Ministers. (2010). The keyhole: healthy choices made easy. Partnership, synergies, activities, future. *ANP*: 779. http://www.diva-portal.org/smash/get/diva2:700822/FULLTEXT01.pdf.

OLDWAYS. (2018a). Asian heritage diet. https://oldwayspt.org/traditional-diets/asian-heritage-diet.

OLDWAYS. (2018b). Introducing the updated Asian diet pyramid. https://oldwayspt.org/blog/introducing-updated-asian-diet-pyramid.

OLDWAYS. (2019a). Mediterranean pantry. https://oldwayspt.org/programs/mediterranean-program/mediterranean-pantry.

OLDWAYS. (2019b). Vegetarian & vegan diet pyramid. https://oldwayspt.org/system/files/atoms/files/VEG101-brochure-PRINT19.pdf.

Rangdrol, S.N. (Translated by Padmakara Translation Group) (2004). *Food of Bodhisattvas: Buddhist Teachings on Abstaining from Meat*. Boulder, CO: Shambhala Publications.

Sarri, K.O., Linardakis, M.K., Bervanaki, F.N. et al. (2004). Greek Orthodox fasting rituals: a hidden characteristic of the Mediterranean diet of Crete. *Br. J. Nutr.* 92 (2): 277–284.

Urban Dharma. (2019). Buddhism and vegetarianism. http://www.urbandharma.org/udharma3/vegi.html.

USDA. (2020). Appendix 4. USDA food patterns: healthy Mediterranean-style eating pattern. In: *2015–2020 Dietary Guidelines for Americans*, 8e, 83–85. https://health.gov/our-work/food-nutrition/2015-2020-dietary-guidelines.

van de Walle, G. (2020). Buddhist diet: How it works and what to eat. *Healthline* (April 14). https://www.healthline.com/nutrition/buddhist-diet.

World Health Organization. (n.d.). Dietary recommendations for the month of Ramadan. http://www.emro.who.int/nutrition/nutrition-infocus/dietary-recommendations-for-the-month-of-ramadan.html.

Food Components of the Mediterranean Diet

Cereals

Cereals represent a major food group of the Mediterranean tradition (Figure C.1). Given their wide produce, variety, low cost, and long-term storage nature, they constituted the basis of the majority of cooking recipes and an essential sustenance able to induce satiety primarily to the lower socioeconomic layers of former Mediterranean populations. Wheat, barley, rye, maize, bread, pasta, rice, couscous, oats, and bulgur, among others, are typical paradigms of cereals.

Cereals have the same structure; they are composed by the germ, in which the genetic material is packed, the endosperm, filled with starch granules, and the pericarp, which constitutes the outer layer of the grain. Their nutritional value lies in the fact that they confer energy, complex carbohydrates (about 75% of the grain), small amounts of vegetable protein (6–15% of the grain), and even smaller amounts of lipids ranging from 1 to 10%, mainly in the form of an essential fatty acid, i.e., linoleic acid. Cereals also contain fibers and various micronutrients like vitamin E, some B complex vitamins (thiamin, riboflavin, niacin), magnesium (Mg), zinc (Zn), and selenium (Se), which contribute to the maintenance of a good health. Refined grains, in contrast to whole grains, refers to grain products that have undergone processing that removes the outer part of the grain and leaves the endosperm or starchy part.

This process lowers the content of beneficial nutrients substantially, such as dietary fibers, vitamins, Mg, iron (Fe), phosphorus (P), and others. The nutritional value of the final product depends on the magnitude of the elimination of these layers – i.e., the less the grain is processed, the higher the fiber and vitamin content will be in the final grain product. The concentration of phytochemicals naturally present in grains, such as lignans, tocopherols, tocotrienoles, carotenoids, and phenolic acids, which have been linked to numerous health benefits, are also decreased after processing.

Complete absence or a decrease in availability of the aforementioned non-nutrients (fibers, phytochemicals, etc.) may increase the health risk. For instance, the ingestion of fibers can mitigate constipation, contribute to diverticulosis prevention, and regulate T2DM and blood lipid profile. Moreover, whole grains are foods with low GI and GL and have been associated with reduced risk of developing T2DM and CHD compared to refined products.

Cereal consumption is omnipresent in all three main meals of the day in the MedD (i.e., breakfast, lunch, supper) in quantities ranging from 1–2 servings per meal, but also throughout the day as a snacking choice. As previously mentioned, the serving is not strictly defined in the context of the MedD, and it is supposed to illustrate the different habits, energy needs, and traditions of each Mediterranean region. Different recommendations are observed across different Mediterranean countries. For instance, in Greece, cereal intake is recommended to be 6–8 servings/day with 1 serving composed of one thin slice of bread (~25 g) or half a cup (~50–60 g) of cooked pasta or rice. The recommendation in Spain and France is that cereals should be present in every meal.

Fruits and Vegetables

Fruits and vegetables belong to the lavish flora of the Mediterranean region, and because the MedD is conceived to be a plant-based dietary pattern, fruits and vegetables play a key role in it. The Mediterranean region is rich with diverse species of fruits and vegetables (Figure C.2a and b) that grow during different seasons of the year following a seasonal pattern. Apples, oranges, pomegranates, cherries, strawberries, figs, grapes, raisins, melons, watermelons, peaches, pears, tangerines, and nectarines are just a few typical examples of fruits thriving in the Mediterranean region.

Regarding vegetables, chicory, dandelion greens, cabbage, spinach, cucumber, tomatoes, peppers, onions, garlic, zucchini, lettuce, cauliflower, broccoli, beetroots, and carrots are only a

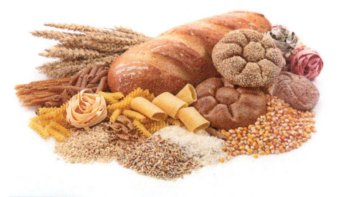

FIGURE C.1 Various kinds of cereals. **Source:** Elena Schweitzer/Shutterstock.

Textbook of Lifestyle Medicine, First Edition. Labros S. Sidossis and Stefanos N. Kales.

(a)   (b)

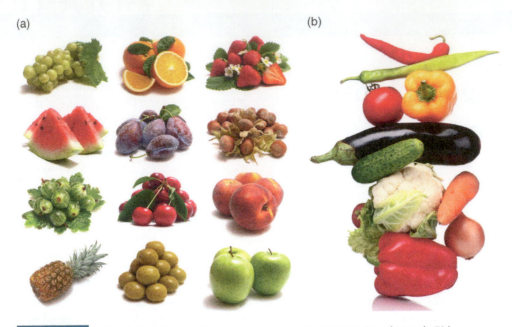

FIGURE C.2   (a) Fruits that thrive in the Mediterranean Basin. **Source:** Spayder pauk_79/ Shutterstock.com. (b) Vegetables that thrive in the Mediterranean Basin. **Source:** serezniy/123 RF.

few among a long list of edible plants growing in Mediterranean countries. They are consumed as an integral part of main meals and throughout the day. The Mediterranean people not only consume the main part of the fruit or vegetable but in some plants also the leaves, seeds, roots, and tubers. For example, beets are root vegetables, but their leaves can be boiled and eaten as a salad. Just like starchy foods, roots and bulbs provide energy and can be stored for extended periods.

Fruits contain sugars, minimal amounts of starch (except bananas), and are rich in dietary fibers. Vegetables are low in energy and sugars, contain small amounts of protein, and are high in dietary fiber, regulating satiation, as some of them cannot be digested by the human small intestine.

Table C.1 summarizes the nutritional value of fruits and vegetables. In addition, fruits and vegetables contain phytochemicals – micronutrients with potential health benefits – in high amounts and various combinations that are shown in

Table C.2. The prevailing phytochemicals in vegetables are beta carotene, lutein, vitamin C, lycopene, folic acid, and phenolic compounds. The consumption of a variety of fruits and vegetables with diverse colors and textures guarantees the daily intake of those vitamins and minerals.

In the MedD, fruits, fresh or dried, are consumed after meals as dessert or during the day as snacks. "Fruit drinks" do not have the benefits of fruit juice, while fruit juices are also considered inferior compared to consuming the whole fruit, as they lack dietary fiber but contain high amounts of simple sugars (because for a glass of orange juice you get the sugar from two to three oranges).

Vegetables are usually seasoned and served with olive oil and lemon or vinegar. In the MedD, 2 servings of vegetables are eaten with lunch and dinner either raw or cooked. One of these 2 servings is suggested to be consumed raw as cooking practices may destroy some water-soluble vitamins. Serving size is not defined consistently across all the Mediterranean countries. In France, the recommendation for fruits and vegetables is limited to the frequency of their intake: 5–6 servings/day. In Spain, it is mentioned that these two food groups should be consumed every day, whereas in Greece, it is recommended that 3 fruit servings and 4 vegetable servings are consumed on a daily basis. The portion of fruits varies according to its kind but usually refers to 120–200 g per serving, while 1 serving of vegetable refers to 1 cup of raw vegetables or half a cup of cooked ones (~150–200 g/serving).

Olive Oil

The cultivation of the olive tree, *Olea europaea*, has been a centuries-old tradition in the Mediterranean region (Figure C.3). Olive oil is extracted by crushing the olives (Figure C.4). The first extract is the extra-virgin olive oil, the best-quality olive oil,

TABLE C.1   **Compositional features of fruits and vegetables.**

g/100 g edible matter	Fruits	Leafy vegetables	Roots and tubers
Water	61.0–89.1	84.3–94.7	62.3–94.6
Protein	0.5–1.1	0.2–3.9	0.1–4.9
Fat	Trace-4.4	0.2–1.4	0.1–0.4
Sugar	4.4–34.8	1.5–4.9	0.5–9.5
Starch	Trace-3.0	0.1–0.8	11.8–31.4
Dietary fiber	2.0–14.8	1.2–4.0	1.1–9.5
Energy (kcal)	90–646	65–177	297–525

Reprinted with permission from Slavin and Lloyd (2012).

TABLE C.2   Phytochemicals: functions and presence in fruits and vegetables.

Phytochemicals	Function	Presence Fruits	Presence Vegetables
Sulfides (allium)			
Diallyl sulfide	Stimulates anticancer enzymes, detoxifies carcinogens; antibacterial activity may inhibit conversion of nitrate to nitrites, thereby reducing formation of nitrosamines, which are thought to be carcinogenic		X
Allyl methyl trisulfide	Stimulates anticancer enzymes, detoxifies carcinogens; antibacterial activity may inhibit conversion of nitrate to nitrites, thereby reducing formation of nitrosamines, which are thought to be carcinogenic		X
Dithiolthiones	Increases activity of enzymes involved in detoxification of carcinogens and other foreign compounds		X
Carotenoids			
α-Carotene	Antioxidant; precursor to vitamin A; inhibits cell proliferation		X
Beta carotene	Antioxidant; precursor to vitamin A; helps in differentiation of normal epithelial cells; inhibits cell proliferation	X	X
Lutein	Antioxidant; protects against cataracts, macular degeneration		X
Lycopene	Antioxidant; promotes oral and bone health, and healthy blood pressure	X	X
Flavonoids			
Quercetin	Antioxidative, anti-inflammatory, antimutagenic, and anticarcinogenic properties; may reduce cell proliferation; extend action of vitamin C; inhibit blood clot formation;	X	X
Kaempferol		X	X
Tangeretin		X	
Nobiletin		X	
Rutin		X	
Glucosinolates/indoles			
Glucobrassicin	Forms indoles		X
Indoles	Protects against estrogen-promoted cancers, induces protective enzymes		X
Phytoestrogens			
Genistein	Antioxidant; inhibits growth of cancer cells; lowers blood cholesterol level and platelet aggregation		X
Biochanin A	Antioxidant; inhibits growth of cancer cells; lowers blood cholesterol level and platelet aggregation		X
Lignans	Antioxidant; may block or suppress cancerous changes	X	X
Isothiocyanates			
Sulphorophane	Exceptionally potent inducer of detoxification enzyme		X
D-Limonene	Increases activity of glutathione transferase, a detoxification enzyme	X	

Reprinted with permission from van Duyn and Pivonka (2000).

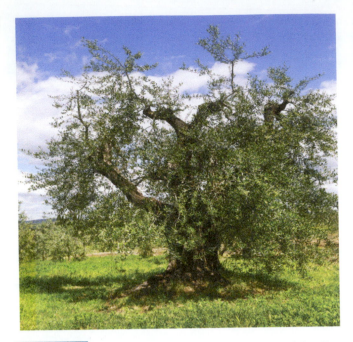

FIGURE C.3 The Mediterranean diet will cease to exist if the olive trees die.

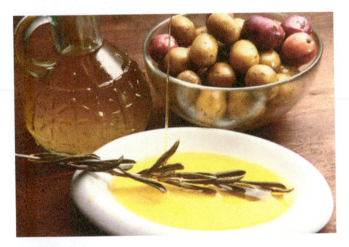

FIGURE C.4 Olive oil and table olives. **Source:** Luca Santilli/Shutterstock.com.

which accrues from absolutely natural procedures: centrifugation and water (cold or hot). If the extraction is performed with cold water, then the product is called "cold pressed, extra virgin olive oil." It is of superior quality but the yield is less compared to extraction with warm water. Successive extractions lead to progressively lower quality of olive oil. Depending on the method of extraction and the integrity of the olives, the quality and the composition of the final product may vary greatly. Although not fully adopted from the USA and Australia, the International Olive Oil Corporation (IOOC) has categorized the qualities of olive oil according to Table C.3.

Olive oil is the core element in the heart of the Mediterranean pyramid. Its high nutritional value is attributed to the energy it provides, the phenolic compounds it contains (primarily hydroxytyrosol, tyrosol, and oleuropein), the types of fatty acids it contains, i.e., mainly the MUFA oleic acid, and its content in α-tocopherol and squalene.

TABLE C.3 Olive oil classification.

Olive oil quality	Sensory characteristics with median defects; median of fruitiness	Free acidity (expressed as oleic acid)
Extra-virgin olive oil (EVOO)	0; >0 (highest quality)	<0.8g/100g
Virgin olive oil (VOO)	0–2.5; >0 (good quality)	<2.0g/100g
Lampante virgin olive oil	>3.5; 0 (intended for refining purposes)	>2.0g/100g
Refined olive oil	Obtained after refinement procedures from VOO, no alterations in the glyceridic structure	
Blended olive oil	Mixture of refined olive oil and VOO	

Reprinted with permission from Delgado et al. (2017).

These compounds make olive oil unique. Due to their structure, MUFAs resist oxidation during thermal processing; this is why olive oil remains chemically stable at high temperatures and offers antioxidant effects. Moreover, olive oil provides fatty acids that constitute precursors for many biologically significant structures and compounds. For instance, the omega-6 linoleic acid plays a crucial role in the lipid structure of cell membranes, and it is implicated in the process of cell signaling. All these characteristics render olive oil the best source of added fat for culinary purposes.

As mentioned above, typical foods of the MedD are combined with olive oil when eaten or during cooking. More than half of the lipids in the MedD are in the form of olive oil.

Spices and Herbs

Herbs and spices have gained the interest of Mediterranean people since antiquity. They were using them in everyday cooking and medicinal practices. Hippocrates, the father of medicine, used physical medications based on garlic, rosemary, and cinnamon. The first Western pharmacological treatise, a listing of herbal plants used in classical medicine, was made in the first century CE by the Greek physician Dioscorides. This ancient monograph comprised the main source of herb selection practices and storage prior to the seventeenth century in the European continent.

According to Tapsell and colleagues, the cooked leaves of a plant are considered to be culinary herbs, while the other parts of the plant, which are usually dried, account for spices. Moreover, they report that "Spices can be the buds (cloves), bark (cinnamon), roots (ginger), berries (peppercorns), aromatic seeds (cumin), and even the stigma of a flower (saffron). Many of the aromatic seeds known as spices are actually gathered from plants when they have finished flowering."

A plethora of herbs and spices are used in various traditional recipes (e.g., stews, rice-based recipes, marinades and dressings, stir-fry dishes, casseroles, and soups), substituting salt, sugar, or other ingredients, and enhancing the palatability of meals (Table C.4).

TABLE C.4   Use of common herbs and spices.

Parsley family

Parsley	Used raw and in cooking with meat, fish, chicken, and vegetables.
Dill	Used in salads, sauces, and with fish, sour cream, and in cheese and potato dishes.
Coriander (cilantro)	Used in marinades, dressings, salsas, and in cooked dishes. Leaves, roots, and seeds are used.

Mint family

Mint	Many varieties with slightly different tastes are used raw and in cooking, dressings, marinades, drinks, yogurt, desserts, sauces, vegetable dishes, and salads.
Basil	Used with tomatoes (fresh and in sauces) and in soups and casseroles with tomato. Also used in salad dressings, pesto, and with pasta, rice, vegetables, meat, chicken, and seafood.
Marjoram	Used in meat, fish, egg, and cheese dishes.
Oregano	Essential for Italian and Greek dishes but also used in cheese and egg dishes.
Sage	Used with veal and in stuffing and cheese dishes.
Thyme	Used in casseroles, soups, and poultry stuffing.
Rosemary	Used in marinades, sauces, and stuffing, and with fish, poultry, and soups.

Allium family

Chives	Used in salad dressings, soups, light sauces, and with egg, cheese, fish, and chicken.
Garlic	Included in almost every cuisine from Asian to Mediterranean. Used in marinades, dressings, sauces, and in stir-fried and slow-cooked dishes.

Other

Bay leaves	Generally used in slow-cooked meat and soup dishes.
Chili	Used with meat, poultry, shellfish, tomato dishes, and curries. Popular also in Asian, Mexican, African, and Caribbean cooking.
Ginger	Used in many Asian dishes but also in cakes, biscuits, desserts, and with fruit and juices.
Lemongrass	Can be used as a tea or beverage and is included in many Asian dishes.
Tarragon	Used with chicken and fish and in salad dressings and egg dishes.

Reprinted with permission from Tapsell et al. (2006).

Marination constitutes a process during which meat or fish is immersed in a liquid seasoned with herbs and spices prior to cooking. This liquid is acidic, and it is mainly vinegar, wine, or lemon juice. Marinades usually contain olive oil, as well. Their purpose is to tenderize the meat and make it more palatable.

Typical paradigms of herbs used in the traditional MedD include thyme, sage, oregano, parsley, marjoram, basil, chives, rosemary, mint, parsley, bay leaf, anise, and fennel, whereas common spices include cumin, cinnamon, garlic, ginger, saffron, and nutmeg (Figures C.5 and C.6). Aromatic plants and spices can be found in different forms (i.e., fresh, whole dried, or pre-ground dried). They are used (fresh or dried) either in seasoning, cooking, or at the end of the cooking, to increase flavor and maintain palatability.

Herbs and spices are also a recognized source of bioactive compounds of various chemical classes, e.g., amides, alkaloids, flavonoids, tannins, saponins, glycosides, terpenoids, and phenols. These compounds have been associated with positive benefits for human health. Some of the most frequently cited biological properties are antioxidant, antimicrobial, antiviral, and anticarcinogenic effects.

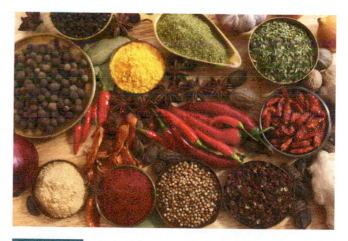

FIGURE C.5 Typical herbs of the Mediterranean land.
Source: Krzysztof Slusarczyk/Shutterstock.com.

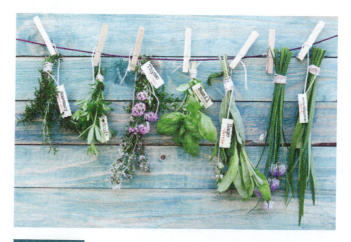

FIGURE C.6 A plethora of spices are used in the Mediterranean region in various combinations to enhance food palatability.
Source: foodandmore/123 RF.

TABLE C.5 Bioactive components of common MedD herbs/spices.

Herb/spice	Bioactive food components
All spice	Eugenol
Basil	Eugenol, apigenin, limonene, ursolic acid, methyl cinnamate, 1,8-cineole, α-terpinene, anthocyanins, β-sitosterol, carvacrol, cintronellol, farnesol, geraniol, kaempherol, menthol, *p*-coumaric acid, quercetin, rosmarinic acid, rutin, safrole, tannin, catechin
Cardamom	Limonene, caffeic acid
Caraway	Carvone, limonene, α-pinene, kaempferol
Cinnamon	Cinnamic aldehyde, 2-hydroxycinnamaldehyde, eugenol
Cloves	Eugenol, isoeugenol, gallic acid
Coriander	Quercetin, caffeic acid, cineole, geraniol, borneol, 1,8-cineole, α-terpinene, β-carotene, β-pinene, β-sitosterol, cinnamic acid, ferrulic acid, γ-terpinene, kaempferol, limonene, myrcene, *p*-coumaric acid, *p*-cymene, quercetin, rutin, vanillic acid
Cumin	α-Pinene, β-pinene, γ-terpinene, *p*-cymene, cuminaldehyde, carvone, 1,8-cineole, β-carotene, β-sitosterol, caffeic acid, carvacrol, carvaol, geranial, kaempferol, limonene, *p*-coumaric acid, quercetin, tannin, thymol
Dill	Carvone, limonene, isorhamnetin, kaempferol, myricetin, quercetin, catechin
Fennel	α-Pinene, β-carotene, limonene, quercetin, benzoic acid, β-sitosterol, caffeic acid, cinnamic acid, ferulic acid, fumaric acid, kaempferol, myristicin, 1,8-cineole, *p*-coumaric acid, quercetin, rutin, vanillic acid, vanillin
Garlic	Allicin, diallyl disulfide, allyl isothiocyanate
Ginger	Zingiberone, zingiberene, ingerol, paradol, curcumin, shagoal
Lemongrass	Farnesol, geraniol
Marjoram	Eugenol, limonene, ursolic acid, 1,8-cineole, α-pinene, α-terpinene, carvacrol, farnesol, geraniol, *p*-cymene, rosmarinic acid, sterols, thymol, apigenin
Mustard	Allyl isothiocyanate, β-carotene
Nutmeg	Caffeic acid, catechin
Onion	Quercetin, dipropyl disulfides
Oregano	Apigenin, luteolin, myricetin, quercetin, caffeic acid, *p*-coumaric acid, rosmarinic acid, carvacrol, thymol
Paprika	α-Tocopherol, capsaicin, dihydrocapsaicin, lutein, β-carotene, ascorbic acid, vitamin E
Parsley	Apigenin, luteolin, kaempferol, myricetin, quercetin, caffeic acid
Pepper, black	Piperidine, piperine, limonene, α-pinene, β-pinene
Pepper, red	Capsaicin, α-tocopherol, lutein, β-carotene, ascorbic acid, vitamin E
Peppermint	Limonene, menthol, eriodictyol, hesperitin, apigenin, luteolin
Rosemary	Carnasol, carnosic acid, cineole, geraniol, α-pinene, β-carotene, apigenin, limonene, naringin, luteolin, caffeic acid, rosmarinic acid, rosmanol, vanillic acid
Saffron	Crocetin, crocin, β-carotene, safranal, all trans retinoic acid
Sage	α-Pinene, β-sitosterol, citral, farnesol, ferulic acid, gallic acid, geraniol, limonene, cineole, perillyl alcohol, β-carotene, catechin, apigenin, luteolin, saponin, ursolic acid, rosemarinic acid, carnosic acid, vanillic acid, caffeic acid, thymol, eugenol
Thyme	Thymol, carvacrol, cineole, α-pinene, apigenin, β-carotene, eugenol, limonene, ursolic acid, luteolin, gallic acid, caffeic acid, rosmarinic acid, carnosic acid, hispidulin, cismaritin
Turmeric	Curcumin, curcuminoids

Reprinted with permission from Kaefer and Milner (2008).

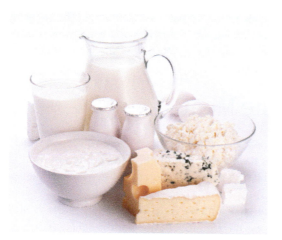

FIGURE C.7 The traditional Mediterranean diet includes primarily fermented dairies. **Source:** Valentyn Volkov/Shutterstock.com.

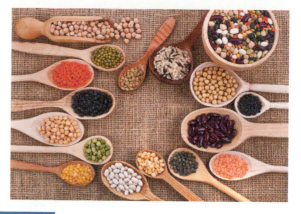

FIGURE C.8 Legumes, a typical component of the Mediterranean diet, when combined with cereals can provide proteins of high biological value. **Source:** Madlen/Shutterstock.com.

Dairy Products

Dairy products in the Mediterranean region come mainly from sheep and goats. They were typically consumed in the form of fermented products, such as cheese and yogurt, rather than in the form of milk (Figure C.7). This is because fresh milk is unstable and carries a substantial high microbial load. To solve these problems, for the past 3000 years people of the Mediterranean region and elsewhere have been turning milk into fermented products, namely, cheese and yogurt, in order to prolong its use and ensure safety.

Dairy provides proteins and carbohydrates and high amounts of Ca, which contributes to bone and heart health. Dairy products also contain fats of animal origin, i.e., SFAs. As mentioned in Chapter 2, the consumption of these products was thought to be positively correlated with the onset of CVD, due to their high content of SFAs. However, newer data have put doubt on this longstanding theory, while suggesting a neutral or even a beneficial association between the consumption of dairy products and the development of several NCDs.

Dairy products contain high amounts of nutraceuticals and probiotics. Milk is the first food that mammals (including humans) eat after they are born. This early lactation milk, called colostrum, provides the newborn with its mother's antibodies, enhancing the offspring's immune system and building its gut microflora. Gut microbiota has emerged as a crucial factor of human health, and the composition of bacterial species can be influenced in a favorable way by the intake of dairy products. The MedD recommends 2 servings of dairies daily. One serving could be roughly defined as 1 cup of milk or yogurt or 30 g of cheese.

Legumes

Lentils, the fava bean, and other legumes (Figure C.8) were critical in terms of energy and nutrients for ancient Mediterranean populations. They are of plant origin, like cereals, fruits, and vegetables. In ancient times, they were thought to be beneficial for diseases such as simple headaches to more life-threatening conditions, e.g., heart disease.

Legumes constitute a significant source of proteins. However, it has been suggested that plant proteins are not of high quality, compared to proteins coming from animal meat and organs or milk. This is because legumes lack certain essential amino acids, and the ratios of the various amino acids in their structure are not optimal for human consumption. Therefore, for many years we believed that for optimal nutrition vegetarians and vegans should carefully combine foods (e.g., legumes with cereals) in every meal. This old idea has been totally refuted. If people following a vegan diet eat a wide variety of legumes, grains, and seeds, then there is no issue about the quality of their protein intake.

In the MedD, legumes are consumed on a weekly basis, in quantities exceeding 2 servings (1 serving is 1 cup or ~100 g), and constitute an ideal alternative to meat-based dishes. Table C.6 summarizes Mediterranean beans and legumes and their protein content.

TABLE C.6	Beans and legumes with high protein content.
Legumes	**Protein content per 100 g of cooked product**
Black-eyed peas (cow peas)	7.7 g
Broad beans (fava beans)	7.6 g
Chick peas (garbanzo beans)	8.9 g
French beans (green beans)	7.1 g
Kidney beans (red beans)	8.7 g
Lentils	9 g
Lupin beans	15.6 g
Pinto beans	9 g
Small white beans	9 g
White beans	9.7 g

From Whitbread (2020).

Fish

The Mediterranean Sea contains a plethora of fish and shellfish species, giving the inhabitants of the region the chance to choose among a great variety of seafood. Like other fresh products, the optimum season for each species varies. For example, cod is primarily consumed in winter, while sardines and smelt in the summer. Table C.7 provides information about the seasonality of fish in the Mediterranean Sea. Some of the most commonly found fish and shellfish include sardines, anchovies, mackerel, bogue, smelt, a few tuna kinds, bream family, mollusks, pandora, dentex, swordfish, squid, shrimps, lobster, and mussels (Figure C.9).

Fish, mainly the oily ones, are rich in omega-3 fatty acids and have been linked to various health benefits. They constitute a great source of protein with high biological value. Traditional dishes containing seafood are usually accompanied by cereals; shrimps and spaghetti with tomato sauce, cuttlefish, and orzo cooked in the oven with tomato sauce, etc.

In the MedD, seafood is consumed on a weekly basis in amounts reaching 2 or more servings. The recommendation varies from one Mediterranean country to another. For example, the Spanish pyramid recommends 2–4 servings of fish per week, while the French at least 2 servings. The Greek pyramid recommends 5–6 servings of fish on a weekly basis with 1 serving weighing approximately 60 g of cooked product.

White Meat

White meat includes primarily poultry, turkey, and duck. These animals have long been domesticated and are used for their meat and eggs production, up to 300 eggs per chicken per year (Figure C.10).

Due to economic and religious reasons, white meat intake was not frequent in the traditional MedD. Prior to and shortly after World War II, meat was saved for special occasions. Feast days were the days on which the reserved meat was consumed in a mood of euphoria, conviviality, and also devoutness, as there were many short- or even long-term periods in which meat consumption was not allowed. The high cost of meat was another reason that people used to eat meat only on holidays or, after the 1960s, mainly on Sundays.

Meat consumption provides energy, high-quality proteins, vitamins, and minerals. In the traditional MedD, white meat is

TABLE C.7   Seasonality of fish in the Mediterranean region.

	January	February	March	April	May	June	July	August	September	October	November	December
Fish												
Smelt	X	X	X	X	X					X	X	X
Anchovy			X	X	X	X	X	X	X	X	X	
Sole	X	X										X
Boce fish						X	X	X	X	X		
Mackerel				X		X	X	X	X	X		
Mullet	X	X	X	X	X					X	X	X
Red snapper	X	X	X	X	X					X	X	X
Barbel								X	X	X		
Swordfish			X		X	X	X	X	X	X		
Sprat				X	X	X	X	X	X	X		
Dentex	X	X	X	X	X					X	X	X
Grouper	X	X	X	X	X					X	X	X
Tuna				X	X	X	X	X	X	X	X	
Dorado						X	X	X	X	X		
Pagrus			X	X	X	X				X	X	

From Barrett (2016).

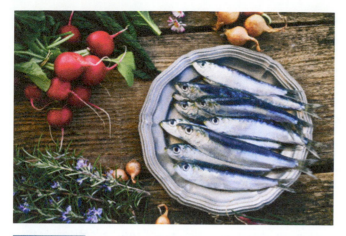

FIGURE C.9   Typical Mediterranean fish species (sardines).
Source: nikkiphoto/123 RF.

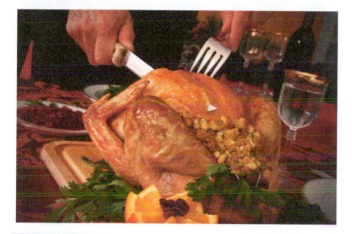

FIGURE C.10   White meat is consumed on a weekly basis in the traditional Mediterranean diet. **Source:** Suhaib Mohsin/Shutterstock.com.

consumed on a weekly basis in quantities reaching 2 servings, with 1 serving consisting of approximately 60 g of cooked lean meat. Eggs are also an important source of animal protein. Taking into account that they are consumed as a whole or as an ingredient of various recipes (e.g., scrambled eggs with tomato, sweets), their consumption ranges from two to four eggs per week.

Red and Processed Meat

Red and processed meat (Figure C.11) used to have only a minor contribution to the traditional MedD. Similarly to white meat, economic and religious reasons kept the Mediterranean people from consuming red meat and its derivatives regularly. Red meat includes beef, veal, pork, goat, and lamb.

This kind of meat constitutes a significant source of energy, high-quality protein, vitamins, and minerals but also lipids in the form of SFAs. Lean cuts of red meat (e.g., eye of round roast and steak, sirloin tip side steak, top round roast and steak, bottom round roast and steak, and top sirloin steak) are preferred, and these are consumed on a weekly basis in amounts smaller than 2 servings, with 1 serving being approximately 60 g of cooked meat.

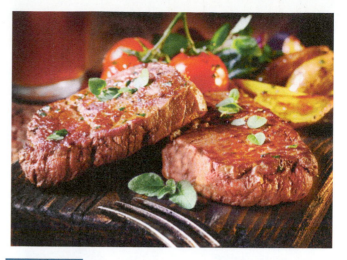

FIGURE C.11   Red meat is rarely consumed within the frame of the traditional Mediterranean diet.

Potatoes

Potato, the common name of *Solanum tuberosum*, is a plant-based starchy vegetable. Its nutrients are starch, dietary fiber, and vitamins C and K. Small amounts of proteins and other water-soluble vitamins are also present. Potatoes contain phytochemicals, like quercetin and chlorogenic acid, with the latter having been attributed with anti-oncogenic potential.

Potatoes became part of the MedD relatively recently, after the discovery of the Americas. The newly discovered land provided new kinds of foods, among them potatoes and tomatoes. The way potatoes are cooked affects their dietary value, since cooking influences the availability of many nutrients and causes changes in molecular structures. Boiled potatoes are rich in digestible starch, whereas French fries are usually high in calories because they are cooked in oil. However, if the oil is of high quality, e.g., extra-virgin olive oil, then French fries, when eaten in moderation, constitute an excellent meal. Oil stability when heated is also very important in maintaining food quality. In the MedD, potatoes usually accompany fish or meat dishes, and they are consumed on a weekly basis in amounts that do not exceed 3 servings, with 1 serving being about 100 g.

Sweets

The less frequently occurring food group within the MedD is that of sweets (Figure C.12). Most sweets are usually high in either simple sugars or lipids or both. As mentioned earlier, excessive sweets consumption has been correlated with adverse health effects, and therefore they should be consumed in moderation.

However, it is worth mentioning that there are many traditional Mediterranean sweets that do not contain fat, such as jams, fruits preserved in syrup (the homemade equivalent of canned fruits), whole-fruit preserves (e.g., the Greek well-known spoon-sweets made of any kind of fruit), Turkish delights

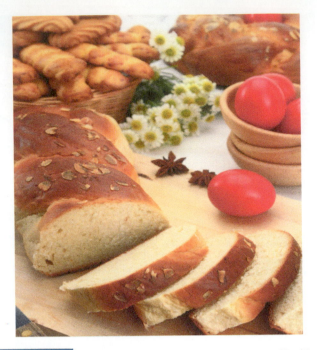

FIGURE C.12 In Greece during Easter people cook *tsoureki,* a kind of sweet brioche, and Easter cookies.

(*loukoumia*) with nuts or plain, macaroons, and sweets usually prepared around Christmas, like *melomakarona, kourampiedes, diples, baklava*, and many others.

Even if sweets contained fat, the quality and quantity of fat determines its nutritional value. Representative homemade sweets from the region include pecan pie, kazan dipi (with milk), custard-filled pastry or *galaktompoureko* (with milk), and *kantaifi*.

Wine and Spirits

Wine, especially the red variety (Figure C.13), holds a special role in the Mediterranean culture and diet, and it is strongly connected with the convivial dimension of food intake. Indeed,

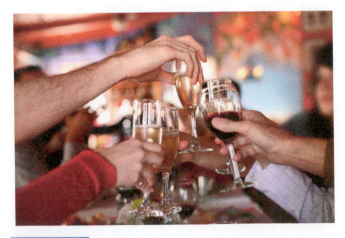

FIGURE C.13 Wine intake in the presence of good company has always strengthened the convivial character of Mediterranean meals.

wine used to accompany all meals in the Mediterranean region, except breakfast.

Wine is produced after the fermentation of grapes, especially of the species *Vitis vinifera*. The 60 species comprising the genus Vitis thrive in zones of the Northern Hemisphere with temperate climate. *Vitis vinifera* is native to the Mediterranean region, central Europe, and southwestern Asia.

The main varieties of wine are the red, white, and rose. White wines are made by fermenting only the grape juice; all skins and seeds are separated immediately after crushing the grapes. The process of making red wines is similar to white wines, except both seeds and skins are left in the juice during fermentation. The seeds and skin give not only the dark color to the wine but impart other flavors and texture, noticeably their tannins. Rose is somewhat between white wine and red wine; after crushing, the grape skins are left with the juices for a few hours. Irrespective of the color, the quality of the final product is strongly determined by the quality of the grapes – this, in turn, depends on the weather conditions during the growing season, the harvest time, and the composition of soil in minerals and acidity.

Wine consists of ethanol, water, polysaccharides, glycerol, and phytochemicals, called polyphenols. Red wine represents a rich source of polyphenols, which have two general classes – flavonoids and phenolic acids. Flavonoids are further divided into flavones, flavanones, flavonols, flavanols, chalcones, and isoflavones. Phenolic acids are generally classified into hydroxybenzoic and hydroxycinnamic acids. Flavonoids account for up to 85% of the polyphenols found in red wine.

In recent years, three more compounds found in wine have attracted attention for their potential health effects: hydroxytyrosol, resveratrol, and melatonin. Hydroxytyrosol and resveratrol have been found in wine in considerable amounts. Melatonin has been found in wine in low amounts. All these compounds show antioxidant, cardioprotective, anticancer, antidiabetic, neuroprotective, and antiaging activities. However, human studies are still in the initial stages and therefore further studies are needed to determine the clinical significance of these compounds on human health.

Current guidelines call for a moderate alcohol consumption that translates into one and two portions of alcoholic beverages per day for women and men, respectively (one portion equals 330 ml of beer, 150 ml of wine, or 40 ml of other beverages). In the context of the MedD, wine can be consumed on a daily basis in moderation and with respect to religious and social norms.

In Greece, *tsipouro* and *raki* constitute alcohol drinks coming from the distillation of grape skins, while *ouzo* comprises a blend of alcohol, water, and various herbs with the predominant one being anise. In France, *absinthe* is a distilled spirit with high alcohol content, deriving from the distillation of several plants, like the flowers of the *Artemisia absinthium* species, fennel, anise, as well as of other herbs. Spanish *sangria* is the drink mostly identifiable with this Mediterranean country. It is a mixture of sweetened red wine, liquor, and, usually, sparkling lemonade.

Bibliography

Angelino, D., Godos, J., Ghelfi, F. et al. (2019). Fruit and vegetable consumption and health outcomes: an umbrella review of observational studies. *Int. J. Food Sci. Nutr.* 70 (6): 652–667.

Barrett, M. (2016). Fish and seafood. Matt Barrett's Travel Guides. www.greecefoods.com/seafood/index.htm.

Casas, R., Estruch, R., and Sacanella, E. (2018). The protective effects of extra virgin olive oil on immune-mediated inflammatory responses. *Endocr. Metab. Immune Disord. Drug Targets* 18 (1): 23–35. doi: 10.2174/1871530317666171114115632.

Chen, G.C., Zhang, R., Martinez-Gonzalez, M.A. et al. (2017). Nut consumption in relation to all-cause and cause-specific mortality: a meta-analysis 18 prospective studies. *Food Funct.* 8 (11): 3893–3905. doi: 10.1039/c7fo00915a.

Cicerale, S., Lucas, L.J., and Keast, R.S.J. (2012). Antimicrobial, antioxidant and anti-inflammatory phenolic activities in extra virgin olive oil. *Curr. Opin. Biotechnol.* 23 (2): 129–135.

Cui, J., Lian, Y., Zhao, C. et al. (2019). Dietary fibers from fruits and vegetables and their health benefits via modulation of gut microbiota. *Compr. Rev. Food Sci. Food Saf.* 18 (5): 1514–1532.

Delgado, A.M., Daniel Vaz Almeida, M., and Parisi, S. (2017). *Chemistry of the Mediterranean Diet*. Basel, Switzerland: Springer.

EFSA Scientific Committee. (2015). Statement on the benefits of fish/seafood consumption compared to the risks of methylmercury in fish/seafood. *EFSA J.* 13 (1): 3982.

George, E.S., Marshall, S., Mayr, H.L. et al. (2019). The effect of high-polyphenol extra virgin olive oil on cardiovascular risk factors: a systematic review and meta-analysis. *Crit. Rev. Food Sci. Nutr.* 59 (17): 2772–2795. doi: 10.1080/10408398.2018.1470491.

Giacosa, A., Barale, R., Bavaresco, L. et al. (2014). Mediterranean way of drinking and longevity. *Crit. Rev. Food Sci. Nutr.* 8398: 37–41.

Gil, A., Ortega, R.M., and Maldonado, J. (2011). Wholegrain cereals and bread: a duet of the Mediterranean diet for the prevention of chronic diseases. *Public Health Nutr.* 14 (12A): 2316–2322.

Ha, V., Sievenpiper, J.L., de Souza, R.J. et al. (2014). Effect of dietary pulse intake on established therapeutic lipid targets for cardiovascular risk reduction: a systematic review and meta-analysis of randomized controlled trials. *CMAJ* 186 (8): E252–262. doi: 10.1503/cmaj.131727.

Iriti, M. and Varoni, E.M. (2014). Cardioprotective effects of moderate red wine consumption: polyphenols vs. ethanol. *J. Appl. Biomed.* 12 (4): 193–202.

Kaefer, C.M. and Milner, J.A. (2008). The role of herbs and spices in cancer prevention. *J. Nutr. Biochem.* 19 (6): 347–361.

Lapuente, M., Estruch, R., Shahbaz, M. et al. (2019). Relation of fruits and vegetables with major cardiometabolic risk factors, markers of oxidation, and inflammation. *Nutrients* 11 (10): 2381. doi: 10.3390/nu11102381.

Martinez-Gonzalez, M.A. and Bes-Rastrollo, M. (2011). Nut consumption, weight gain and obesity: epidemiological evidence. *Nutr. Metab. Cardiovasc. Dis.* 21 Suppl 1: S40–45. doi: 10.1016/j.numecd.2010.11.005.

McKevith, B. (2004). Nutritional aspects of cereals. *Nutr. Bull.* 29 (2): 111–142.

Minzer, S., Estruch, R., and Casas, R. (2020). Wine intake in the framework of a Mediterranean diet and chronic non-communicable diseases: a short literature review of the last 5 years. *Molecules* 25 (21): 5045. doi: 10.3390/molecules25215045.

Nakbi, A., Tayeb, W., Dabbou, S. et al. (2012). Hypolipidimic and antioxidant activities of virgin olive oil and its fractions in 2,4-diclorophenoxyacetic acid-treated rats. *Nutrition* 28 (1): 81–91.

Ruiz-Canela, M. and Martinez-Gonzalez, M.A. (2011). Olive oil in the primary prevention of cardiovascular disease. *Maturitas* 68 (3): 245–250. doi: 10.1016/j.maturitas.2010.12.002.

Slavin, J. and Lloyd, B. (2012). Health benefits of fruits and vegetables. *Adv. Nutr.* 3 (4): 506–516.

Tapsell, L.C., Hemphill, I., Cobiac, L. et al. (2006). Health benefits of herbs and spices: the past, the present, the future. *Med. J. Aust.* 185 (4 Suppl): S1–S24.

Tieri, M., Ghelfi, F., Vitale, M. et al. (2020). Whole grain consumption and human health: an umbrella review of observational studies. *Int. J. Food Sci. Nutr.* 71: 1–10.

Van Duyn, M.A.S. and Pivonka, E. (2000). Overview of the health benefits of fruit and vegetable consumption for the dietetics professional. *J. Am. Diet. Assoc.* 100 (12): 1511–1521.

Waterman, E. and Lockwood, B. (2007). Active components and clinical applications of olive oil. *Altern. Med. Rev.* 12 (4): 331–342.

Wells, E.M., Kopylev, L., Nachman, R. et al. (2020). Seafood, wine, rice, vegetables, and other food items associated with mercury biomarkers among seafood and non-seafood consumers: NHANES 2011–2012. *J. Expo. Sci. Environ. Epidemiol.* 30 (3): 504–514.

Whitbread, D. (2020). Top 10 beans and legumes highest in protein. *My Food Data* (December 9). www.healthaliciousness.com/articles/beans-legumes-highest-protein.php.

Willett, W.C. and Ludwig, D.S. (2020). Milk and health. *N. Engl. J. Med.* 382 (7): 644–654. doi: 10.1056/NEJMra1903547.

Appendix D

Assessment Tools for the Various Lifestyle Components

1. 24-Hour Dietary Recall

Time	Food/beverage	Brand	Quantity	Place, parallel activities, alone or with company

Instructions

1. Make a proper introduction. Example: "In the next few minutes, I would like you to try and remember all the foods and beverages you consumed yesterday. Let's start with what time you woke up in the morning and what was the first food or beverage you had. . .." If yesterday was not a typical day, ask the patient to recall a recent typical day.

2. Ask the patient for a quick list of all foods and beverages consumed during the past 24 hours, i.e., from yesterday morning to this morning (first pass).

3. Starting with the first food item, ask for details of all the foods and beverages consumed, including the exact hour of consumption, type, amount, preparation/cooking method, additions/toppings, and meal conditions, such as place of consumption, if they ate alone or with company, and parallel activities (second pass). Make sure to collect all important information on foods and beverages that reflects the patient's actual dietary habits. For example, "chicken with salad" is a very vague description. A more accurate description would be: "200 g of roasted chicken (breast without skin) and 2 cups of raw green salad (lettuce and rocket) with 2 tablespoons of olive oil." To facilitate an accurate portion size evaluation, ask the patient to report quantities of individual foods and beverages consumed in typical household objects (e.g., teaspoons, tablespoons, cups, etc.) and other commonly known items and size approximations (e.g., matchbox, cell phone, card deck, palm, etc.). For complex food recipes and when common measures are not helpful, use a booklet with multiple photos of different portion sizes for several food items and ask the patient to indicate portion sizes using the available photos.

4. Make a review of all foods and beverages reported and give the patient the opportunity to correct any inaccurate data or add previously ignored data (third pass).

Textbook of Lifestyle Medicine, First Edition. Labros S. Sidossis and Stefanos N. Kales.
© 2022 John Wiley & Sons Ltd. Published 2022 by John Wiley & Sons Ltd.

2. Food Frequency Questionnaire

How often did you consume the following foods/beverages during the last month? Please answer, keeping in mind the indicated reference portion size for each food/beverage.

Food or beverage	Reference portion size	Frequency of consumption
DAIRY		
Full-fat milk/yogurt	1 cup (240 ml)	never/rarely, 1–3 t/mo, 1–2 t/wk, 3–6 t/wk, 1 t/d, ≥2 t/d
Low-fat milk/yogurt	1 cup (240 ml)	never/rarely, 1–3 t/mo, 1–2 t/wk, 3–6 t/wk, 1 t/d, ≥2 t/d
Yellow cheese/cream cheese	30 g	never/rarely, 1–3 t/mo, 1–2 t/wk, 3–6 t/wk, 1 t/d, ≥2 t/d
White cheese (e.g., feta cheese)	30 g	never/rarely, 1–3 t/mo, 1–2 t/wk, 3–6 t/wk, 1 t/d, ≥2 t/d
Low-fat cheese (light/cottage)	30 g	never/rarely, 1–3 t/mo, 1–2 t/wk, 3–6 t/wk, 1 t/d, ≥2 t/d
Egg (boiled, fried, omelet)	50 g	never/rarely, 1–3 t/mo, 1–2 t/wk, 3–6 t/wk, 1 t/d, ≥2 t/d
CEREALS, STARCHY FOODS		
White bread/toast	1 slice (30 g)	never/rarely, 1–3 t/mo, 1–2 t/wk, 3–6 t/wk, 1 t/d, ≥2 t/d
Whole-meal bread/rusk	1 slice (30 g), 2 pieces	never/rarely, 1–3 t/mo, 1–2 t/wk, 3–6 t/wk, 1 t/d, ≥2 t/d
Burger-bread	1 piece (60 g)	never/rarely, 1–3 t/mo, 1–2 t/wk, 3–6 t/wk, 1 t/d, ≥2 t/d
Crisp breads	2 thin pieces (20 g)	never/rarely, 1–3 t/mo, 1–2 t/wk, 3–6 t/wk, 1 t/d, ≥2 t/d
Cereal/cereal bars	½ cup (20 g), 1 piece	never/rarely, 1–3 t/mo, 1–2 t/wk, 3–6 t/wk, 1 t/d, ≥2 t/d
White rice	1 cup (160 g)	never/rarely, 1–3 t/mo, 1–2 t/wk, 3–6 t/wk, 1 t/d, ≥2 t/d
Brown rice	1 cup (195 g)	never/rarely, 1–3 t/mo, 1–2 t/wk, 3–6 t/wk, 1 t/d, ≥2 t/d
Pasta/pearl barley	1 cup (140 g)	never/rarely, 1–3 t/mo, 1–2 t/wk, 3–6 t/wk, 1 t/d, ≥2 t/d
Whole-meal pasta	1 cup (140 g)	never/rarely, 1–3 t/mo, 1–2 t/wk, 3–6 t/wk, 1 t/d, ≥2 t/d
Potatoes boiled/baked/mashed	1 medium (90 g)	never/rarely, 1–3 t/mo, 1–2 t/wk, 3–6 t/wk, 1 t/d, ≥2 t/d
French fried potatoes	½ portion (70 g)	never/rarely, 1–3 t/mo, 1–2 t/wk, 3–6 t/wk, 1 t/d, ≥2 t/d
MEAT		
Veal (steak, filet)	150 g	never/rarely, 1–3 t/mo, 1–2 t/wk, 3–6 t/wk, 1 t/d, ≥2 t/d
Burger/meat balls/minced-meat	120 g	never/rarely, 1–3 t/mo, 1–2 t/wk, 3–6 t/wk, 1 t/d, ≥2 t/d
Chicken/turkey (all kinds)	150 g	never/rarely, 1–3 t/mo, 1–2 t/wk, 3–6 t/wk, 1 t/d, ≥2 t/d
Pork (steak, filet)	150 g	never/rarely, 1–3 t/mo, 1–2 t/wk, 3–6 t/wk, 1 t/d, ≥2 t/d
Lamb/goat/game/lambchops	150 g	never/rarely, 1–3 t/mo, 1–2 t/wk, 3–6 t/wk, 1 t/d, ≥2 t/d
Cold sliced meats	1 slice (30 g)	never/rarely, 1–3 t/mo, 1–2 t/wk, 3–6 t/wk, 1 t/d, ≥2 t/d
Sausage/bacon	1 medium, 2 slices (30 g)	never/rarely, 1–3 t/mo, 1–2 t/wk, 3–6 t/wk, 1 t/d, ≥2 t/d
Light/no-fat cold sliced meats	30 g	never/rarely, 1–3 t/mo, 1–2 t/wk, 3–6 t/wk, 1 t/d, ≥2 t/d
FISH		
Small fish	150 g	never/rarely, 1–3 t/mo, 1–2 t/wk, 3–6 t/wk, 1 t/d, ≥2 t/d
Large fish	150 g	never/rarely, 1–3 t/mo, 1–2 t/wk, 3–6 t/wk, 1 t/d, ≥2 t/d
Seafood (octopus, sleeve-fish, prawns)	150 g	never/rarely, 1–3 t/mo, 1–2 t/wk, 3–6 t/wk, 1 t/d, ≥2 t/d
LEGUMES, TRADITIONAL DISHES		
Pulses (lentils, beans, chickpeas)	1 portion (300 g)	never/rarely, 1–3 t/mo, 1–2 t/wk, 3–6 t/wk, 1 t/d, ≥2 t/d
Spinach-rice/cabbage-rice	1 portion (250 g)	never/rarely, 1–3 t/mo, 1–2 t/wk, 3–6 t/wk, 1 t/d, ≥2 t/d
Pastitsio/moussaka/papoutsakia	1 portion (150 g)	never/rarely, 1–3 t/mo, 1–2 t/wk, 3–6 t/wk, 1 t/d, ≥2 t/d
VEGETABLES		
Petit pois (peas), green beans, okra, artichoke	200 g	never/rarely, 1–3 t/mo, 1–2 t/wk, 3–6 t/wk, 1 t/d, ≥2 t/d
Tomato, cucumber, carrot, pepper	100 g	never/rarely, 1–3 t/mo, 1–2 t/wk, 3–6 t/wk, 1 t/d, ≥2 t/d

Food or beverage	Reference portion size	Frequency of consumption
Lettuce, cabbage, spinach, rocket	80 g	never/rarely, 1–3 t/mo, 1–2 t/wk, 3–6 t/wk, 1 t/d, ≥2 t/d
Broccoli, cauliflower, courgette	100 g	never/rarely, 1–3 t/mo, 1–2 t/wk, 3–6 t/wk, 1 t/d, ≥2 t/d
Greens, celery, spinach	90 g	never/rarely, 1–3 t/mo, 1–2 t/wk, 3–6 t/wk, 1 t/d, ≥2 t/d
FRUITS, NUTS		
Orange	1 medium (170 g)	never/rarely, 1–3 t/mo, 1–2 t/wk, 3–6 t/wk, 1 t/d, ≥2 t/d
Apple, pear	1 medium (140 g)	never/rarely, 1–3 t/mo, 1–2 t/wk, 3–6 t/wk, 1 t/d, ≥2 t/d
Other winter fruits	1 piece, ½ cup (150 g)	never/rarely, 1–3 t/mo, 1–2 t/wk, 3–6 t/wk, 1 t/d, ≥2 t/d
Banana	1 medium (100 g)	never/rarely, 1–3 t/mo, 1–2 t/wk, 3–6 t/wk, 1 t/d, ≥2 t/d
Other summer fruits	1 piece, ½ cup (150 g)	never/rarely, 1–3 t/mo, 1–2 t/wk, 3–6 t/wk, 1 t/d, ≥2 t/d
Fruit juice	1 glass (240 g)	never/rarely, 1–3 t/mo, 1–2 t/wk, 3–6 t/wk, 1 t/d, ≥2 t/d
Dried fruits	1/4 cup (35 g)	never/rarely, 1–3 t/mo, 1–2 t/wk, 3–6 t/wk, 1 t/d, ≥2 t/d
Nuts	1 coffee cup (50 g)	never/rarely, 1–3 t/mo, 1–2 t/wk, 3–6 t/wk, 1 t/d, ≥2 t/d
SNACKS		
Homemade pies (e.g., cheese-pie, spinach-pie)	1 piece (150 g)	never/rarely, 1–3 t/mo, 1–2 t/wk, 3–6 t/wk, 1 t/d, ≥2 t/d
Pies	1 piece (150 g)	never/rarely, 1–3 t/mo, 1–2 t/wk, 3–6 t/wk, 1 t/d, ≥2 t/d
Toasted sandwich, sandwich	1 piece (200 g)	never/rarely, 1–3 t/mo, 1–2 t/wk, 3–6 t/wk, 1 t/d, ≥2 t/d
SWEETS, SAVORY SNACKS		
Sweets made in tray	1 piece (150 g)	never/rarely, 1–3 t/mo, 1–2 t/wk, 3–6 t/wk, 1 t/d, ≥2 t/d
Sweet preserves, stewed fruit, fruit – jelly	1 portion (100 g)	never/rarely, 1–3 t/mo, 1–2 t/wk, 3–6 t/wk, 1 t/d, ≥2 t/d
Gateau, tart	1 piece (150 g)	never/rarely, 1–3 t/mo, 1–2 t/wk, 3–6 t/wk, 1 t/d, ≥2 t/d
Croissant, gofer, cake, biscuits	1 item, 1 slice, 3–4 pieces	never/rarely, 1–3 t/mo, 1–2 t/wk, 3–6 t/wk, 1 t/d, ≥2 t/d
Chocolate	1 medium (60 g)	never/rarely, 1–3 t/mo, 1–2 t/wk, 3–6 t/wk, 1 t/d, ≥2 t/d
Ice cream, milkshake, cream, rice pudding	1 piece	never/rarely, 1–3 t/mo, 1–2 t/wk, 3–6 t/wk, 1 t/d, ≥2 t/d
Chips, pop-corn	1 bag (70 g)	never/rarely, 1–3 t/mo, 1–2 t/wk, 3–6 t/wk, 1 t/d, ≥2 t/d
Honey, marmalade, sugar	1 tsp. (5 g)	never/rarely, 1–3 t/mo, 1–2 t/wk, 3–6 t/wk, 1 t/d, ≥2 t/d
Olives	10 small/5 large	never/rarely, 1–3 t/mo, 1–2 t/wk, 3–6 t/wk, 1 t/d, ≥2 t/d
BEVERAGES		
Wine	1 glass (125 ml)	never/rarely, 1–3 t/mo, 1–2 t/wk, 3–6 t/wk, 1 t/d, ≥2 t/d
Beer	1 glass (240 ml)	never/rarely, 1–3 t/mo, 1–2 t/wk, 3–6 t/wk, 1 t/d, ≥2 t/d
Other alcohol drink	1 glass (30 ml)	never/rarely, 1–3 t/mo, 1–2 t/wk, 3–6 t/wk, 1 t/d, ≥2 t/d
Soft drinks	1 can (330 ml)	never/rarely, 1–3 t/mo, 1–2 t/wk, 3–6 t/wk, 1 t/d, ≥2 t/d
Light soft drinks	1 can (330 ml)	never/rarely, 1–3 t/mo, 1–2 t/wk, 3–6 t/wk, 1 t/d, ≥2 t/d
Coffee	1 cup (240 ml)	never/rarely, 1–3 t/mo, 1–2 t/wk, 3–6 t/wk, 1 t/d, ≥2 t/d
Tea, other teas	1 cup (240 ml)	never/rarely, 1–3 t/mo, 1–2 t/wk, 3–6 t/wk, 1 t/d, ≥2 t/d
FATS		
Mayonnaise, sauce	1 Tbsp (15 g)	never/rarely, 1–3 t/mo, 1–2 t/wk, 3–6 t/wk, 1 t/d, ≥2 t/d
Light mayonnaise, light sauce	1 Tbsp (15 g)	never/rarely, 1–3 t/mo, 1–2 t/wk, 3–6 t/wk, 1 t/d, ≥2 t/d
Olive oil	3 Tbsp (45 g)	never/rarely, 1–3 t/mo, 1–2 t/wk, 3–6 t/wk, 1 t/d, ≥2 t/d
Seed oil	3 Tbsp (45 g)	never/rarely, 1–3 t/mo, 1–2 t/wk, 3–6 t/wk, 1 t/d, ≥2 t/d
Margarine	1 Tbsp (15 g)	never/rarely, 1–3 t/mo, 1–2 t/wk, 3–6 t/wk, 1 t/d, ≥2 t/d
Butter	1 Tbsp (15 g)	never/rarely, 1–3 t/mo, 1–2 t/wk, 3–6 t/wk, 1 t/d, ≥2 t/d

t/mo: times per month; t/wk: times per week; t/d: times per day.
Source: Adapted with permission from Bountziouka et al. (2012).

3. The Mediterranean Diet Score (MedDietScore)

How often do you consume the following:	Frequency of consumption (servings/week or as otherwise stated)					
Nonrefined cereals	Never	1–6	7–12	13–18	19–31	>32
	0	1	2	3	4	5
Potatoes	Never	1–4	5–8	9–12	13–18	>18
	0	1	2	3	4	5
Fruits	Never	1–4	5–8	9–15	16–21	>22
	0	1	2	3	4	5
Vegetables	Never	1–6	7–12	13–20	21–32	>33
	0	1	2	3	4	5
Legumes	Never	<1	1–2	3–4	5–6	>6
	0	1	2	3	4	5
Fish	Never	<1	1–2	3–4	5–6	>6
	0	1	2	3	4	5
Red meat and products	≤1	2–3	4–5	6–7	8–10	>10
	5	4	3	2	1	0
Poultry	≤3	4–5	5–6	7–8	9–10	>10
	5	4	3	2	1	0
Full-fat dairy products	≤10	10–15	16–20	21–28	29–30	>30
	5	4	3	2	1	0
Olive oil in cooking (times/week)	Never	Rarely	<1	1–3	3–5	Daily
	0	1	2	3	4	5
Alcoholic beverages (ml/day) 100 ml = 12 g ethanol	<300	300	400	500	600	>700
	5	4	3	2	1	0

Scoring

The MedDietScore takes into account the habitual consumption of 9 food groups (i.e., unrefined cereals, potatoes, fruits, vegetables, legumes, full-fat dairy products, fish, poultry, and red meat and products), as well as the use of olive oil in cooking and consumption of alcohol. Based on the recommendations of the Mediterranean diet, the consumption of each of the 11 components of the index is scored using a scale that ranges from 0 to 5. For foods that are considered part of the Mediterranean diet, i.e., unrefined cereals, potatoes, fruits, vegetables, legumes, fish, and olive oil, scoring ranges from 0 to 5, 0 denoting very rare consumption and 5 very frequent consumption. The opposite scale (i.e., 0 for a very frequent to 5 for a very rare consumption) is used for foods not typically consumed in the Mediterranean diet, i.e., full-fat dairy products, poultry, and red meat products. Alcohol consumption receives a score of 0 for no consumption or consumption of >7 standardized servings per day, and scores of 1 to 5 for the consumption of 6–7, 5–6, 4–5, 3–4, and <3 standardized servings per day, respectively (1 standardized serving equals to 12 g of ethanol, i.e., 12 oz of regular beer – 5% alcohol, 5 oz of wine – 12% alcohol, or 1.5 oz of distilled spirits – 40% alcohol). The total MedDietScore ranges from 0 to 55, with higher values indicating a greater level of adherence to the Mediterranean diet.

For the calculation of MedDietScore, in a rough approximation, 1 serving equals to ½ of the portion as defined in market regulations, i.e., ½ of the portion served in restaurants. Examples:

- 1 slice of bread (25 g)
- 100 g of potatoes
- ½ cup (i.e., 50–60 g) of cooked rice or pasta
- 1 cup of raw leafy vegetables or ½ cup of other vegetables, cooked or chopped (i.e., 100 g)
- 1 apple (80 g), 1 small banana (60 g), 1 orange (100 g), 200 g of melon or watermelon, 30 g of grapes
- 1 cup of milk or yogurt
- 30 g of cheese
- 1 egg
- 60 g of cooked meat and fish
- 1 cup (100 g) of cooked dry beans

Source: Adapted with permission from Panagiotakos et al. (2006).

4. The 14-Item Mediterranean Diet Adherence Screener

Questions	Criteria for 1 point
1. Do you use olive oil as the main culinary fat?	Yes
2. How much olive oil do you consume in a given day (including oil used for frying, salads, out-of-house meals, etc.)?	≥4 tbsp
3. How many vegetable servings do you consume per day? (1 serving: 200 g [consider side dishes as half a serving])	≥2 (≥1 portion raw or as a salad)
4. How many fruit units (including natural fruit juices) do you consume per day?	≥3
5. How many servings of red meat, hamburger, or meat products (ham, sausage, etc.) do you consume per day? (1 serving: 100–150 g)	<1
6. How many servings of butter, margarine, or cream do you consume per day? (1 serving: 12 g)	<1
7. How many sweet or carbonated beverages do you drink per day?	<1
8. How much wine do you drink per week?	≥7 glasses
9. How many servings of legumes do you consume per week? (1 serving: 150 g)	≥3
10. How many servings of fish or shellfish do you consume per week? (1 serving 100–150 g of fish or 4–5 units or 200 g of shellfish)	≥3
11. How many times per week do you consume commercial sweets or pastries (not homemade), such as cakes, cookies, biscuits, or custard?	<3
12. How many servings of nuts (including peanuts) do you consume per week? (1 serving: 30 g)	≥3
13. Do you preferentially consume chicken, turkey, or rabbit meat instead of veal, pork, hamburger, or sausage?	Yes
14. How many times per week do you consume vegetables, pasta, rice, or other dishes seasoned with sofrito (sauce made with tomato and onion, leek, or garlic and simmered with olive oil)?	≥2

Scoring

The 14-item Mediterranean Diet Adherence Screener was developed in a Spanish case–control study of myocardial infarction, where the best cut-off points for discriminating between cases and controls were identified for selected foods or food groups. With this first step, 9 of the 14 score items were obtained. Five additional items relevant to the traditional Mediterranean diet were subsequently added. Each item is scored with 0 or 1, based on whether the established criteria for Mediterranean dietary habits are fulfilled. The total score ranges from 0 to 14, with higher values indicating a greater level of adherence to the Mediterranean diet. Source: Adapted with permission from Martinez-Gonzalez et al. (2004) and Schroder et al. (2011).

5. The Short-Form International Physical Activity Questionnaire (IPAQ)

The following questions will ask you about the time you spent being physically active in the last 7 days. Please answer each question even if you do not consider yourself to be an active person. Please think about the activities you do at work, at your house and your yard, moving from place to place, and the activities you perform in your spare time for recreation, exercise, or sport.

Think about all the vigorous activities that you did in the last 7 days. Vigorous activities refer to activities that require a lot of physical effort and make you breathe much harder than normal. Think only about those activities that you did for at least 10 minutes at a time.

1. During the last 7 days, on how many days did you do vigorous physical activities like heavy lifting, digging, aerobics, running, or fast bicycling?

_____ days per week   If no vigorous physical activities, skip to question 3.

2. How much time did you usually spend doing vigorous physical activities on one of those days?

_____ minutes per day   Don't know/Not sure

Think about all the moderate activities that you did in the last 7 days. Moderate activities refer to activities that take moderate physical effort and make you breathe somewhat harder than normal. Think only about those activities that you did for at least 10 minutes at a time.

3. During the last 7 days, on how many days did you do moderate physical activities like carrying light loads, bicycling at a regular pace, or doubles tennis? Do not include walking.

_____ days per week   If no moderate physical activities, skip to question 5.

4. How much time did you usually spend doing moderate physical activities on one of those days?

_____ minutes per day   Don't know/Not sure

Think about the time you spent walking in the last 7 days. This includes walking from place to place, and any other walking that you have done solely for recreation, sport, exercise, or leisure.

5. During the last 7 days, on how many days did you walk for at least 10 minutes at a time?

_____ days per week   If no walking, skip to question 7.

6. How much time did you usually spend walking on one of those days?

_____ minutes per day   Don't know/Not sure

The last question is about the time you spent sitting on weekdays during the last 7 days. Include time spent at work, at home, while doing course work, and during leisure time. This may include time spent sitting at a desk, visiting friends, reading, or sitting or lying down to watch television.

7. During the last 7 days, how much time did you spend sitting on a weekday?

_____ minutes per day   Don't know/Not sure

Scoring

The short-form IPAQ provides raw data about walking and moderate-intensity and high-intensity activities during a typical week, in terms of frequency (days/week) and duration (min/d). Weekly time (min) spent in each activity category can be calculated as [(days/week (number) × time per day (min)]. The total weekly time (min) of physical activity can be calculated by adding the weekly time spent in all three activity categories. The average daily time spent in physical activity can be calculated as [total weekly time (min) of physical activity ÷ 7].

According to the IPAQ scoring guidelines, each activity category corresponds to a mean metabolic equivalent of task (MET) value (i.e., 3.3 for walking, 4 for moderate-intensity activities, and 8 for high-intensity activities). Based on these values, weekly minutes of metabolic equivalent of tasks (METmins) for each physical activity category can be calculated as [days per week (number) × time per day (min) × MET value], and total weekly exercise METmins can be calculated by adding the weekly METmins of all three physical activity categories.

Category 1: Low

This is the lowest level of physical activity. Those individuals who do not meet criteria for categories 2 or 3 are considered inactive.

Category 2: Moderate

Any one of the following three criteria:

- 3 or more days of vigorous activity of at least 20 minutes per day OR
- 5 or more days of moderate-intensity activity or walking for at least 30 minutes per day OR
- 5 or more days of any combination of walking, moderate-intensity, or vigorous-intensity activities achieving at least 600 METmins/week.

Category 3: High

Any one of the following two criteria:

- 3 or more days of vigorous activity achieving at least 1500 METmins/week OR
- 7 days of any combination of walking, moderate-intensity, or vigorous-intensity activities achieving at least 3000 METmins/week

Source: Adapted with permission from Craig et al. (2003).

6. The Athens Physical Activity Questionnaire (APAQ)

Please record your physical activity during the last 7 days.

SECTION 1: PHYSICAL ACTIVITY AT WORK
What is your main occupation?

Did you work during the last 7 days?
No   → Proceed to Section 2
Yes   How many days did you work in the last 7 days?   _____days
How many hours per day did you work?   _____hours per day
– Of those hours, how much time did you spend on:

hours per day of work	
sitting	(1.5)
standing	(2.3)
walking	(3.0)
carrying loads	(4.0)
total working time	

How long did it take you to commute to work during these days?   _____min per day
Of that time, how much did you
a. walk?   _____min per day (4.0)
b. drive?   _____min per day (2.0)

SECTION 2: PHYSICAL ACTIVITY AT HOME
During the last 7 days, how many hours per day did you:
        sleep (including naps, if any)?   _____hours per day (0.9)
        watch TV/video?   _____hours per day (1.0)
During the last 7 days, how many hours in total did you spend on:
        light housework (e.g., cooking, washing dishes etc.)?   _____hours per week (2.5)
        heavy housework (e.g., hand-washing clothes, mopping etc.)?   _____hours per week (4.0)
        reading and working on a computer (excluding occupation)?   _____hours per week (1.5)

SECTION 3: RECREATIONAL PHYSICAL ACTIVITY
During the last 7 days, how many hours in total did you:

hours per week	
dance	(4.0)
stand or sit in a coffee shop, bar, tavern, restaurant, theater	(1.5)
walk for recreation (window-shopping, in the park, etc.) and for transportation (apart from work)	(2.5)

Did you exercise during the last 7 days?   Yes   No
If yes, what did you do exactly and for how many hours per week in total:

Type of exercise	hours per week

Scoring

Energy expenditure from the APAQ can be calculated as follows: for each activity, energy expenditure (kcal/min) is calculated by multiplying the corresponding metabolic equivalents of task (MET) by the patient's body weight (kg) divided by 60. The MET value appears in parenthesis next to each activity of the questionnaire. A detailed list of MET values for various activities can be found at: https://sites.google.com/site/compendiumofphysicalactivities/home. To estimate the energy expenditure of each activity per week, the reported time of each activity is extrapolated to time (min) per week and then multiplied by the corresponding energy expenditure (kcal/min). The total weekly energy expenditure is calculated as the sum of the weekly energy expenditure of all activities. The mean daily energy expenditure is then calculated as [total weekly energy expenditure (kcal) ÷ 7].
Source: Adapted with permission from Kavouras et al. (2016).

7. The Pittsburgh Sleep Quality Index (PSQI)

Instructions: The following questions relate to your usual sleep habits during the past month only. Your answers should indicate the most accurate reply for the majority of days and nights in the past month. Please answer all questions.

1. During the past month, what time have you usually gone to bed at night?

2. During the past month, how long (in minutes) has it usually taken you to fall asleep each night?

3. During the past month, what time have you usually gotten up in the morning?

4. During the past month, how many hours of actual sleep did you get at night? (This may be different than the number of hours you spent in bed.)

5. During the past month, how often have you had trouble sleeping because you. . .

	Not during the past month	Less than once a week	Once or twice a week	Three or more times a week
a. cannot get to sleep within 30 minutes?				
b. wake up in the middle of the night or early morning?				
c. have to get up to use the bathroom?				
d. cannot breathe comfortably?				
e. cough or snore loudly?				
f. feel too cold?				
g. feel too hot?				
h. have bad dreams?				
i. have pain?				
j. other reason(s); please describe:				

6. During the past month, how often have you taken medicine to help you sleep (prescribed or "over the counter")?

Not during the past month	Less than once a week	Once or twice a week	Three or more times a week

7. During the past month, how often have you had trouble staying awake while driving, eating meals, or engaging in social activity?

Not during the past month	Less than once a week	Once or twice a week	Three or more times a week

8. During the past month, how much of a problem has it been for you to keep up enough enthusiasm to get things done?

No problem at all	Only a very slight problem	Somewhat of a problem	A very big problem

9. During the past month, how would you rate your sleep quality overall?

Very good	Fairly good	Fairly bad	Very bad

10. Do you have a bed partner or roommate?

No bed partner or roommate	Partner or roommate in other room	Partner in same room but not same bed	Partner in same bed

If you have a roommate or bed partner, ask them how often in the past month you have had:

	Not during the past month	Less than once a week	Once or twice a week	Three or more times a week
a. loud snoring				
b. long pauses between breaths while asleep				
c. legs twitching or jerking while you sleep				
d. episodes of disorientation or confusion during sleep				
e. other restlessness while you sleep; please describe:				

Scoring

The first nine items contribute to the total score. In scoring the PSQI, seven component scores are derived, each scored 0 (no difficulty) to 3 (severe difficulty). The component scores are summed to produce a global score (range 0 to 21). Higher scores indicate worse sleep quality.

Component 1: Subjective sleep quality – question #9

Response to question #9	Component 1 score
Very good	0
Fairly good	1
Fairly bad	2
Very bad	3

Component 1 score: _____

Component 2: Sleep latency – questions #2 and #5a

Response to question #2	Component 2/question #2 subscore
< 15 minutes	0
16–30 minutes	1
31–60 minutes	2
> 60 minutes	3

Response to question #5a	Component 2/question #5a subscore
Not during past month	0
Less than once a week	1
Once or twice a week	2
Three or more times a week	3

Sum of q #2 and q #5a subscores	Component 2 score
0	0
1–2	1
3–4	2
5–6	3

Component 2 score: _____

Component 3: Sleep duration – question #4

Response to question #4	Component 3 score
> 7 hours	0
6–7 hours	1
5–6 hours	2
< 5 hours	3

Component 3 score: _____

Component 4: Sleep efficiency – questions #1, #3, and #4

Sleep efficiency = (# hours slept/# hours in bed) × 100%

hours slept – question #4

hours in bed – calculated from responses to questions #1 and #3

Sleep efficiency	Component 4 score
> 85%	0
75–84%	1
65–74%	2
< 65%	3

Component 4 score:_____

Component 5: Sleep disturbance – questions #5b - #5j

Questions #5b to #5j should be scored as follows:

Not during past month	0
Less than once a week	1
Once or twice a week	2
Three or more times a week	3

Sum of q #5b to q #5j scores	Component 5 score
0	0
1–9	1
10–18	2
19–27	3

Component 5 score: _____

Component 6: Use of sleep medication – question #6

Response to question #6	Component 6 score
Not during past month	0
Less than once a week	1
Once or twice a week	2
Three or more times a week	3

Component 6 score: _____

Component 7: Daytime dysfunction – questions #7 and #8

Response to question #7	Component 7/question #7 subscore
Not during past month	0
Less than once a week	1
Once or twice a week	2
Three or more times a week	3

Response to question #8	Component 7/question #8 subscore
No problem at all	0
Only a very slight problem	1
Somewhat of a problem	2
A very big problem	3

Sum of q #7 and q #8 subscores	Component 7 score
0	0
1–2	1
3–4	2
5–6	3

Component 7 score: _____

Global PSQI score (sum of seven component scores): _____

Source: Adapted with permission from Buysse (1989).

8. The Berlin Questionnaire

Please choose the correct response to each question.
Complete the following:
Height (m): _____ Weight (kg): _____ Age: _____ Gender:_____

1. Do you snore?

a. Yes   b. No   c. Don't know

2. If you answered "yes," your snoring is:

a. Slightly louder than breathing   b. As loud as talking   c. Louder than talking

3. How often do you snore?

a. Almost every day   b. 3–4 times per week   c. 1–2 times per week   d. 1–2 times per month   e. Rarely or never

4. Has your snoring ever bothered other people?

Yes   No   Don't know

5. Has anyone noticed that you stop breathing during your sleep?

a. Almost every day   b. 3–4 times per week   c. 1–2 times per week   d. 1–2 times per month   e. Rarely or never

6. How often do you feel tired or fatigued after your sleep?

a. Almost every day   b. 3–4 times per week   c. 1–2 times per week   d. 1–2 times per month   e. Rarely or never

7. During your waking time, do you feel tired, fatigued, or not up to par?

a. Almost every day   b. 3–4 times per week   c. 1–2 times per week   d. 1–2 times per month   e. Rarely or never

8. Have you ever nodded off or fallen asleep while driving a vehicle?

a. Yes   b. No

9. If you answered "yes," how often does this occur?

a. Almost every day   b. 3–4 times per week   c. 1–2 times per week   d. 1–2 times per month   e. Rarely or never

10. Do you have high blood pressure?

a. Yes   b. No   c. Don't know

Scoring

The questionnaire consists of three categories related to the risk of having sleep apnea. Patients can be classified into high risk or low risk based on their responses to the individual items and their overall scores in the symptom categories.

Category 1: items 1, 2, 3, 4, and 5

Item 1: If the response is "yes," assign 1 point.

Item 2: If the response is "c" or "d," assign 1 point.

Item 3: If the response is "a" or "b," assign 1 point.

Item 4: If the response is "a," assign 1 point.

Item 5: If the response is "a" or "b," assign 2 points.

Add points. Category 1 is positive if the total score is 2 or more points.

Category 2: items 6, 7, and 8

Item 6: If the response is "a" or "b," assign 1 point.

Item 7: If the response is "a" or "b," assign 1 point.

Item 8: If the response is "a," assign 1 point.

Add points. Category 2 is positive if the total score is 2 or more points.

Category 3 is positive if the answer to item 10 is "a" or if the BMI of the patient is greater than $30 \, kg/m^2$ (BMI is defined as weight (kg) divided by height (m) squared, i.e., kg/m^2).

High risk: If there are two or more categories where the score is positive.

Low risk: If there is only one or no categories where the score is positive.

   Additional question: Item 9 does not contribute to the total Berlin score but can be assessed individually to evaluate the severity of daytime sleepiness.

Source: Adapted with permission from Netzer et al. (1999).

9. The STOP-BANG Questionnaire

Snoring	Do you snore loudly (loud enough to be heard through closed doors or your bed-partner elbows you for snoring at night)?	Yes	No
Tired	Do you often feel tired, fatigued, or sleepy during the daytime (such as falling asleep during driving or talking to someone)?	Yes	No
Observed	Has anyone observed you stop breathing or choking/gasping during your sleep?	Yes	No
Pressure	Do you have or are you being treated for high blood pressure?	Yes	No
BMI	Do you have a body mass index (BMI) of more than 35 kg/m²? (BMI is defined as weight (kg) divided by height (m) squared).	Yes	No
Age	Are you older than 50 years of age?	Yes	No
Neck	Is your neck size large? (Measured around Adam's apple.) Is your shirt collar 16 in./40 cm or larger?	Yes	No
Gender	Are you male?	Yes	No

Scoring

Obstructive sleep apnea (OSA) – low risk: Yes to 0–2 questions
OSA – intermediate risk: Yes to 3–4 questions
OSA – high risk: Yes to 5–8 questions
or Yes to 2 or more of 4 STOP questions + male gender
or Yes to 2 or more of 4 STOP questions + BMI >35 kg/m²
or Yes to 2 or more of 4 STOP questions + neck circumference ≥ 16 in./40 cm
Source: Adapted with permission from Chung et al. (2008).

10. The Perceived Stress Scale (PSS)

The questions below ask you about your feelings and thoughts during the last month. In each case, you will be asked to indicate by circling how often you felt or thought a certain way.
0 = Never; 1 = Almost never; 2 = Sometimes; 3 = Fairly often; 4 = Very often
In the last month, how often have you:

1. been upset because of something that happened unexpectedly?	0 1 2 3 4
2. felt that you were unable to control the important things in your life?	0 1 2 3 4
3. felt nervous and "stressed"?	0 1 2 3 4
4. felt confident about your ability to handle your personal problems?	0 1 2 3 4
5. felt that things were going your way?	0 1 2 3 4
6. found that you could not cope with all the things that you had to do?	0 1 2 3 4
7. been able to control irritations in your life?	0 1 2 3 4
8. felt that you were on top of things?	0 1 2 3 4
9. been angered because of things that were outside of your control?	0 1 2 3 4
10. felt difficulties were piling up so high that you could not overcome them?	0 1 2 3 4

Scoring

PSS scores are obtained by reversing responses (e.g., 0 = 4, 1 = 3, 2 = 2, 3 = 1, and 4 = 0) to the four positively stated items (items 4, 5, 7, and 8) and then summing across all scale items.
Scores ranging 0–13 denote low perceived stress.
Scores ranging 14–26 denote moderate perceived stress.
Scores ranging 27–40 denote high perceived stress.
Source: Adapted with permission from Cohen et al. (1983).

11. The Zung Self-Rating Anxiety Scale (SAS)

For each item below, please check the column that best describes how often you felt or behaved this way during the past several days.

1 = A little of the time; 2 = Some of the time; 3 = Good part of the time; 4 = Most of the time

1. I feel more nervous and anxious than usual.	1 2 3 4
2. I feel afraid for no reason at all.	1 2 3 4
3. I get upset easily or feel panicky.	1 2 3 4
4. I feel like I'm falling apart and going to pieces.	1 2 3 4
5. I feel that everything is all right and nothing bad will happen.	1 2 3 4
6. My arms and legs shake and tremble.	1 2 3 4
7. I am bothered by headaches, neck and back pain.	1 2 3 4
8. I feel weak and get tired easily.	1 2 3 4
9. I feel calm and can sit still easily.	1 2 3 4
10. I can feel my heart beating fast.	1 2 3 4
11. I am bothered by dizzy spells.	1 2 3 4
12. I have fainting spells or feel like it.	1 2 3 4
13. I can breathe in and out easily.	1 2 3 4
14. I get numbness and tingling in my fingers and toes.	1 2 3 4
15. I am bothered by stomachaches or indigestion.	1 2 3 4
16. I have to empty my bladder often.	1 2 3 4
17. My hands are usually dry and warm.	1 2 3 4
18. My face gets hot and blushes.	1 2 3 4
19. I fall asleep easily and get a good night's rest.	1 2 3 4
20. I have nightmares.	1 2 3 4

Scoring

Add the raw score values for all questions and calculate the total raw score. Compare the raw score to the anxiety index on the conversion table and record the anxiety index.

Raw score	Anxiety index	Raw score	Anxiety index	Raw score	Anxiety index
20	25	40	50	60	75
21	26	41	51	61	76
22	28	42	53	62	78
23	29	43	54	63	79
24	30	44	55	64	80
25	31	45	56	65	81
26	33	46	58	66	83
27	34	47	59	67	84
28	35	48	60	68	85
29	36	49	61	69	86
30	38	50	63	70	88
31	39	51	64	71	89
32	40	52	65	72	90
33	41	53	66	73	91

Raw score	Anxiety index	Raw score	Anxiety index	Raw score	Anxiety index
34	43	54	68	74	92
35	44	55	69	75	94
36	45	56	70	76	95
37	46	57	71	77	96
38	48	58	73	78	98
39	49	59	74	79	99
				80	100

Anxiety index	Interpretation
<45	Anxiety within normal range
45–59	Minimal to moderate anxiety
60–74	Marked to severe anxiety
≥75 and over	Most extreme anxiety

Source: Adapted with permission from Zung (1971).

References

Bountziouka, V., Bathrellou, E., Giotopoulou, A. et al. (2012). Development, repeatability and validity regarding energy and macronutrient intake of a semi-quantitative food frequency questionnaire: methodological considerations. *Nutr. Metab. Cardiovasc. Dis.* 22 (8): 659–667.

Buysse, D.J., Reynolds, C.F. 3rd, Monk, T.H. et al. (1989). The Pittsburgh Sleep Quality Index: a new instrument for psychiatric practice and research. *Psychiatry Res.* 28 (2): 193–213.

Chung, F., Yegneswaran, B., Liao, P. et al. (2008). STOP questionnaire: a tool to screen patients for obstructive sleep apnea. *Anesthesiology* 108 (5): 812–821.

Cohen, S., Kamarck, T., and Mermelstein, R. (1983). A global measure of perceived stress. *J. Health Soc. Behav.* 24 (4): 385–396.

Craig, C.L., Marshall, A.L., Sjostrom, M. et al. (2003). International Physical Activity Questionnaire: 12-country reliability and validity. *Med. Sci. Sports Exerc.* 35 (8): 1381–1395.

Kavouras, S.A., Maraki, M.I., Kollia, M. et al. (2016). Development, reliability and validity of a physical activity questionnaire for estimating energy expenditure in Greek adults. *Sci. Sport.* 31 (3): e47–e53.

Martinez-Gonzalez, M.A., Fernandez-Jarne, E., Serrano-Martinez, M. et al. (2004). Development of a short dietary intake questionnaire for the quantitative estimation of adherence to a cardioprotective Mediterranean diet. *Eur. J. Clin. Nutr.* 58 (11): 1550–1552.

Netzer, N.C., Stoohs, R.A., Netzer, C.M. et al. (1999). Using the Berlin questionnaire to identify patients at risk for the sleep apnea syndrome. *Ann. Intern. Med.* 131 (7): 485–491.

Panagiotakos, D.B., Pitsavos, C., and Stefanadis, C. (2006). Dietary patterns: a Mediterranean diet score and its relation to clinical and biological markers of cardiovascular disease risk. *Nutr. Metab. Cardiovasc. Dis.* 16 (8): 559–568.

Schroder, H., Fito, M., Estruch, R. et al. (2011). A short screener is valid for assessing Mediterranean diet adherence among older Spanish men and women. *J. Nutr.* 141 (6): 1140–1145.

Zung, W.W. (1971). A rating instrument for anxiety disorders. *Psychosomatics* 12 (6): 371–379.

Glossary

Anthropometry: The estimation of the size and proportions of the human body. It encompasses a variety of techniques, ranging from simple measurements of height and weight to advanced body composition analyses methods. Depending on the method, it allows the estimation of total body mass, total lean body mass, muscle mass, bone tissue, total body water, extracellular and intracellular water, total body fat mass and its individual compartments, such as the subcutaneous, visceral, and intramuscular adipose tissue, as well as the fat deposited on various organs, such as the liver or kidneys.

Asian diet: The diet adopted by most Asian countries, including Bangladesh, Cambodia, China, India, Indonesia, Japan, Laos, Malaysia, Mongolia, Myanmar, Nepal, North Korea, South Korea, Philippines, Singapore, Taiwan, Thailand, and Vietnam. It is characterized by high consumption of rice, foods of plant origin (e.g., soy products), fish and seafood, fruits and vegetables, and tea. The majority of foods are boiled, steamed, or grilled without the addition of culinary fat, or fried with minimum quantities of seed oils, or consumed raw.

Basal metabolic rate (BMR): The rate at which the body uses energy while at rest to maintain vital functions, such as breathing and blood flow. It accounts for approximately 60% of the total daily energy expenditure. Indirect calorimetry is the gold standard for measuring BMR; however, it is not routinely used in clinical practice due to complexity, high cost, and need for special equipment and skilled staff. Alternatively, BMR can be estimated using population-specific equations that take into account simple variables, such as age, sex, and body weight.

Body mass index (BMI): An easy, quick, and practical estimate of adiposity. It correlates positively with body fat and health risk and is widely used in clinical practice to provide a rough assessment of body weight status. BMI is calculated as [weight (kg) ÷ height^2 (m^2)]. Values ≤18.5, 18.5–25, ≥25, and ≥30 kg/m^2 classify an adult in the category of underweight, healthy weight, overweight, and obese, respectively.

Body weight history: A history of changes of body weight over the years. Such a history should include the assessment of the minimum and maximum body weight, the identification of critical periods and events that led to significant changes in body weight, and a record of previous weight loss or weight gain efforts. An easy way to get all the necessary information is to ask the patient to draw a graph of important changes in body weight during adulthood and note the facts/events that correlate with significant changes in body weight. These changes are usually accompanied by changes in lifestyle habits.

Cognitive–behavioral therapy (CBT): A blend of cognitive therapy and behavioral therapy that aims to help patients modify their insight and understanding of thoughts and beliefs concerning health issues, including weight regulation, obesity, and its consequences. It also directly addresses behaviors that require change for successful regulation of body weight (i.e., weight gain or loss and maintenance of the new body weight). CBT includes several components, such as self-monitoring (e.g., dietary record), evaluation of readiness and self-efficacy for change, problem solving, techniques controlling the process of eating, stimulus control and reinforcement, as well as cognitive and relaxation techniques.

Conventional medicine: The type of medicine using medications as the core treatment for diseases. It is usually provided by health professionals who operate independently and treat patients as passive recipients of care with little consideration of their environment and lifestyle choices.

Diet: The word *diet* originates from the Greek word δίαιτα (*diaita*) meaning "way of living," "lifestyle."

Diet history: Any dietary assessment that prompts the respondent to report about past dietary habits. It can vary in content and structure and usually refers to dietary assessment methods that ascertain a person's usual food intake and meal patterns. Details about characteristics of commonly consumed foods are assessed in addition to the frequency and amount of food consumed and other dietary habits and practices.

Dietary Approaches to Stop Hypertension (DASH) diet: It originated in the 1990s from a study funded by the National Institutes of Health, aiming to identify dietary interventions that could be useful in treating hypertension. Since then, it has been advocated as the first-line dietary therapy for hypertension, and several studies have confirmed its beneficial effects on blood pressure, total cardiovascular risk, morbidity, and mortality. The DASH diet emphasizes the intake of plant-based products, such as fruits, vegetables, whole grains, legumes, nuts, and seeds, as well as lean animal products, such as low-fat dairy products, poultry, and fish. It is a low-fat (especially saturated fat) dietary pattern rich in potassium, magnesium, calcium, and dietary fiber.

Dietary fiber: The edible parts of plants that are resistant to digestion and absorption in the human small intestine with complete or partial fermentation in the large intestine. They are classified into (i) soluble fiber (i.e., dissolves in water), which is fermented in the colon by gut microbiota into gases and physiologically active byproducts, such as short-chain fatty acids; examples are beta-glucans, fructans, pectins, raffinose, and inulin; and (ii) insoluble fiber (i.e., does not dissolve in water), which is inert to digestive enzymes in the gastrointestinal tract and triggers the secretion of mucus in the large intestine, providing bulking; examples are cellulose chitin, lignin, and resistant starch. Dietary fiber promotes beneficial physiological effects, including laxation, blood cholesterol attenuation, and blood glucose control.

Dietary pattern: The quantity, variety, and combination of different foods and beverages in a diet and the frequency at which they are habitually consumed. Evaluating the impact of a single dietary factor independently of any other changes in the diet is problematic. As foods are mixtures of different nutrients that have synergistic or antagonistic interactions, it is not appropriate to attribute the health effects of a diet to only one of its components. Moreover, if total energy intake is kept constant, eating less of one nutrient or food implies eating more of others, and the quality of the replacement can influence the effect observed. In recent years, nutrition research and epidemiology focus on the relationship between health/disease and dietary patterns, rather than single nutrients or foods.

Dietary recall: A dietary assessment tool in which the respondent is asked to report all the

Textbook of Lifestyle Medicine, First Edition. Labros S. Sidossis and Stefanos N. Kales.
© 2022 John Wiley & Sons Ltd. Published 2022 by John Wiley & Sons Ltd.

meals consumed in the past 24 hours, exact quantities, cooking methods, location and conditions for each meal, and the brand names for packaged foods. The recall is typically conducted by personal interview, either in print or in a computer-assisted form.

Dietary record: A dietary assessment tool in which the respondent records the foods/beverages and the amount of each consumed over a period of several days. The amounts consumed may be measured with a food scale or household measures or estimated using food models.

Food: Any nourishing substance that is eaten, drunk, or otherwise taken into the body to sustain life, provide energy, and promote growth. Foods are categorized in food groups, i.e., collections of foods that share similar nutritional and biological properties. There are six major food groups: (i) fruits (apple, orange, strawberry, etc.); (ii) vegetables (tomato, carrot, zucchini, etc.); (iii) grains (bread, pasta, rice, etc.); (iv) meat products (chicken, pork, veal, etc.); (v) dairy products (milk, yogurt, cheese, etc.); and (vi) fats and oils (olive oil, butter, nuts, etc.).

Food frequency questionnaire (FFQ): A dietary assessment tool in which the respondent is asked to report the usual frequency of consumption of each food/beverage from a list of foods for a specific period (usually ≥1 month). Only information on frequency and sometimes quantity is collected, with little detail on other characteristics, such as cooking methods or food combinations in meals and other dietary practices.

Globesity: The worldwide public health crisis caused by excessive weight gain.

Glycemic index (GI): A ranking of foods on a scale from 0 to 100 according to the extent to which they raise blood glucose levels after consumption, compared to the same quantity of a reference food, usually white bread or glucose. Foods with a high GI are rapidly digested, absorbed, and metabolized and result in marked fluctuations in blood glucose levels, while low-GI foods produce smaller fluctuations in blood glucose and insulin levels and promote normoglycemia.

Glycemic load (GL): An index that evaluates the glycemic response of a food, taking into account the consumed portion size of the food and its glycemic index. The GL is used to compare the blood glucose raising effects of different quantities of foods and is calculated as [glycemic index × carbohydrate (g) content per portion (minus the dietary fiber) ÷ 100]. Adopting a low-GL diet can have a positive impact on glycemic control, especially in insulin-resistant and diabetic patients.

Health: A state of complete physical, mental, and social well-being and not merely the absence of disease or infirmity.

Lifestyle medicine: The use of a whole food, plant-predominant dietary pattern, regular physical activity, restorative sleep, stress management, avoidance of risky substances, and positive social connection as a primary therapeutic modality for the prevention and treatment of chronic disease. Lifestyle medicine is provided by a multidisciplinary team of health professionals from many fields: medicine, nutrition, exercise, psychology, sleep, and others. In this setting, the patient is no longer a passive recipient of care but an active partner who makes decisions and assumes responsibility for the changes that need to take place in his/her life to improve health and wellness. This can be achieved through a patient-centered counseling style, focused on increasing motivation, health efficacy, and health literacy.

Meditation: An ancient form of stress relief that has recently been accepted as a complementary practice in modern medical science. It results in alterations in human physiology associated with a decrease in stress and anxiety and has been associated with improvements in mental health both in healthy and chronically ill individuals.

Mediterranean diet (MedD): The dietary pattern adopted in the olive-growing areas of the Mediterranean region in the late 1950s and early 1960s, when the region was recovering from the effects of World War II. The MedD has evolved throughout time and currently is defined as a dietary pattern characterized by high consumption of extra-virgin olive oil (as the main edible fat), vegetables, legumes, whole grains, fruits and nuts; moderate consumption of poultry and fish (varying with proximity to the sea); low consumption of full-fat dairy, red meat products, sweets, and processed foods; and moderate consumption of wine as the main source of alcohol consumed with meals.

Mediterranean lifestyle (MedL): The lifestyle paradigm encompassing the various components of the daily life of the people living in the Mediterranean basin; a plant-based diet characterized by moderation, seasonality, participation in culinary activities and conviviality, daily engagement in physical activity as an inherent feature of everyday life, healthy sleeping practices, stress management practices, adequate rest, engagement in spiritual activities, active social life, and the rich cultural heritage transmitted from one generation to the next.

Metabolic syndrome (MetS): A constellation of interconnected physiological, biochemical, clinical, and metabolic factors that directly increase the risk of several adverse health outcomes related to noncommunicable diseases. It is defined as the coexistence of three or more of the five following components: (i) increased sex-specific waist circumference values, indicative of central obesity; (ii) increased fasting glucose levels or use of antidiabetic medication or presence of type 2 diabetes mellitus; (iii) decreased sex-specific high-density-lipoprotein cholesterol levels or use of relevant medication; (iv) increased triglyceride levels or use of lipid-lowering medication; (v) increased blood pressure levels or use of antihypertensive medication.

Motivational interviewing (MI): A technique in which the health professional becomes a helper in the change process and expresses acceptance of the patient. It is a way to interact with patients and a style of counseling that can help resolve the ambivalence that prevents patients from realizing, achieving, and maintaining personal goals. The role of a health professional in MI is directive, with a goal of eliciting self-motivational statements and behavioral change from the patient in addition to creating patient discrepancy to enhance motivation for positive change. Essentially, MI activates a person's capacity for beneficial change.

Noncommunicable diseases (NCDs): Diseases with a prolonged course that are not cured spontaneously and result from a combination of genetic, physiological, environmental, and behavioral factors. NCDs include cardiovascular diseases, cancer, chronic respiratory disease, diabetes, chronic neurologic disorders, and musculoskeletal diseases.

Nordic diet: The dietary pattern adopted around the Nordic regions, namely, northern European countries, such as Denmark, Finland, Norway, Sweden, and Iceland. The Nordic diet is characterized by high consumption of fruits (e.g., berries, apples, and pears), vegetables (e.g., root vegetables, cabbage, potatoes, carrots), wild mushrooms, pulses (e.g., beans, peas), nuts, whole-grains foods (e.g., rye, barley, oats), rapeseed oil, oily fish (e.g., mackerel, salmon, herring), shellfish, and seaweed, while emphasis is given to low-fat choices of meat, low-fat dairy, salt restriction, and avoidance of sugar-sweetened products.

Nutrient: A substance that provides nourishment essential for the maintenance of life and for growth. Nutrients are classified into two major categories: (i) macronutrients, i.e., nutrients the body needs in larger amounts, namely, carbohydrates, proteins, and fats; and (ii) micronutrients, i.e., nutrients the body needs in smaller amounts, namely, vitamins and minerals. Macronutrients are sources of energy for the human body, while micronutrients are essential to human metabolism.

Obesity: A chronic disease involving the excessive accumulation of fat in the body, which poses health risks and leads to a reduced life expectancy.

Physical activity (PA): Any bodily movement produced by skeletal muscles that requires energy expenditure. It can be classified as incidental or structured. Incidental PA is not planned and usually is the result of daily activities at work, at home, or during transportation. Structured PA, also called exercise or exercise training, is a component of leisure-time PA and can be defined as planned, structured, repetitive, and purposeful activity, in the sense that it is performed to improve or maintain one or more components of physical fitness.

Physical fitness (PF): The ability to carry out daily tasks with vigor and alertness, without undue fatigue, and with ample energy to enjoy leisure-time pursuits and to meet unforeseen emergencies. It comprises cardiorespiratory endurance, muscle endurance and muscle strength, flexibility, balance, agility, and coordination. PF represents the ability of an individual to perform physical activity efficiently.

Saturated fatty acids (SFAs): The simplest fatty acids; they are unbranched, linear chains of CH2 groups linked by carbon–carbon single bonds. Examples include butyric acid (found in butter), lauric acid (found in coconut oil), myristic acid (found in dairy products), palmitic acid (found in palm oil and meat), and stearic acid (found in meat and cocoa butter).

Siesta: An afternoon rest or short nap, usually taken during the hottest hours of the day in hot climates. It is a typical practice in many populations in the Mediterranean region, other countries in southern Europe, South America, the Philippines, and Mainland China.

Sleep: The natural, easily reversible periodic state of many living beings, marked by the absence of wakefulness and by the loss of consciousness of one's surroundings. Sleep is not just the simple absence of wakefulness but a physiologically active state in which specific processes and metabolic pathways take place that are essential for the regulation of daytime functioning and overall well-being.

Spirituality: A lifelong guiding principle that involves feelings and beliefs of a religious nature, rather than the physical parts of life. Firmly held spiritual values have the potential to enhance incentives, abilities, and hope, and in this way, they can help people to confront insulin-resistant and disease states.

Stress: A condition in which expectations, whether genetically programmed, established by prior learning, or deduced from circumstances, do not match current or anticipated perceptions of the internal or external environment. This mismatch between what is observed or sensed and what is expected or programmed evokes patterned, compensatory mechanisms and reactions, known as the "stress response." The effects of stress mediators, although essential for the survival of an organism, can have negative effects, especially in the case of chronic exposure to stressful stimuli.

Therapeutic Lifestyle Changes (TLC) diet: A diet recommended by the National Cholesterol Education Program Expert Panel for the management of high blood cholesterol. The TLC diet is a relatively low-fat (especially saturated fat and cholesterol) diet, focusing on an adequate intake of dietary fiber (especially soluble) and plant sterols/stanols.

Trans fatty acids (TFAs): A type of unsaturated fatty acid formed as a result of the hydrogenation process, having a trans arrangement of the carbon atoms adjacent to its double bonds. Hydrogenation aims at stabilizing polyunsaturated fatty acids to prevent them from becoming rancid and keep them solid at room temperature. Dietary sources of TFA include baked goods, such as cakes, cookies, and pies, fast-food fried products, including French fries and doughnuts, and stick margarine. Frequent consumption of TFA increases the risk for cardiovascular diseases and should be avoided.

Unsaturated fatty acids: Fatty acids whose carbon chain has one or more double or triple bonds. The term *unsaturated* indicates that the carbon atoms do not have the maximum possible hydrogen atoms bound to carbon atoms. As a result, unsaturated fatty acids can undergo hydrogenation, resulting in saturated fatty acids. Monounsaturated fatty acids, such as oleic acid, have only one unsaturated carbon bond and are found in abundance in olive oil, nuts, and avocado. Polyunsaturated fatty acids have more than one unsaturated carbon bond and include omega-3 and omega-6 fatty acids. Omega-3 fatty acids are found in fish–seafood (as eicosapentaenoic acid and docosahexaenoic acid) and some plant-based foods, such as soybean oil, canola oil, walnuts, and flaxseed (as α-linolenic acid). Omega-6 fatty acids are found mostly in liquid vegetable oils like soybean oil, corn oil, and safflower oil. Substituting saturated with mono- and polyunsaturated fatty acids has been associated with anti-inflammatory actions and cardiovascular benefits.

Vegetarian diet: A dietary pattern based predominantly on plant-origin products.

Waist circumference (WC): It should ideally be measured to the nearest 0.1 cm between the lowest rib and the superior border of the iliac crest at the end of normal expiration, using a nonelastic measuring tape positioned parallel to the floor and with the patient standing. When the specific anatomic points are hard to distinguish, the maximum circumference in the abdomen can be measured instead. For Caucasians, WC values >94 cm (men) and >80 cm (women) are considered high, while values >102 cm (men) and >88 cm (women) are considered very high. WC is a rough estimate of the body's abdominal fat stores, which is a significant risk factor for cardiometabolic diseases.

Wellness: The optimal state of health of individuals and groups, with two focal concerns: the realization of the individual's fullest potential physically, socially, spiritually, and economically, and the fulfillment of one's role expectations in the family, community, place of worship, workplace, and other settings.

Index